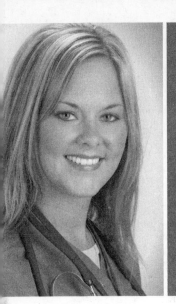

"I immediately went to my nurse manager after I failed the NCLEX® and she referred me to ATI. I was able to discover the areas I was weak in, and focused on those areas in the review modules and online assessments.

I was much more prepared the second time around!"

Terim Richards
Nursing student

Danielle Platt

Nurse Manager • Children's Mercy Hospital • Kansas City, MO

"The year our hospital did not use the ATI program, we experienced a 15% decrease in the NCLEX® pass rates. We reinstated the ATI program the following year and had a 90% success rate."

"As a manager, I have witnessed graduate nurses fail the NCLEX® and the devastating effects it has on their morale. Once the nurses started using ATI, it was amazing to see the confidence they had in themselves and their ability to go forward and take the NCLEX® exam."

Mary Moss

Associate Dean of Nursing - Service and Health Division • Mid-State Technical College • Wisconsin Rapids, WI

"I like that ATI lets students know what to expect from the NCLEX®, helps them plan their study time and tells them what to do in the days and weeks before the exam. It is different from most of the NCLEX® review books on the market."

Editor

Jeanne Wissmann, PhD, RN, CNE
Director Nursing Curriculum and Educational Services
Assessment Technologies Institute®, LLC

Associate Editors

Audrey Knippa, MS, MPH, RN, CNE
Curriculum Project Coordinator

Sally Swenson, MA, RN
Consulting Associate Editor

Erika Knoblock, BS Education
Product Developer

Brant Stacy, BS Journalism
Product Developer

Copyright Notice

Important Notice to the Reader of this Publication

Preface

Overview

The overall goal of this Assessment Technologies Institute®, LLC (ATI) Content Mastery Series module is to provide nursing students with an additional resource for the focused review of "Fundamentals for Nursing" content relevant to NCLEX® preparation and entry-level nursing practice. Content within this review module is provided in a key-point plus rationale format in order to focus recall and application of relevant content. Unit and chapter selections are reflective of the fundamentals nursing-relevant content categories and explanations of the RN/PN NCLEX® test plans, the ATI "Fundamentals for Nursing" assessment test plans, and standard nursing curricular content. Each chapter begins with an overview of some of the topic-relevant nursing activities outlined by the RN/PN NCLEX® test plans in an effort to guide the learner's review and application of chapter content.

Contributors

ATI would like to extend appreciation to the nurse educators and nurse specialists who contributed content for this review module. The names of contributors are noted in the chapter bylines. We would also like to thank those talented individuals who reviewed, edited, and developed this module. In the summer and fall of 2005, two focus groups of committed nurse educators gave invaluable input and feedback regarding the format and purposes of review modules. Their input and ideas were instrumental to the development of this review module, and we are very appreciative. Additionally, we would like to recognize and extend appreciation to the multiple nursing students and educators who have contacted us in the past year with comments and ideas regarding the content of this review module. And finally, we want to recognize and express appreciation to all of the contributors, reviewers, production developers, and editors of previous editions of this Content Mastery Series module.

Suggestions for Effective Utilization

Δ   Understanding the organizational framework of this review module will facilitate focused review. Each unit focuses on a specific aspect of nursing fundamentals. Unit 1 focuses on foundations of practice; Unit 2 focuses on health assessment; Unit 3 focuses on basic nursing care; Unit 4 focuses on supporting psychosocial, family, cultural and spiritual health; and Unit 5 focuses on physiological needs. The chapters are organized with headings to include Key Points, Key Factors, Assessment, NANDA Nursing Diagnoses, Nursing Interventions, and Complications and Nursing Implications.

Δ   Some suggested uses of this review module include:

- As a review of NCLEX®-relevant nursing fundamentals content in developing and assessing your readiness for the NCLEX®.

- As a focused-review resource based on the results of an ATI "Nursing for Fundamentals" or "Comprehensive Predictor" assessment. "Topics to Review" identified upon completion of these assessments can be used to focus your efforts to a review of content within specific chapter(s) of this review module. For example, an identified "Topic to Review" of "Medication Administration: Legal Responsibilities" suggests that a review of chapter 44, "Safe Medication Administration and Error Prevention," and completion of the application exercises at the end of the chapter, would be helpful.

Δ   To foster long-term recall and development of an ability to apply knowledge to a variety of situations, learners are encouraged to take a comprehensive approach to topic review. Using this review module along with other resources (class notes, course textbooks, nursing reference texts, instructors, and ATI DVD series), consider addressing questions for each aspect of nursing fundamentals.

- For **foundations of practice** ask questions such as:

◊   What are the basic concepts of the foundation of practice?

◊   What key points should the nurse know?

◊ Who makes up the interdisciplinary team?

◊ How does the registered nurse interact with the members of the interdisciplinary team?

◊ How is the nursing process used in the delivery of nursing care?

◊ What should the nurse do to communicate effectively?

◊ What are some of the legal and ethical responsibilities of nursing care?

◊ How does the developmental stage of the client impact nursing care?

• For **health assessment** ask questions such as:

◊ What is the body's normal physiological response to changes in temperature, pulse, respirations, and blood pressure?

◊ What are normal ranges for these vital signs?

◊ How are vital signs obtained?

◊ What are complications and nursing implications for the client experiencing an abnormality in one of the vital signs?

◊ What are the components of each body system assessment?

◊ How is each assessment performed?

◊ For what normal findings should the nurse observe?

• For **basic nursing care** ask questions such as:

◊ What tasks are included in providing basic nursing care?

◊ What assessments should be done prior to performing a skill?

◊ What is the correct procedure?

◊ What are basic principles of medication error prevention?

◊ How are dosages calculated using a specific method?

• For **supporting psychosocial, family, cultural and spiritual health** ask questions such as:

◊ What psychosocial aspects of health must be supported for the client?

◊ What are common nursing diagnoses identified for clients experiencing an altered response to a health care issue?

• For **physiological needs** ask questions such as:

◊ What are the various physiological needs the client may have?

◊ What does the nurse assess when the client has such a need?

◊ What are some possible nursing diagnoses for the client with such a need?

◊ How does the nurse intervene?

Δ   Complete application exercises at the end of each chapter after a review of the topic. Answer questions fully and note rationales for answers. Complete exercises initially without looking for the answers within the chapter or consulting the answer key. Use these exercises as an opportunity to assess your readiness to apply knowledge. When reviewing the answer key, in addition to identifying the correct answer, examine why you missed or answered correctly each item. Was it related to ability to recall, recognition of a common testing principle, or perhaps attention to key words?

Feedback

All feedback is welcome – suggestions for improvement, reports of mistakes (small or large), and testimonials of effectiveness. Please address feedback to: comments@atitesting.com

Unit 2 Health Assessment

Section: Vital Signs

Section: System-Specific Assessment

Unit 3 Basic Nursing Care

Section: Admission, Transfer, and Discharge Processes

Section: Medication Administration and Error Prevention

Section: Safety

Unit 5 Supporting Physiologic Needs

Unit 1   **Foundations for Practice**

Section: Health Care Delivery

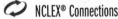

Chapter 1:   **Health Care Delivery Systems**

Contributor: Patricia A Girczyc, EdD(c), MPH, FNP

 NCLEX® Connections

> **Learning Objective**: Review and apply knowledge within "**Health Care Delivery Systems**" in readiness for performance of the following nursing activities as outlined by the NCLEX® test plans:
>
> Δ   Identify the components of health care systems and the roles within healthcare.
>
> Δ   Discuss the various levels of health care and identify activities that take place within each level.
>
> Δ   Recognize the various levels of care needed throughout a client's life to maintain wellness and independence.

Key Points

Δ   Health care delivery systems are comprised of interactions between health care providers and clients within the constraints of financing mechanisms and regulatory agencies.

Δ   Health care systems are comprised of the individuals who participate, the settings in which health care takes place, the agencies that regulate health care, and mechanisms that provide financial support.

Δ   Multiple settings exist to provide health care services and vary from community to community.

Δ   Different levels of health care exist, and clients are directed to the most appropriate levels and intensity of care based on their needs.

Key Factors

Components of Health Care Systems	

People – participants in the health care system	• **Consumers (clients)**
	• **Providers**
	  ◊ Licensed providers such as:
	    ° Registered nurses
	    ° Licensed vocational/practical nurses
	    ° Advanced practice nurses
	    ° Medical doctors
	    ° Pharmacists
	    ° Dentists
	    ° Physical, respiratory, and occupational therapists
	  ◊ Unlicensed providers such as assistive personnel

Settings – where health care is provided	• Hospitals • Homes • Skilled-nursing, assisted-living, and extended-care facilities • Community/health departments • Adult day care centers • Schools • Hospices
Regulatory agencies – enforce regulations for practice	• United States Department of Health and Human Services • Federal Drug Administration (FDA) • State and local public health agencies • State licensing boards – to ensure that health care providers and agencies comply with state regulations • The Joint Commission (formerly JCAHO) – to set quality standards for accreditation of hospitals • Professional Standards Review Organizations (PSROs) • Utilization review committees – to monitor for appropriate diagnosis and treatment of the hospitalized client

Components of Health Care Systems	

Health care financing mechanisms – how health care is paid	• Public federally funded programs:
	◊ Medicare is for clients over 65 years of age. Premiums can be applied to one of two mechanisms:
	  ° Insurance program – reimburses providers based on diagnosis-related groups (DRGs).
	  ° Managed care organizations (MCOs) – enrolled clients receive comprehensive care overseen by a primary care provider.
	◊ Medicaid is for the client with a low income.
	  ° It is federally funded.
	  ° Individual states determine eligibility requirements.
	• Private plans
	◊ Traditional insurance reimburses for services on a fee-for-service basis.
	◊ MCOs – comprehensive care is overseen by a primary care provider and focuses on prevention. Providers receive a fixed fee every month for each client.
	◊ Preferred provider organizations (PPOs) – the client chooses from a list of contracted providers. Using noncontracted providers increases the client out-of-pocket costs.
	◊ Exclusive provider organizations (EPOs) – the client chooses from a list of providers within a contracted organization.
	◊ Long-term care insurance – this provides for long-term care expenses and is in addition to Medicare.

Δ **Levels of Health Care**

- **Preventive** health care focuses on educating and equipping the client to **reduce and control risk factors** of disease. Examples include immunization programs, stress management classes, and advocating seat belt use.

- **Primary** health care includes **routine care with periodic screenings** designed to detect disease at its earliest stage. This level of care is based on a sustained partnership between the client and primary care provider. Examples include office or clinic visits and scheduled school or work-centered screenings (e.g., vision, hearing, obesity).

- **Secondary** health care includes the **diagnosis and treatment** of emergency or acute illness. Examples include care that is given in hospital settings or emergency departments.

- **Tertiary** health care involves the provision of specialized highly technical care for the client. Examples include oncology centers, burn centers, and psychiatric facilities.

- **Restorative** health care involves **intermediate follow-up care** for restoring health. Examples include home health care, rehabilitation centers, and skilled nursing facilities.

- **Continuing** health care is designed to address long-term or chronic health care needs. Examples include hospice, adult day care, and in-home respite care.

Δ **Relationship between health care systems and levels of care**

- **People** – The level of care provided depends on the needs of the client. Licensed and unlicensed health care personnel work in every level of care.

- **Setting** – The settings for secondary and tertiary care are usually within a hospital or specific facility/agency. Other levels of care can occur in a variety of settings.

- **Regulatory agencies** are involved with ensuring the quality and quantity of health care, and the protection of the health care consumer.

- **Health care finance** influences the quality and type of care by setting parameters for cost containment and reimbursement.

Primary Reference:

Potter, P. A., & Perry, A. G. (2005). *Fundamentals of nursing* (6th ed.). St. Louis, MO: Mosby.

Additional Resources:

NANDA International (2004). *NANDA nursing diagnoses: Definitions and classification 2005-2006.* Philadelphia: NANDA.

For information about Medicare Prescription Drug Coverage, go to *www.medicare.gov./*

Chapter 1: Health Care Delivery Systems

Application Exercises

1. Match the type of service with the appropriate health care level.

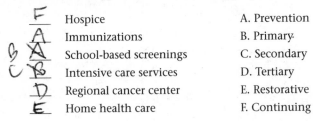

F	Hospice	A. Prevention
A	Immunizations	B. Primary
A	School-based screenings	C. Secondary
B	Intensive care services	D. Tertiary
D	Regional cancer center	E. Restorative
E	Home health care	F. Continuing

2. Which of the following are health care regulatory agencies? (Select all that apply.)

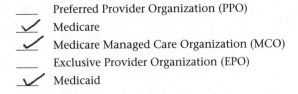

_____ American Nurses Association (ANA)

✓ The Joint Commission (formerly JCAHO)

✓ State Boards of Nursing

_____ National League of Nursing (NLN)

✓ Federal Drug Administration (FDA)

3. Which of the following health care financing mechanisms is federally funded? (Select all that apply.)

_____ Preferred Provider Organization (PPO)

✓ Medicare

✓ Medicare Managed Care Organization (MCO)

_____ Exclusive Provider Organization (EPO)

✓ Medicaid

4. A hospital conducts a community blood pressure screening in its lobby. This is an example of what level of care?

A. Preventive

B. Primary

C. Secondary

D. Tertiary

5. A client in a managed care organization (MCO) requires hospitalization. The admission must first be approved by the

       A. emergency department physician.

       B. utilization review committee.

       C. primary care provider.

       D. managed care administrator.

Chapter 1: Health Care Delivery Systems

Application Exercises Answer Key

1. Match the type of service with the appropriate health care level.

__F__	Hospice	A. Prevention
__A__	Immunizations	B. Primary
__B__	School-based screenings	C. Secondary
__C__	Intensive care services	D. Tertiary
__D__	Regional cancer center	E. Restorative
__E__	Home health care	F. Continuing

2. Which of the following are health care regulatory agencies? (Select all that apply.)

_____ American Nurses Association (ANA)

__X__ **The Joint Commission (formerly JCAHO)**

__X__ **State Boards of Nursing**

_____ National League of Nursing (NLN)

__X__ **Federal Drug Administration (FDA)**

JCAHO, State Boards of Nursing, and the FDA are all health care regulatory agencies. ANA and NLN are both professional nursing organizations. Even though ANA and NLN function to maintain high nursing practice standards, they do not regulate health care agencies.

3. Which of the following health care financing mechanisms is federally funded? (Select all that apply.)

_____ Preferred Provider Organization (PPO)

__X__ **Medicare**

__X__ **Medicare Managed Care Organization (MCO)**

_____ Exclusive Provider Organization (EPO)

__X__ **Medicaid**

4. A hospital conducts a community blood pressure screening in its lobby. This is an example of what level of care?

> A. Preventive
>
> **B. Primary**
>
> C. Secondary
>
> D. Tertiary

A screening is an attempt to diagnose an undiagnosed disease at its earliest stage, and is an example of primary care. Preventive care includes immunizations or education for minimizing risk factors for illness. Secondary care includes hospital-based care that is performed on emergency department or hospitalized clients. Tertiary care includes specialized care usually located regionally, such as burn or cancer centers.

5. A client in a managed care organization (MCO) requires hospitalization. The admission must first be approved by the

> A. emergency department physician.
>
> B. utilization review committee.
>
> **C. primary care provider.**
>
> D. managed care administrator.

In an MCO, the primary care provider oversees all of the client's care including hospitalizations. The emergency department physician may consult with the primary care provider regarding a client, but the decision to admit the client is left to the primary care provider in order for the admission and services to be reimbursed. Utilization review committees and the managed care administrator may review the appropriateness of the primary care provider's treatment decisions, but they do not make admission decisions.

Unit 1   Foundations for Practice
Section: Health Care Delivery

Chapter 2:   Roles and the Interdisciplinary Team
Contributor: Patricia A Girczyc, EdD(c), MPH, FNP

 NCLEX® Connections:

Learning Objective: Review and apply knowledge within "**Roles and the Interdisciplinary Team**" in readiness for performance of the following nursing activities as outlined by the NCLEX® test plans:

Δ   Identify the role of the nurse as a member of the interdisciplinary health care team.

Δ   Assess the need for and collaborate with the interdisciplinary team in the development of interdisciplinary client care plans.

Δ   Use knowledge of roles and responsibilities of the members of the interdisciplinary health care team to make appropriate referrals.

Δ   Compare and contrast roles and responsibilities of advanced practice nurses, registered nurses, and licensed practical nurses.

Δ   Obtain and communicate information regarding the client to members of the nursing and interdisciplinary health care team to plan and provide care.

 Key Points

Δ   The interdisciplinary health care team works collaboratively to provide holistic care to the client.

Δ   The interdisciplinary health care team consists of health care providers including nurses, physicians, specialty area clinicians (e.g., physical, occupational, respiratory therapists), and assistive personnel.

Δ   The nurse is most often the manager of care and must understand the roles and responsibilities of other health care team members in order to collaborate in the care of the client and make appropriate referrals.

Δ   The roles and responsibilities of nurses are based on knowledge and skill acquisition that is regulated by state nurse practice acts. Nursing care delivery models provide various formats for nurses to meet the needs of the client.

Key Factors

Δ   Interdisciplinary Personnel (non-nursing)

Title	Job description	Example of when to refer
Clergy	Provide spiritual care to the client (e.g., pastors, rabbis, priests).	The client requests for communion, or the family asks for prayer prior to the client undergoing a procedure.
Registered dietitian	• Assess, plan for, and educate the client regarding nutrition needs. • Direct care of nutritional aides.	The client has a low albumin level and has experienced a recent unexplained weight loss.
Laboratory technician	Obtain specimens of the client's body fluids and perform the necessary diagnostic tests.	Primary care provider orders a complete blood count (CBC) to be performed immediately.
Occupational therapist	• Assess and plan for the client to regain activities of daily living skills, especially motor skills of the upper extremities. • Direct care of occupational therapy assistants.	A client has difficulties using an eating utensil with her dominant hand following a stroke.
Pharmacist	Provide and monitor medications for the client as prescribed by the primary care provider.	A client is concerned about whether or not a new medication will interact with any of his other medications.
Physical therapist	• Assess and plan for the client to increase musculoskeletal function, especially of the lower extremities, to maintain mobility. • Direct care of physical therapy assistants.	Following a hip replacement, a client requires assistance learning to ambulate and regain strength.
Primary care provider	• Assess, diagnose, and treat the client for disease and/or injury. • Supervise care delivered by physician assistants.	A client experiences a change in vital signs. Temperature is 39° C (102.2° F). Client is achy, shaking, and reports "feeling cold."
Radiology technician	Position the client and perform x-rays and other imaging procedures for primary care providers to review for diagnosis of disorders of various body parts.	A client reports severe pain in his hip after a fall, and the primary care provider orders an x-ray of the client's hip.
Respiratory therapist	Assess respiratory status and provide prescribed respiratory treatments.	A client with respiratory disease is short of breath and requests a nebulizer treatment that has been ordered "as needed."

Title	Job description	Example of when to refer
Social worker	Work with the client and the client's family by coordinating inpatient and community resources to meet psychosocial and environmental needs that are necessary for recovery and/or discharge.	A client who is dying of cancer wishes to go home but is no longer able to perform many activities of daily living. The spouse needs medical equipment in the home to care for the client.
Speech therapist	• Evaluate and make recommendations regarding the functions of speech, language, and swallowing impacted by various client disorders or injuries. • Teach the client techniques and exercises to improve function when possible.	A client is having difficulty swallowing a regular diet after trauma to the head and neck.

Δ Nursing Personnel

- The nursing team is responsible for working together to advocate for and meet the needs of the client within the health care delivery system.

- The registered nurse is the lead team member, soliciting input from all nursing team members, setting priorities, sharing information with other disciplines, and coordinating the care of the client.

Title	Educational preparation	Roles/responsibilities
Registered Nurse (RN)	• Varies – must meet requirements for licensure set by each state board of nursing • Required completion of a diploma program, an associate degree, or baccalaureate degree in nursing prior to taking the licensure exam (licensed)	• Function legally under state nurse practice acts. • Perform assessments; establish nursing diagnoses, goals, and interventions; and conduct ongoing client evaluations. • Participate in developing interdisciplinary plans for client care. • Share appropriate information among team members, initiate referrals for client assistance, including health education, and identify community resources.

Title	Educational preparation	Roles/responsibilities
Licensed Vocational/ Practical Nurse (LVN/ LPN)	• Varies – must meet requirements set by each state board of nursing • Vocational or community college education required prior to taking the licensure exam (licensed)	• Work under the supervision of the RN. • Collaborate within the nursing process, coordinate the client plan of care, consult with other team members, and recognize the need for referrals to assist the client with actual or potential problems. • Possess technical knowledge and skills. • Participate in the delivery of nursing care, using the nursing process as a framework.
Assistive Personnel (AP) including Certified Nurse Assistants (CNAs) and Certified Medical Assistants (CMAs)	• Varies – formal or informal training requirements as set by each state • Specialized roles: nutritional aides, monitor technicians, and physical therapy aides • Requirement by most states for training and examination to attain CNA status • Usually under the direct supervision of an RN	• Specific tasks are usually outlined in a position description in the employing facility/agency. • Tasks may include feeding clients, preparing nutritional supplements, lifting, basic care (e.g., grooming, bathing, transferring, toileting, positioning), measuring and recording vital signs, and ambulating clients.

Δ   **Expanded nursing roles**

- An **Advanced Practice Nurse (APN)** has a great deal of autonomy. APNs usually possess a minimum of a master's degree in nursing (or related field), advanced education in pharmacology and physical assessment, and certification in a specialized area of practice. Included in this role is the:

  ◊   **Clinical Nurse Specialist (CNS)** – typically specializes in a practice setting or a disease field.

  ◊   **Nurse Practitioner (NP)** – collaborates with one or more providers to provide nonemergency primary health care in a variety of settings.

  ◊   **Certified Nurse-Midwife (CNW)** – collaborates with one or more providers to provide care to maternal-newborn clients and their families.

◊ **Certified Registered Nurse Anesthetist (CRNA)** – administers anesthesia and provides care to the client during procedures. The RNA is under the supervision of an anesthesiologist.

◊ **Nurse Educator** – may teach at the associate degree, baccalaureate, master's, or doctoral level.

◊ **Nurse Administrator** – provides leadership to nursing departments within a health care facility/agency.

◊ **Nurse Researcher** – conducts research that will provide more nursing knowledge to improve the quality of client care.

Primary Reference:

Potter, P. A., & Perry, A. G. (2005). *Fundamentals of nursing* (6th ed.). St. Louis, MO: Mosby.

Additional Resources:

NANDA International (2004). *NANDA nursing diagnoses: Definitions and classification 2005-2006.* Philadelphia: NANDA.

For information about labor statistics, go to the U.S. Department of Labor's Bureau of Labor Statistics Web site, *http://www.bls.gov/,* and choose *Occupational Outlook Handbook.*

Chapter 2: Roles and the Interdisciplinary Team

Application Exercises

1. A nursing team comprised of an RN team leader, a LPN/LVN, and a CNA, is assigned to nine clients on a medical surgical unit. One of the nine clients has leg stasis ulcers and requires wound care. Which of the following team members should be assigned to complete this task?

> A. The CNA who is 2 months away from completing her RN program
> B. The RN who is licensed to perform this task
> C. The LPN/LVN who has worked on the unit for 6 years
> D. A wound care nurse specialist

2. The nursing team is directed by the

> A. assistive personnel.
> B. LPN/LVN.
> C. registered nurse.
> D. nutrition aide.

3. Match the following job title to the activity the team member might perform.

D	Occupational therapist	A. Evaluates the client's nutritional status
G	Physical therapist	B. Dispenses medications as prescribed by the primary care provider
E	Speech therapist	C. Draws blood specimens
F	Radiology technician	D. Provides the client a fork with an enlarged handle
C	Laboratory technician	E. Observes the client swallow gelatin
A	Registered dietician	F. Removes the client's wristwatch prior to a magnetic resonance imaging (MRI) scan
B	Pharmacist	G. Teaches the client how to use a walker to ambulate

4. An older adult client who lives alone is to be discharged in 3 to 4 days. He is assigned a prescribed diet but states that it is difficult to prepare adequate nutritious meals at home for just one person. Which of the following members of the health care team should he be referred to?

> A. Registered dietician
> B. Occupational therapist
> C. Speech therapist
> D. Social worker

Chapter 2: Roles and the Interdisciplinary Team

Application Exercises Answer Key

1. A nursing team comprised of an RN team leader, a LPN/LVN, and a CNA is assigned to nine clients on a medical surgical unit. One of the nine clients has leg stasis ulcers and requires wound care. Which of the following team members should be assigned to complete this task?

    A. The CNA who is 2 months away from completing her RN program

    B. The RN who is licensed to perform this task

    C. The LPN/LVN who has worked on the unit for 6 years

    D. Wound care nurse specialist.

    The LPN/LVN collaborates within the nursing process and is qualified to perform wound care. Wound care is not within the scope of practice of a CNA, even if this particular person learned how to perform wound care in her RN educational setting. As the team leader, the RN is ultimately responsible for the care, but can delegate the intervention to the LPN/LVN. A wound care specialist may be preferable; however, wound care is within the scope of practice of both an RN and LPN/LVN.

2. The nursing team is directed by the

    A. assistive personnel.

    B. LPN/LVN.

    C. registered nurse.

    D. nutrition aide.

    The RN is ultimately responsible for the care given to clients. Both AP and LPNs are supervised by the nurse. The LPN collaborates within the nursing process; AP are usually assigned specific tasks to complete. The nutrition aide is a member of the health care team but not the nursing team.

3. Match the following job title to the activity the team member might perform.

D	Occupational therapist	A. Evaluates the client's nutritional status
G	Physical therapist	B. Dispenses medications as prescribed by the primary care provider
E	Speech therapist	C. Draws blood specimens
F	Radiology technician	D. Provides the client a fork with an enlarged handle
C	Laboratory technician	E. Observes the client swallow gelatin
A	Registered dietician	F. Removes the client's wristwatch prior to a magnetic resonance imaging (MRI) scan
B	Pharmacist	G. Teaches the client how to use a walker to ambulate

4. An older adult client who lives alone is to be discharged in 3 to 4 days. He is assigned a prescribed diet but states that it is difficult to prepare adequate nutritious meals at home for just one person. Which of the following members of the health care team should he be referred to?

    A. Registered dietician

    B. Occupational therapist

    C. Speech therapist

    D. Social worker

A social worker can make arrangements for Meals on Wheels to deliver nutritious meals daily, or recommend a congregate meal site near the client's home. The registered dietician usually performs the assessment of a client's nutritional status and provides teaching concerning appropriate diet. The occupational therapist can assist the client who is having problems manipulating eating/drinking utensils. The speech therapist can assist the client who is having swallowing problems.

Unit 1   Foundations for Practice
Section: Health Care Delivery

Chapter 3:	Delegation of Nurse-Related Tasks

Contributor: Linda Turchin, MSN, RN

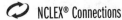 NCLEX® Connections

Learning Objective: Review and apply knowledge within "**Delegation of Nurse Related Tasks**" in readiness for performance of the following nursing activities as outlined by the NCLEX® test plans:

RN Role

Δ   Identify tasks that can be delegated to licensed professional nurses (LPNs)/assistive personnel (AP) by the registered nurse.

Δ   Plan and provide care by assigning, delegating, and supervising LPNs/AP, based on level of care needed.

Δ   Assess and ensure ability (e.g., knowledge, skill level, experience) of health care team members when delegating responsibilities.

Δ   Provide accurate, concise reports to assist health care team members in their performance of delegated tasks, and instruct when to seek assistance immediately.

Δ   Delegate tasks to LPNs/AP consistent with all regulatory requirements, including the five rights of delegation.

Δ   Evaluate delegated care given by LPNs/AP.

LPN Role

Δ   Assign client care to AP after comparing the abilities of AP with the client's care needs.

Key Points

Δ   **Delegating** is the transfer of responsibility for the performance of a task or activity while retaining accountability for its outcome.

Δ   To delegate a task, the nurse directs another person to perform nursing-related tasks and activities.

Δ The risk of liability with delegation relates to the appropriateness of the **delegation** to an individual and the monitoring of the performance.

Δ Nurses need to use informed judgment when decisions are made regarding the delegation process.

Key Factors

Δ State nurse practice acts hold the RN **responsible** and **accountable** for providing client care.

Δ The RN decides on the **appropriateness** of delegating direct client care.

Δ Parts of nursing care can be delegated, but the RN **cannot delegate** the care related to the **nursing process.**

Δ **Effective communication skills** are needed by the RN and other health care team members.

Δ Professional judgment and critical thinking skills are used when implementing the **five rights** of delegation.

- **Right task** – "a task that is delegable for a specific patient." A right task is repetitive, requires little supervision, and/or is relatively noninvasive for a certain client.

Right Task	Wrong Task
Delegate LPN to perform a dressing change on a client with cellulitis.	Delegate LPN to develop the care plan for a client with cellulitis.

- **Right circumstances** – the appropriate client setting, available resources, and other relevant factors are considered. If the circumstances have not been assessed or are deemed too complicated, the nurse takes the responsibility and does not delegate a task to AP.

Right Circumstance	Wrong Circumstance
Delegate AP to take and record routine check-in vital signs of office clients.	Delegate AP to take vital signs on a client receiving IV therapy for hypovolemic shock.

- **Right person** – the right person is delegating the right task to the right person to be performed on the right person.

Right Person	Wrong Person
Delegate LPN to perform tracheostomy care on a client.	Delegate AP to perform tracheostomy care on a client.

- **Right direction/communication** – a clear, concise description of the task is conveyed, including its objective, limits, expectations, and when to report concerns/assessment findings. Very specific, clear directions are essential for delegation to work well.

Right Direction/Communication	Wrong Direction/Communication
Delegate AP the task of obtaining a clean-catch urine specimen from the client in room 423, bed 2.	Delegate AP the task of obtaining a urine specimen on a client in room 423, but not informing her of what type of urine specimen, or which specific client in the room needs the specimen.

- **Right supervision** – "appropriate monitoring, evaluation, intervention, as needed, and feedback." The nurse remains accountable for the tasks that were delegated and for making clinical judgments.

Right Supervision	Wrong Supervision
An RN delegates to an LPN the task of administering enteral feedings to a client (after the RN performs a physical assessment to evaluate the client's tolerance to feedings thus far).	An RN delegates to an LPN the task of providing client teaching to a client without a written care plan in place.

Nursing Interventions

Δ   Under their direction, RNs may delegate to LPNs/AP (provided agency policies and state practice guidelines permit) tasks such as:

Tasks Delegated to LPNs	Tasks Delegated to AP
<ul><li>Monitoring client findings (as input to the RN's ongoing assessment of the client)</li><li>Reinforcement of client teaching from a standard care plan</li><li>Tracheostomy care</li><li>Suctioning</li><li>Checking nasogastric tube patency</li><li>Administration of enteral feedings</li><li>Insertion of a urinary catheter</li><li>Medication administration (excluding intravenous medications, in several states)</li></ul>	<ul><li>Activities of daily living (ADLs)</li><li>Bathing</li><li>Grooming</li><li>Dressing</li><li>Toileting</li><li>Ambulating</li><li>Feeding (without swallowing precautions)</li><li>Positioning</li><li>Bed making</li><li>Specimen collection</li><li>Intake and output (I&O)</li><li>Vital signs</li></ul>

Primary Reference:

Potter, P. A., & Perry, A. G. (2005). *Fundamentals of nursing* (6th ed.). St. Louis, MO: Mosby.

Additional Resources:

NANDA International (2004). *NANDA nursing diagnoses: Definitions and classification 2005-2006*. Philadelphia: NANDA.

Trossman, S. (2006, October). Issues up close: Getting a clearer picture on delegation. *American Nurse Today, 1*, 54.

Chapter 3: Delegation of Nurse-Related Tasks

Application Exercises

1. Which of the following tasks may be delegated to AP? (Select all that apply.)

_____ Establishing an intravenous route

_____ Transcribing a medical order

_____ Assisting a client to take a shower

_____ Providing fresh water to a client tolerating a clear liquid diet started 2 hr ago

_____ Assessing vital signs on a client who is expected to be discharged later in the day

2. What information should be shared by the nurse delegating the ambulation of a client who had a left knee replaced 5 days ago to AP? (Select all that apply.)

_____ The client is in room 203 – Bed B.

_____ The roommate is up independently.

_____ The client ambulates with his gray slippers on over his antiembolic stockings.

_____ The client uses the front-wheeled walker when ambulating.

_____ The client had pain medication 30 min ago.

_____ The client is allergic to codeine.

_____ The client needs to try and ambulate at least 50 ft.

_____ The client ate 50% of his breakfast this morning.

_____ The client mainly needs assistance getting in and out of bed.

Chapter 3: Delegation of Nurse-Related Tasks

Application Exercises Answer Key

1. Which of the following tasks may be delegated to AP? (Select all that apply.)

_____ Establishing an intravenous route

_____ Transcribing a medical order

__X__ **Assisting a client to take a shower**

__X__ **Providing fresh water to a client tolerating a clear liquid diet started 2 hr ago**

__X__ **Assessing vital signs on a client who is expected to be discharged later in the day**

Assisting a client to take a shower, providing fresh water, and assessing vital signs are all tasks that may be delegated to AP. Establishing an intravenous route and transcribing a medical order must be performed by a licensed nurse.

2. What information should be shared by the nurse delegating the ambulation of a client who had a left knee replaced 5 days ago to AP? (Select all that apply.)

__X__ **The client is in room 203 – Bed B.**

_____ The roommate is up independently.

__X__ **The client ambulates with his gray slippers on over his antiembolic stockings.**

__X__ **The client uses the front-wheeled walker when ambulating.**

__X__ **The client had pain medication 30 min ago.**

_____ The client is allergic to codeine.

__X__ **The client needs to try and ambulate at least 50 ft.**

_____ The client ate 50% of his breakfast this morning.

__X__ **The client mainly needs assistance getting in and out of bed.**

Right direction/communication is necessary for safe delegation. The information checked is necessary for the AP to perform the task safely. The other information is not necessary to know for the task to be performed safely.

Unit 1   Foundations for Practice
Section: Health Care Delivery

Chapter 4:   Health Promotion and Disease Prevention
Contributor: Patricia A Girczyc, EdD(c), MPH, FNP

 NCLEX® Connections:

Learning Objective: Review and apply knowledge within "**Health Promotion and Disease Prevention**" in readiness for performance of the following nursing activities as outlined by the NCLEX® test plans:

Δ   Assess/monitor/evaluate the client's and family's understanding of, and participation in, health promotion behaviors/activities.

Δ   Identify lifestyle practices and genetic risk factors that may impact the health of the client and the family.

Δ   Instruct/reinforce teaching of clients and families on ways to promote health and age appropriate actions to maintain health and prevent disease.

 Key Points

Δ   Nurses can contribute greatly to the health of clients and population groups using health promotion and disease prevention strategies.

Δ   Levels of prevention address health related activities and are classified as primary, secondary, and tertiary. Levels of prevention are not the same as levels of care (*Refer to chapter 1, Health Care Delivery Systems.*).

Δ   Health promotion and disease prevention activities occur throughout the health care delivery system.

Key Factors

Level of prevention	Examples of prevention activities
Primary prevention addresses the needs of healthy clients to promote health and prevent disease with specific protections.	• Immunization programs • Child car seat education • Nutrition and fitness activities • Health education in schools
Secondary prevention focuses on early identification of individuals or communities experiencing illness, providing treatment, and conducting activities that are geared to prevent a worsening health status.	• Communicable disease screening and case finding • Early detection and treatment of diabetes • Exercise programs for older adult clients who are frail
Tertiary prevention aims to prevent the long-term consequences of a chronic illness or disability and to support optimal functioning.	• Prevention of pressure ulcers as a complication of spinal cord injury • Promoting independence for the client with traumatic brain injury • Providing case management services for victims of a disaster

Δ   **Risk factor** assessment includes:

- **Genetics** – There can be a predisposition for various illnesses that can be attributed to heredity (e.g., family history of heart disease, cancers, certain mental illnesses).

- **Gender** – Gender differences can be seen in increased risks for certain health concerns (e.g., males having a higher suicide rate, breast cancer being more common in females).

- **Physiologic factors** – Various physiologic states place the client at an increased risk for health problems (e.g., body mass index [BMI] > than 25, pregnancy).

- **Environmental factors** – The presence of toxic substances and chemicals can impact health in the places where clients live and work. Water quality, pesticide exposure, and air pollution should be commonly assessed.

- **Lifestyle-risk behaviors** – Risk behaviors for which to screen include stress, substance abuse, diet, exercise habits, and sun exposure.

- **Age** – Early disease detection and intervention is facilitated by following screening guidelines developed in a joint effort of the American Diabetes Association, the American Heart Association, and the American Cancer Society. Ages may vary based on individual practices (e.g., a female client who has become sexually active before the age of 20 should start screenings at the age when sexual activity begins.).

Test	Female	Male
Blood pressure	Starting at age 20 – each routine healthcare visit, minimum of every 2 years	Starting at age 20 – each routine health care visit, minimum of every 2 years
Body mass index (BMI)	Starting at age 20 – each routine healthcare visit	Starting at age 20 – each routine health care visit
Blood cholesterol	Starting at age 20 – a minimum of every 5 years	Starting at age 20 – a minimum of every 5 years
Blood glucose	Starting at age 45 – a minimum of every 3 years	Starting at age 45 – a minimum of every 3 years
Colorectal screening	Starting at age 50 – every 1 to 10 years depending on test used by primary care provider	Starting at age 50 – every 1 to 10 years depending on test used by primary care provider
Pap test	• Starting at age 20 (or earlier if sexually active) – yearly, • After age 30 – every 1 to 3 years, depending on test used by primary care provider	
Clinical breast exam	• Starting at age 20 – every 3 years • Starting at age 40 – yearly	
Mammogram	Starting at age 40 – yearly	
Clinical testicular exam		Starting at age 20 – with every routine health visit
Prostate-specific antigen test and digital rectal exam		Starting at age 50 – as indicated by the primary care provider

Nursing Interventions

Δ   Facilitate health behavior changes.

- Provide health information.

- Adopt **mutually agreed upon goals,** and identify supports to attain goals (e.g., client will give up unhealthy behaviors and/or adopt healthy behaviors).

- Identify and make appropriate referrals to educational/community/support resources, based upon assessment information.

Δ   Use behavior-change strategies.

- Identify the client's readiness to receive and act upon health information.

- Identify interventions acceptable to the client.

- Help motivate the client to change by setting realistic timelines.

- Reinforce steps the client makes toward change.

- Encourage the client to maintain the change.

Δ   Promote healthy lifestyle behaviors.

- Minimize or reduce stress.

- Get adequate sleep and rest.

- Eat a nutritious diet to achieve and maintain a healthy weight.

- Participate in physical activity at least 30 min/day.

- Respect the sun's rays by wearing protective clothing, using sunscreen, and avoiding exposure between 10 a.m. and 4 p.m.

- Wear safety gear (e.g., bike helmets, knee and elbow pads) when participating in physical activity.

- Avoid substances such as tobacco products, alcohol, and illegal drugs.

- Practice safe sex.

- Seek medical care when necessary, and visit primary care provider for routine screenings.

Primary Reference:

Potter, P. A., & Perry, A. G. (2005). *Fundamentals of nursing* (6th ed.). St. Louis, MO: Mosby.

Additional Resources:

American Cancer Society (2006). *Guidelines for the early detection of cancer.* Retrieved Sept. 8, 2006 from http://www.cancer.org/docroot/home/index.asp

American Heart Association (2006). *A common agenda for health from the American Cancer Society, American Diabetes Association, and the American Heart Association.* Retrieved Sept. 8, 2006 from www.americanheart.org/presenter.jhtml?identifier=1200000

NANDA International (2004). *NANDA nursing diagnoses: Definitions and classification 2005-2006.* Philadelphia: NANDA.

Chapter 4: Health Promotion and Disease Prevention

Application Exercises

1. Match the appropriate level of health care prevention with the preventive activity. Each level can be used more than once.

1. Primary prevention

2. Secondary prevention

3. Tertiary prevention

_____ Blood pressure screening at senior center

_____ Driver's education

_____ Monitored exercise therapy at a cardiac rehabilitation center

_____ Community cholesterol screening

_____ Teaching self-catheterization to a client with a spinal cord injury

_____ Newborn immunizations

2. A 19-year-old female client has come to the college health clinic for a Pap test. It is her first visit. Which of the following interventions should the nurse perform first to determine the client's need for health promotion and disease prevention?

   A. Take the client's vital signs.

   B. Stress the need for HIV screening.

   C. Assess the client's risk factors.

   D. Instruct the client to use condoms for birth control.

3. Which of the following risk factors should the nurse address when providing education to a client at a routine health care visit? (Select all that apply.)

   _____ Age

   _____ Use of tobacco

   _____ Lack of physical activity

   _____ Gender

   _____ Diet high in fats

4. A 21-year-old college student presents to the health clinic for a sore throat. He tells the nurse that he has not seen a doctor since high school. What health screening should the nurse anticipate will be performed for this client?

Chapter 4: Health Promotion and Disease Prevention

Application Exercises Answer Key

1. Match the appropriate level of health care prevention with the preventive activity. Each level can be used more than once.

1. Primary prevention

2. Secondary prevention

3. Tertiary prevention

  2   Blood pressure screening at senior center

  1   Driver's education

  3   Monitored exercise therapy at a cardiac rehabilitation center

  2   Community cholesterol screening

  3   Teaching self-catheterization to a client with a spinal cord injury

  1   Newborn immunizations

2. A 19-year-old female client has come to the college health clinic for a Pap test. It is her first visit. Which of the following interventions should the nurse perform first to determine the client's need for health promotion and disease prevention?

    A. Take the client's vital signs.

    B. Stress the need for HIV screening.

    C. Assess the client's risk factors.

    D. Instruct the client to use condoms for birth control.

Assessment of risk factors must occur before health promotion or disease prevention interventions are developed. The nurse should conduct an interview with the client before performing any physical exam. This allows the nurse time to establish rapport with the client prior to any invasive procedures. Stressing the need for HIV screening and instructing the client in the use of birth control assumes that certain risk factors already exist.

3. Which of the following risk factors should the nurse address when providing education to a client at a routine health care visit? (Select all that apply.)

    _____ Age

    X   **Use of tobacco**

    X   **Lack of physical activity**

    _____ Gender

    X   **Diet high in fats**

Age and gender are nonmodifiable risk factors. A client can change health behaviors related to tobacco use, physical activity, and diet.

4. A 21-year-old college student presents to the health clinic for a sore throat. He tells the nurse that he has not seen a doctor since high school. What health screening should the nurse anticipate will be performed for this client?

The nurse can expect that the client will be screened for blood pressure, BMI, blood cholesterol, and testicular cancer.

Unit 1   Foundations for Practice
Section: Health Care Delivery

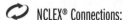

Chapter 5:   Nursing Care of the Individual, Family, and Community
Contributor: Patricia A Girczyc, EdD(c), MPH, FNP

 NCLEX® Connections:

> **Learning Objective**: Review and apply knowledge within "**Nursing Care of the Individual, Family, and Community**" in readiness for performance of the following nursing activities as outlined by the NCLEX® test plans:
>
> Δ   Develop a therapeutic relationship with clients of diverse ages and backgrounds.
>
> Δ   Promote, maintain, and restore the health of individuals, families, and communities.

Key Points

Δ   A foundational therapeutic relationship should be established and maintained with the client.

Δ   Clients include individuals, as well as families and communities.

Δ   This dynamic and constantly changing interaction occurs as the nurse and the individual, family, and/or community develop mutual approaches to promote, maintain, and restore health.

Key Factors

Δ   Elements of a therapeutic relationship

Steps	With individuals	With families	With communities
Establishing Trust	• The nurse sets the tone of the initial interaction, knowing that future interactions will be more in-depth as the client develops trust in the nurse's abilities and willingness to help. • Techniques include being present, demonstrating empathy and warmth, active listening, and being nonjudgmental.	• The nurse suspends all preconceived notions in order to develop an understanding of the unique relationships within each family, as well as the perspectives and concerns of the individuals as members of the family. • The nurse identifies who is a family member, what role each family member undertakes, and the dynamic interactions within the family.	• The nurse assesses the elements of the community and the dynamics internal and external to the community. • The nurse suspends judgment, gathers pertinent health statistic data, and seeks information through the perspective of community members.
Sharing Concern about the Well-being of the Client	The nurse gets to know the client and asks reflective questions to deepen an understanding of the client's experience and priorities.	The nurse listens attentively and uses therapeutic communication techniques of reflection and restatement to clarify the family concerns.	The nurse analyzes and summarizes the findings of the community assessment to accurately reflect community concerns.
Establishing Mutual Goals	The nurse understands the goals of the client and adds her own knowledge and experience to promote wellness.	The nurse establishes mutual goals and adds experience and knowledge to the concerns of the family to develop a mutual set of goals and plans.	The nurse blends knowledge and experience to suggest the establishment of realistic goals that address the concerns of the community.

Steps	With individuals	With families	With communities
Evaluation	• The nurse evaluates progress of goal achievement. • The nurse brings closure to the relationship or an easy transition to other care providers as health is restored or goals are met.	The nurse evaluates goals within the context of the family unit, which includes checking back to ensure that goals are realistic and achievable, or that new goals are established.	The nurse evaluates progress within the community setting and re-establishes goals as necessary.

Interventions

Δ   Examples of therapeutic relationships in promoting, maintaining, and restoring health

Client	Promoting health	Maintaining health	Restoring health
Individual	Teaching what comprises a healthy weight based on the client's height	Well child check-up	Referral to a smoking cessation program
Family	Teaching injury prevention in the home	Teaching the family how to improve communication with an adolescent child	Family therapy to deal with the chronic illness of a family member
Community	Replacing soda pop machines with water/juice machines in the school cafeteria	Tuberculosis screening for employees of a long-term care facility.	Providing counselors at the school after the death of a classmate

Primary Reference:

Potter, P. A., & Perry, A. G. (2005). *Fundamentals of nursing* (6th ed.). St. Louis, MO: Mosby.

Additional Resources:

NANDA International (2004). *NANDA nursing diagnoses: Definitions and classification 2005-2006.* Philadelphia: NANDA.

Stanhope, M. & Lancaster, J. (2004*). Community and public health nursing* (6th ed.). St. Louis, MO: Mosby.

Chapter 5: Nursing Care of the Individual, Family, and Community

Application Exercises

1. Which of the following behaviors demonstrated by the nurse will facilitate establishment of trust with individual clients, families, and communities? (Select all that apply.)

_____ Asking reflective questions

_____ Favoring the opinions of one family member

_____ Assisting a community to make realistic goals

_____ Demonstrating empathy and competency

_____ Communicating a nonjudgmental attitude

_____ Changing the subject when a family member expresses anger at another family member

2. Which of the following interventions is specific to working with communities?

A. Use clarification to gain a deeper understanding of the health problems.

B. Reflect and restate health concerns.

C. Maintain eye contact and listen actively.

D. Accurately analyze and summarize assessment data from numerous sources.

3. A nurse is making the first home visit to a family of a newborn for a well-infant check. The family includes the 17-year-old mother of the newborn, her 2-year-old daughter, and the grandmother of the two young children. Which of the following interventions will be the most beneficial in establishing a therapeutic relationship with this family?

A. Tell the family members not to worry about any concerns they may have.

B. Include all the family members in the discussion about the infant's exam.

C. Present a nonjudgmental attitude.

D. Give written information regarding well-infant checks.

4. What is the key to successful goal setting in the therapeutic relationship?

Chapter 5: Nursing Care of the Individual, Family, and Community

Application Exercises Answer Key

1. Which of the following behaviors demonstrated by the nurse will facilitate establishment of trust with individual clients, families, and communities? (Select all that apply.)

   __X__   **Asking reflective questions**

   _____   Favoring the opinions of one family member

   __X__   **Assisting a community to make realistic goals**

   __X__   **Demonstrating empathy and competency**

   __X__   **Communicating a nonjudgmental attitude**

   _____   Changing the subject when a family member expresses anger at another family member

   Asking reflective questions, assisting to set realistic goals, and demonstrating empathy and competency will all help establish trust between the nurse and the client, family, and community. Therapeutic communication requires the nurse to remain objective and not show favoritism. Changing the subject when the topic is uncomfortable will not facilitate conflict resolution.

2. Which of the following interventions is specific to working with communities?

   A. Use clarification to gain a deeper understanding of the health problems.

   B. Reflect and restate health concerns.

   C. Maintain eye contact and listen actively.

   D. Accurately analyze and summarize assessment data from numerous sources.

   When sharing concerns with a community, a nurse must analyze and summarize extensive data from available statistics and members of the community. With individuals and families, the information comes primarily from the clients themselves or from their other primary care providers.

3. A nurse is making the first home visit to a family of a newborn for a well-infant check. The family includes the 17-year-old mother of the newborn, her 2-year-old daughter, and the grandmother of the two young children. Which of the following interventions will be the most beneficial in establishing a therapeutic relationship with this family?

A. Tell the family members not to worry about any concerns they may have.

B. Include all the family members in the discussion about the infant's exam.

C. Present a nonjudgmental attitude.

D. Give written information regarding well-infant checks.

Presenting a nonjudgmental attitude is the most beneficial in establishing a therapeutic relationship with a new family. False reassurance dismisses feelings that family members may have. Further assessment is necessary before deciding to include all family members in the discussion. Giving written information is important but is not the most beneficial at the first visit.

4. What is the key to successful goal setting in the therapeutic relationship?

Goal setting should be a mutual activity with the client and nurse working together.

Unit 1   Foundations for Practice
Section: Health Care Delivery

Chapter 6:   Complementary Alternative Therapies
                    Contributor: Patricia A Girczyc, EdD(c), MPH, FNP

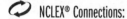 NCLEX® Connections:

Learning Objective: Review and apply knowledge within "**Complementary Alternative Therapies**" in readiness for performance of the following nursing activities as outlined by the NCLEX® test plans:

Δ   Assess/monitor the client's need and use of complementary alternative therapies.

Δ   Plan and/or provide complementary alternative therapies that are within the scope of nursing practice when appropriate.

Δ   Instruct/reinforce teaching of clients and families in the use of available complementary alternative therapies, and make referrals as necessary.

Δ   Evaluate the effectiveness of complementary alternative therapies being used by the client.

 Key Points

Δ   There is a growing interest in the use of complementary and alternative therapies. These therapies are also referred to as **complementary alternative medicine (CAM)** throughout the world.

Δ   Categories of CAM include:

•   **Alternative medical philosophy** (e.g., traditional oriental medicine, acupuncture, homeopathy).

•   **Biological and botanical therapies** (e.g., diets, vitamins, minerals, herbal medicines).

•   **Body manipulation** (e.g., massage, touch, chiropractic therapy).

•   **Mind-body therapies** (e.g., biofeedback, art therapy, meditation, therapeutic touch, psychotherapy).

Δ   An important principle for implementing complementary alternative therapies is the client's acceptance of and involvement in the therapeutic intervention.

Key Factors

    Δ   **Role of the nurse and CAM**

- Possess knowledge about the varieties of therapies available.

- Be receptive to learn about the alternative health beliefs and practices of the client (e.g., home remedies, cultural practices, vitamin use, modification of prescriptions).

- Identify the client's needs for possible complementary alternative therapies.

- Incorporate and provide complementary alternative therapies into the client's care plan as nursing interventions.

    Δ   Specialized licensed or certified practitioners may provide complementary alternative therapies. These include:

Therapy	Characteristics
Acupuncture/pressure	Needles or pressure are exerted along meridians to alter body function.
Homeopathic medicine	Small doses of substances (remedies) that would produce symptoms of the disease state in a well person are given to the ill client to bring about healing.
Naturopathic medicine	Diet, exercise, environment, and herbal remedies are used to promote the natural healing of the body.
Chiropractic medicine	The client is treated through manipulation of the spine.
Massage therapy	Relaxation and circulation are improved through the manipulation of the skin and underlying muscles.
Biofeedback	Technology is used to increase the client's awareness of various neurological body responses to minimize extremes.
Therapeutic touch	Practitioners use their hands to help bring the client's energy fields into balance.

Δ **Nursing interventions** can incorporate aspects of complementary alternative therapies into client care plans. Such nursing interventions include:

Therapy	Characteristics
Guided imagery/visualization therapy	Encourages healing and relaxation of the body by having the mind focus on images
Prayer	Focuses on the power and resources of a higher being to deal with the stress of procedures and/or illness
Breath work	Type of relaxation therapy that teaches various breathing patterns to help the client feel less stressed and more energized
Humor	<ul><li>A coping mechanism that can have a positive effect on the physiological and emotional state of the client</li><li>Used to reduce tension and to keep situations from getting too serious</li></ul>
Meditation	A technique used to calm the mind and body
Touch	Communicates presence with the client and acceptance
Music Therapy	<ul><li>Type of movement and relaxation therapy that includes distraction from pain</li><li>Sessions should last a minimum of 15 min</li><li>Use of earphones can increase concentration</li></ul>
Therapeutic communication	Allows the client to verbalize and become aware of emotions and fears in a safe, nonjudgmental environment

Δ Nurses evaluate the outcomes of complementary alternative therapies and revise the nursing care plan as necessary.

Primary Reference:

Potter, P. A., & Perry, A. G. (2005). *Fundamentals of nursing* (6th ed.). St. Louis, MO: Mosby.

Additional Resources:

NANDA International (2004). *NANDA nursing diagnoses: Definitions and classification 2005-2006.* Philadelphia: NANDA.

For information, go to the National Center for Complementary and Alternative Medicine Web site, *www.nccam.nih.gov.*

Chapter 6: Complementary Alternative Therapies

Application Exercises

1. A nurse admits a 68-year-old client for abdominal surgery. The client's initial vital signs are: temperature 37° C (98.6° F), pulse 98/min, respirations 20/min, and blood pressure 148/88 mm Hg. The nurse notices that the client is anxious and restless. The client states, "I am really worried. This is the first surgery I have ever had!" Which of the following is an appropriate use of a complementary alternative intervention?

   A. Offer information and ask the client if he is interested in trying a relaxation technique.

   B. Call the primary care provider and get permission to use relaxation techniques with the client.

   C. Provide reassurance and information to the client about the procedure.

   D. Give the client a therapeutic back massage and tell him to try to relax.

2. A client presents to a health clinic with back pain. The client tells the nurse that a friend recommended she go to a chiropractor. She asks the nurse what a chiropractor does to relieve back pain. Which of the following statements by the nurse is correct?

   A. "Chiropractors use their hands to manipulate the spine to treat back pain."

   B. "Chiropractors insert needles or pressure along meridians in the back."

   C. "Chiropractors use herbal remedies to treat back pain."

   D. "Chiropractors use their hands to balance the energy fields in the back."

3. Massage therapy is an example of what category of alternative therapy?

   A. Alternative medical philosophy

   B. Biological therapy

   C. Body manipulation

   D. Mind-body therapy

4. Match the following complementary alternative therapies with the appropriate requirements needed to perform the technique.

_____ Relaxation techniques   A. Within the scope of nursing practice

_____ Therapeutic touch

_____ Humor   B. Additional certification or license required

_____ Acupuncture

_____ Chiropractic techniques

_____ Therapeutic communication

5. A complementary alternative therapy that helps to reduce tension, lighten the mood, and improve physiologic function is _____.

Chapter 6: Complementary Alternative Therapies

Application Exercises Answer Key

1. A nurse admits a 68-year-old client for abdominal surgery. The client's initial vital signs are: temperature 37° C (98.6° F), pulse 98/min, respirations 20/min, and blood pressure 148/88 mm Hg. The nurse notices that the client is anxious and restless. The client states, "I am really worried. This is the first surgery I have ever had!" Which of the following is an appropriate use of a complementary alternative intervention?

   A. Offer information and ask the client if he is interested in trying a relaxation technique.

   B. Call the primary care provider and get permission to use relaxation techniques with the client.

   C. Provide reassurance and information to the client about the procedure.

   D. Give the client a therapeutic back massage and tell him to try to relax.

   Providing information and obtaining consent by the client gives him information with which to make an informed decision. A provider's order is not required for relaxation therapy. Providing reassurance may negate the client's fear. Providing more information without validating this as a need may increase his anxiety. The nurse should not give any therapy without informing the client and obtaining his consent. Telling him to relax does not acknowledge his anxiety.

2. A client presents to a health clinic with back pain. The client tells the nurse that a friend recommended she go to a chiropractor. She asks the nurse what a chiropractor does to relieve back pain. Which of the following statements by the nurse is correct?

   A. "Chiropractors use their hands to manipulate the spine to treat back pain."

   B. "Chiropractors insert needles or pressure along meridians in the back."

   C. "Chiropractors use herbal remedies to treat back pain."

   D. "Chiropractors use their hands to balance the energy fields in the back."

   Chiropractors use their hands to manipulate the spine. Acupuncture uses needles or pressure. Naturopathic medicine uses herbal remedies, and therapeutic touch practitioners use their hands to balance the energy fields in the back.

3. Massage therapy is an example of what category of alternative therapy?

        A. Alternative medical philosophy

        B. Biological therapy

        C. Body manipulation

        D. Mind-body therapy

Massage therapy is one type of body manipulation therapy. Alternative medical philosophy includes acupuncture and homeopathy. Biological therapy includes diet, vitamin and mineral supplementation, and herbal remedies. Mind-body therapy includes biofeedback, meditation, and psychotherapy.

4. Match the following complementary alternative therapies with the appropriate requirements needed to perform the technique.

   A Relaxation techniques   A. Within the scope of nursing practice

   B Therapeutic touch

   A Humor   B. Additional certification or license required

   B Acupuncture

   B Chiropractic techniques

   A Therapeutic communication

5. Fill in the blank: A complementary alternative therapy that helps to reduce tension, lighten the mood, and improve physiologic function is _____.

Humor

Unit 1   Foundations for Practice
Section: Thinking Strategies for Nursing Practice

Chapter 7:	Nursing Process

Contributor: Linda Turchin, MSN, RN

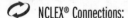 **NCLEX® Connections:**

Learning Objective: Review and apply knowledge within **"Nursing Process"** in readiness for performance of the following nursing activities as outlined by the NCLEX® test plans:

Δ   Use knowledge from the biologic and social sciences in assessing/monitoring, identifying nursing diagnoses, setting priorities, implementing interventions, and evaluating care for the client/family/community.

Δ   Gain awareness of the use of data collection/client assessment for developing problem lists and nursing diagnoses.

Δ   Prioritize the care required by the client using appropriate critical thinking strategies.

Δ   Plan and/or provide care appropriate to the client's mental and physiologic needs.

Δ   Evaluate the client's response to the care provided in order to make adjustments in the plan of care as needed.

 Key Points

Δ   The **Nursing Process**:

•   Uses critical thinking to organize and deliver nursing care through the identification, diagnosis, and treatment of the client's response to health and illness.

•   Provides a framework in which nurses can apply their knowledge, experience, attitudes, and skills, as well as the established Standards of Nursing Practice to the formulation of a plan of nursing care. This plan is applicable to any client system, including individuals, families, groups, or communities.

- Includes five sequential, but overlapping steps that include assessment, diagnosis, planning, implementation, and evaluation. Use of the nursing process results in a comprehensive, individualized, client-centered plan of nursing care that can be delivered in a timely, reasonable manner.

- Allows nurses to creatively integrate critical thinking to make nursing judgments based on reason.

- Promotes the professionalism of nursing while differentiating the practice of nursing from the practice of medicine and other health care professionals.

Δ The North American Nursing Diagnosis Association (NANDA) has developed a standardized terminology or taxonomy for identifying client problems (Nursing Diagnosis). The Center for Nursing Classification and Clinical Effectiveness at the University Of Iowa College Of Nursing has developed standardized terminology for nursing outcomes (Nursing Outcomes Classification [NOC]) and for nursing interventions (Nursing Interventions Classification [NIC]).

Δ The nursing process is sequential with each step depending on the satisfactory completion of the preceding step(s). The nurse must have accurate assessment data in order to select the correct nursing diagnosis, appropriate client outcomes, and nursing interventions. Implementation and evaluation are directly impacted by the accuracy and thoroughness of the preceding phases.

Key Factors

Δ **Assessment**

- Client data can be collected during an initial assessment (baseline data), a focused assessment, and ongoing assessments.

- Methods of data collection include observation, interviewing, physical examination, and collaboration.

- **Subjective** data (**symptoms**) are usually obtained during a **nursing history** and include the client's own feelings, perceptions, and descriptions of her health status. Subjective data are described, verified, and apparent only to the client.

- **Objective** data (**signs**) are usually obtained during a **physical examination**. The data are observable and measurable. Objective data is felt, seen, heard, or smelled by the nurse through observation or physical assessment of the client.

Sources of data	Subjective	Objective
Primary sources of data	What the client tells the nurse: "My shoulder is really, really sore."	Data the nurse obtains through observation and examination: The client is observed grimacing when attempting to brush her hair with her left arm.
Secondary sources of data	What others tell the nurse based on what the client has told them: "She told me that her shoulder is sore every morning."	Data collected from other sources (e.g., family, friends, caregivers, health care professionals, literature review, medical records): Physical therapy note in chart indicates that the client has decreased range of motion of shoulder.

- During this step, the nurse will validate, interpret, and cluster data.

- Documentation of the assessment data must be thorough, concise, and accurate. State nurse practice acts in all states, the American Nurses Association Policy Statement (2003), and the Standards of Clinical Nursing Practice (1998) mandate accurate data collection and recording as independent functions essential to the role of the professional nurse.

Δ **Diagnosis**

- The nurse uses critical thinking skills (a diagnostic reasoning process) to identify the client's health status or problem(s), interpret the assessment database in order to identify nursing diagnoses, and provide direction for nursing care.

- Analysis requires the nurse to look at the data and

  ◊ Recognize patterns or trends.

  ◊ Compare the data with normal standards.

  ◊ Arrive at diagnostic conclusions.

- A nursing diagnosis:

  ◊ Specifically describes the client's actual or potential reaction to a health problem that the nurse is licensed and skilled to treat.

- The following "formula" is used to construct a nursing diagnosis:

  ◊ **Problem statement** r/t (related to) **etiology** AEB (as evidenced by) **defining characteristics**.

Problem Statement or Diagnostic Label	Etiology	Defining Characteristics
• Standardized terminology created by NANDA – the definition of each label clarifying the meaning • Brief phase or term describing the client's response to actual or potential health problems • Directs the development of desired client outcomes • Descriptors or modifiers limiting or defining the diagnostic label (e.g., impaired, imbalanced, dysfunctional)	• One or more probable causes of the health problem • Factors causing or contributing to the health problem • Related or risk factors of the health problem • Biological, psychological, social, developmental, treatment-related, and situational factors contributing to the cause of the problem	• Subjective and objective data obtained from client assessment • Cues and inferences that point to the existence of a particular diagnostic label

Actual Nursing Diagnosis	At-risk Nursing Diagnosis
• Client problem exists at time of nursing assessment. • Diagnosis is based on identification of defining characteristics. • Nursing care focuses on relief or resolution of the problem.	• Presence of risk factors indicates likelihood of problem developing. • Diagnosis is based on presence of risk factors rather than defining characteristics. • Nursing care focuses on reduction of risk factors to prevent the problem from occurring.

- A **syndrome nursing diagnosis** signifies a problem that has common signs and symptoms that almost always present together.

- A **wellness diagnosis** signifies a state of a client/family/community ready for improved health status.

Δ **Planning** – The nurse **sets priorities**, determines **client outcomes,** and selects specific **nursing interventions**.

- The nurse participates in **priority setting** when a preferential order of client problems is identified. This guides the delivery of nursing care. The nurse can use guidelines to set priorities, such as Maslow's hierarchy of basic needs.

- The nurse works with the client to identify **goals and client outcomes.**

  ◊ The goal will identify the desired client status, whereas the client outcome will identify the observable criterion that will determine success or failure of the goal.

  ◊ Often these terms are used interchangeably. Nurses need to follow their health care facility/agency protocol. Regardless of the format used, the goal/client outcome must be **client-centered, singular, observable, measurable, time-limited, mutually agreed upon, and reasonable.**

◊ Concise, measurable goals allow the nurse and client to evaluate progress toward the desired outcome and the effectiveness of nursing care.

◊ Each outcome identified in the **Nursing Outcomes Classification** (NOC) includes a definition, measurement scale, and indicators.

• The nurse identifies nursing actions or **nursing interventions** that will assist in achievement of client outcomes. Nursing interventions are any treatment or action that the nurse performs to enhance/achieve the client's outcomes.

◊ Nursing interventions are based on scientific principles that give the rationale for the action to be taken.

◊ Each nursing intervention identified in the **Nursing Interventions Classifications** (NIC) includes a label (name), definition, and a list of activities and rationales.

◊ Interventions include:

° **Nurse initiated/independent interventions** – autonomous action based on scientific rationale that is expected to benefit the client. It is initiated by the nurse based on the client's nursing diagnosis, health care needs, and within the nurse's scope of practice as identified by the ANA Standards of Practice, state nurse practice acts, and healthcare facility/agency policies. The nurse performs or delegates the interventions. The nurse is accountable for these interventions, such as turning a client every 2 hr to prevent skin breakdown.

° **Physician initiated/dependent interventions** – interventions that the nurse initiates as a result of a primary care provider's order (written, standing, or verbal) or facility/agency protocol, such as blood administration procedure.

° **Collaborative interventions** – interventions the nurse carries out in collaboration with other health care team professionals, such as assuring that the client receives and eats his evening snack.

• The nursing care plan (NCP) is the end product of the planning step. The NCP is organized for quick identification of the client's nursing diagnosis, outcomes, and the interventions that need to be implemented.

Δ **Implementation**

• The nurse will use intellectual skills (problem solving, critical, and creative thinking), interpersonal skills (therapeutic communication), and technical skills (psychomotor performance) when implementing nursing interventions.

• During implementation, the nurse may reassess the client, implement nursing actions, delegate tasks, supervise other health care personnel, and document care given and client responses.

Δ   Evaluation

- The nurse determines the effectiveness of the nursing care plan. The nurse collects data from the client based on the outcome criteria determined. The nurse will compare what actually happened to the desired client outcome. This assists the nurse to determine what further actions need to be taken.

- Questions the nurse should ask herself include:

   ◊   "Were the desired client outcomes met?"

   ◊   "Were the nursing interventions appropriate/effective?"

   ◊   "Do the outcomes and/or interventions need to be modified?"

- Client outcomes that are stated in specific, measurable terms are easier to evaluate.

- Factors that can lead to lack of goal achievement include:

   ◊   Incomplete database.

   ◊   Unrealistic client outcomes.

   ◊   Nonspecific nursing interventions.

   ◊   Inadequate time for client to achieve outcome.

Primary Reference:

Potter, P. A., & Perry, A. G. (2005). *Fundamentals of nursing* (6th ed.). St. Louis, MO: Mosby.

Additional Resources:

Ackley, G. & Ladwig, B. (2004). *Nursing diagnosis handbook: A guide to planning care.* St. Louis, MO: Mosby.

NANDA International (2004). *NANDA nursing diagnoses: Definitions and classification 2005-2006.* Philadelphia: NANDA.

Chapter 7: Nursing Process

Application Exercises

1. Identify each of the following statements as subjective data (S) or as objective data (O).

	Respiratory rate of 22/min that is even and unlabored
	"I can only walk 3 blocks before my legs start to hurt."
	Pain rated at 3 on a scale of 1 to 10
	Skin pink, warm, and dry
	Urine output of 300 mL/8 hr
	"My wife doesn't come to visit very often."
	Dressing clean, dry, and intact

2. By the second postoperative day a client has not achieved satisfactory pain relief. Based on this evaluation, what should the nurse do next based on the nursing process?

    A. Reassess the client to determine the reason satisfactory pain relief has not been achieved.

    B. Wait to see if the pain lessens over the next 24 hr.

    C. Change the plan to ensure that the client achieves adequate pain relief.

    D. Teach the client about the plan of care that is being implemented to manage his pain.

3. When a nurse evaluates the care he has given a client, the client's responses to care are compared with the

    A. assessment data.

    B. nursing diagnosis.

    C. client outcomes.

    D. medical diagnosis.

4. The cues and inferences that the nurse uses to choose a nursing diagnosis label are considered the

    A. probable causes.

    B. defining characteristics.

    C. nursing interventions.

    D. goals.

5. In evaluation, the nurse must gather information about the client to

        A. judge whether or not the client outcomes have been met.

        B. organize resources to proceed with implementing interventions.

        C. establish client-centered outcomes that are measurable and realistic.

        D. determine the priority nursing diagnoses and appropriate interventions.

6. For each of the following nursing interventions, identify if the intervention is a nurse-initiated intervention (N) or a primary-care-provider-initiated intervention (P).

	Give morphine sulfate 1 to 2 mg IV every 1 hr as needed for pain.
	Insert nasogastric tube.
	Apply moist heat to left arm.
	Listen actively to client's concerns.
	Perform daily bath after evening meal.
	Infuse 0.9% normal saline at 125 mL/hr.

7. Determine the correct nursing process step for each of the following statements.

	Assess	Diagnose	Plan	Implement	Evaluate
Identify the client's health problem.					
Call the social worker to visit the client for discharge needs.					
Develop a care plan.					
Client has crackles in the left lower lobe.					
Develop a therapeutic relationship.					
Activity intolerance is related to prolonged immobility.					
Client will walk to the bathroom twice daily.					
Client states, "I don't sleep well at night."					
Place all supplies for dressing change at bedside.					
Bathe the client in the evening.					
Nurse interprets data.					
Client has active bowel sounds and is tolerating clear liquids well.					
Expected outcomes are to be met within the first week.					
Turn the client every 2 hr for the first 24 hr.					
Transfer the client with the help of three staff members.					
Client is unable to walk to the bathroom this morning.					

Chapter 7: Nursing Process

Application Exercises Answer Key

1. Identify each of the following statements as subjective data (S) or as objective data (O).

O	Respiratory rate of 22/min that is even and unlabored
S	"I can only walk 3 blocks before my legs start to hurt."
S	Pain rated at 3 on a scale of 1 to 10
O	Skin pink, warm, and dry
O	Urine output of 300 mL/8 hr
S	"My wife doesn't come to visit very often."
O	Dressing clean, dry, and intact

2. By the second postoperative day a client has not achieved satisfactory pain relief. Based on this evaluation, what should the nurse do next based on the nursing process?

> **A. Reassess the client to determine the reason satisfactory pain relief has not been achieved.**
>
> B. Wait to see if the pain lessens over the next 24 hr.
>
> C. Change the plan to ensure that the client achieves adequate pain relief.
>
> D. Teach the client about the plan of care that is being implemented to manage his pain.

The nurse should reassess the client to determine why the client has not achieved satisfactory pain relief. Various factors may be influencing the lack of pain relief. By the second postoperative day, the interventions implemented should have achieved the desired client outcome. Changing the plan may be necessary, but the nurse first needs to reassess the client to determine the reason for lack of outcome achievement. The current plan is not working, so teaching the client about this plan is providing false reassurance and does not address the client's current pain.

3. When a nurse evaluates the care he has given a client, the client's responses to care are compared with the

    A. assessment data.

    B. nursing diagnosis.

    C. client outcomes.

    D. medical diagnosis.

The nurse will compare the client's responses (what actually happened) to the desired client outcome. This compares what the client actually achieved to what was desired. The assessment data is used to identify the original client outcomes, the nursing diagnosis is the problem statement; and the medical diagnosis is determined by the primary care provider to plan treatment.

4. The cues and inferences that the nurse uses to choose a nursing diagnosis label are considered the

    A. probable causes.

    B. defining characteristics.

    C. nursing interventions.

    D. goals.

The defining characteristics are the subjective and objective data obtained from the client assessment. The probable causes are the etiology of the nursing diagnosis. The goals are what the nurse will help the client achieve by implementing nursing interventions.

5. In evaluation, the nurse must gather information about the client to

    A. judge whether or not the client outcomes have been met.

    B. organize resources to proceed with implementing interventions.

    C. establish client-centered outcomes that are measurable and realistic.

    D. determine the priority nursing diagnoses and appropriate interventions.

Evaluation involves gathering information about the client to judge whether or not client outcomes have been met. Organizing resources takes place during the implementation step. Establishing client-centered outcomes and establishing priorities of care take place in the planning step.

6. For each of the following nursing interventions, identify if the intervention is a nurse-initiated intervention (N) or a primary-care-provider-initiated intervention (P).

P	Give morphine sulfate 1 to 2 mg IV every 1 hr as needed for pain.
P	Insert nasogastric tube.
P	Apply moist heat to left arm.
N	Listen actively to client's concerns.
N	Perform daily bath after evening meal.
P	Infuse 0.9% normal saline at 125 mL/hr.

7. Determine the correct nursing process step for each of the following statements.

	Assess	Diagnose	Plan	Implement	Evaluate
Identify the client's health problem.		X			
Call the social worker to visit the client for discharge needs.				X	
Develop a care plan.			X		
Client has crackles in the left lower lobe.	X				
Develop a therapeutic relationship.	X				
Activity intolerance is related to prolonged immobility.		X			
Client will walk to the bathroom twice daily.			X		
Client states, "I don't sleep well at night."	X				
Place all supplies for dressing change at bedside.				X	
Bathe the client in the evening.			X		
Nurse interprets data.		X			
Client has active bowel sounds and is tolerating clear liquids well.					X
Expected outcomes are to be met within the first week.			X		
Turn the client every 2 hr for the first 24 hr.			X		
Transfer the client with the help of three staff members.			X		
Client is unable to walk to the bathroom this morning.					X

Unit 1　Foundations for Practice

Section:　Thinking Strategies for Nursing Practice

Chapter 8:　Critical Thinking

Contributor: Linda Turchin, MSN, RN

 NCLEX® Connections:

Learning Objective: Review and apply knowledge within **"Critical Thinking"** in readiness for performance of the following nursing activities as outlined by the NCLEX® test plans:

Δ　Gain an awareness of the impact critical thinking has on nursing practice.

Δ　Use critical thinking to assess, diagnose, plan, implement, and evaluate nursing care.

Δ　Use critical thinking in consulting with other health care providers, make appropriate referrals, and provide continuity in client care.

Δ　Consider potential hazards and take measures to ensure safety in client care and the work environment.

Δ　Evaluate the performance of self and others with the purpose of taking measures to improve the quality of care being given.

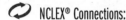 Key Points

Δ　In nursing, critical thinking is an active, organized, cognitive process used to scrutinize one's thinking and the thinking of others by the application of knowledge and experience, problem solving, and decision making resulting in a nursing judgment.

Δ　In order to positively impact the client's health status, a professional nurse must be able to think critically, correctly identify problems, and both identify and implement the best solutions (interventions). Critical thinking discourages the nurse from forming judgments that lead to quick, single-focused solutions.

Δ　Critical thinking incorporates reflection, language, and intuition, and it evolves through three distinct levels as the nurse gains knowledge and experience while maturing into a competent nursing professional.

Δ　The components of critical thinking include knowledge, experience, critical thinking competencies, attitudes, and intellectual and professional standards.

Δ Critical thinking requires lifelong learning and the acquisition of relevant experiences that are continuously being reflected on for the purpose of producing appropriate nursing judgments.

Key Factors

Δ **Reflection**: purposefully thinking back or recalling a situation to discover its meaning in order to gain insight regarding the event. The nurse should ask herself:

- "Why did I say that or do this?"

- "Was the original plan of care achieved?"

  ◊ If so – "Which interventions were successful?"

  ◊ If not – "Which interventions were unsuccessful?"

Δ **Language**: precise, clear language reflecting focused thinking and communicating unambiguous messages and expectations to both the client and other health care team members. The nurse should ask herself:

- "Was the language used appropriate for the client?"

- "Was the message communicated clearly to the primary care provider?"

Δ **Intuition**: an inner sensing that something is not currently supported with fact. Intuition should spark the nurse to consciously search the data to confirm or disprove the "feeling." The nurse should ask herself:

- "Did the vital signs reflect any changes that would account for the client's acute confusion?"

- "Since the client experienced confusion when she had a urinary infection last month, does her confusion reflect another possible infection?"

Levels of Critical Thinking

Δ **Basic Critical Thinking**

- The nurse trusts the experts and thinking is concrete and based on the "rules."

- Basic critical thinking results from limited nursing knowledge and experience, as well as inadequate critical thinking experience.

  ◊ Example: The client complains of pain 1 hr after receiving a pain medication. Instead of reassessing the client's pain, the nurse tells the client he must wait 2 more hours before another dose can be given.

Δ **Complex Critical Thinking**

- The nurse begins to express autonomy by analyzing and examining data to determine the best alternative.

- Complex critical thinking results from increased nursing knowledge, experience, intuition, and more flexible attitudes.

  ◊ Example: The nurse realizes that the client is not ambulating as often as ordered because of a fear of missing her daughter's phone call. The nurse reassures the client that the staff will listen for and answer her phone when she is out of her room.

Δ **Commitment**

- The nurse anticipates the need to make choices without the assistance of others and fully assumes the responsibility for those choices.

- Commitment results from expert level of knowledge, experience, developed intuition, and reflective, flexible attitudes.

  ◊ Example: The nurse increases the rate of IV fluid infusion when the client's blood pressure is consistent with hypovolemic shock 24 hr post surgery.

Components of Critical Thinking

Δ **Knowledge**: Information specific to nursing acquired through:

- Basic nursing education.

- Continuing education courses.

- Advanced degrees and certifications.

Δ **Experience**: decision making ability derived from opportunities to observe, sense, and interact with clients followed by active reflection. The nurse:

- Demonstrates understanding of clinical situations.

- Recognizes and analyzes cues for relevance.

- Incorporates experience into intuition.

Δ **Competence**: cognitive processes a nurse uses to make nursing judgments, such as:

- **General critical thinking.**

  ◊ Scientific method

  ◊ Problem solving

  ◊ Decision making

  ◊ Diagnostic reasoning and inference

  ◊ **Clinical decision making** – collaboration

- **Specific critical thinking in nursing.**

◊ The nursing process:

The Nursing Process	Critical Thinking Skills
Assessment – Identify human responses to health and illness.	• Observe. • Differentiate between relevant and irrelevant data and between important and unimportant data. • Organize, categorize, and validate data.
Diagnosing – Analyze and interpret assessment data.	• Identify clusters and cues. • Detect inferences. • Recognize the problem. • Defer from making judgments.
Planning – Determine the best approach to address and resolve the client's health problem(s).	• Make generalizations. • Take knowledge and apply to more than one situation. • Create outcome criteria. • Theorize.
Implementation – Form conclusions, make decisions, and draw inferences about the care plan.	• Use knowledge base. • Test theories.
Evaluation – Interpret evaluative findings to judge both the client's current health status and whether or not outcomes were achieved.	• Determine accuracy of theories. • Evaluate based on outcome criteria.

Δ **Attitudes**: Mindset(s) that affect how a nurse approaches a problem. Attitudes of critical thinkers include:

- Confidence – feels sure of abilities.

- Independence – analyzes ideas for logical reasoning.

- Fairness – is objective, nonjudgmental.

- Responsibility – practices according to standards of practice.

- Risk taking – takes calculated chances in finding better solutions to problems.

- Discipline – develops a systematic approach to thinking.

- Perseverance – continues to work at a problem until it is resolved.

- Creativity – uses imagination to find solutions to unique client problems.

- Curiosity – requires more information about clients and problems.

- Integrity – practices truthfully and ethically.

- Humility – acknowledges weaknesses.

Δ   **Standards**: Model to which care is compared in order to determine acceptability, excellence, or appropriateness.

- Intellectual standards ensure the thorough application of critical thinking.

- Professional standards include:

    ◊   Nursing judgment based on ethical criteria.

    ◊   Evaluation that relies on evidence-based practice.

    ◊   Demonstration of professional responsibility.

Primary Reference:

Potter, P. A., & Perry, A. G. (2005). *Fundamentals of nursing* (6th ed.). St. Louis, MO: Mosby.

Additional Resources:

NANDA International (2004). *NANDA nursing diagnoses: Definitions and classification 2005-2006*. Philadelphia: NANDA.

Chapter 8: Critical Thinking

Application Exercises

Scenario: A nurse is caring for a 35-year-old man who is 24 hr postoperative for an inguinal hernia. The client is tolerating clear liquids well, has normal bowel sounds, and is expressing a desire for "real food." Preoperatively, he was cooperative and pleasant. Now, he is easily agitated. The nurse has explained the importance of coughing, deep breathing, and dangling. However, he refuses to comply for the most part. The client has pain medication ordered every 4 to 6 hr as needed. He has been accepting it every 6 to 7 hr. His vital signs taken prior to his last pain medication were heart rate 100/min, respiratory rate 16/min, temperature 37° C (98.6° F), and blood pressure 136/80 mm Hg. His surgical dressing is dry and intact.

1. The nurse tells the client that she will call the primary care provider to see whether or not he can have the ice cream and tomato soup that he is requesting. The provider gives her an order for a full liquid diet. This is an example of which level of critical thinking? Provide rationale.

2. The nurse suspects that the client is experiencing pain. Analyze the above situation and provide data to support or refute that judgment.

3. Analyze the client's seeming noncompliance and provide alternative possibilities for the lack of cooperation.

4. A client is experiencing hypertension, and the primary care provider orders a newly approved antihypertensive medication. Prior to administering the medication, the nurse gathers information about the medication using an electronic data base. The nurse is using which of the following components of critical thinking when reviewing the medication information?

   A. Knowledge

   B. Experience

   C. Intuition

   D. Competence

5. A nurse receives an order to administer an antibiotic to a 35-year-old man with cellulitis. The nurse checks the client's chart, discovers that the client is allergic to the antibiotic, and phones the primary care provider to obtain a different antibiotic. What critical thinking attitude did the nurse exhibit?

> A. Fairness
>
> B. Responsibility
>
> C. Risk taking
>
> D. Creativity

6. Match the critical thinking attitude with the appropriate example.

_____	Confidence	A. A nurse mistakenly gives the wrong dose of medication to a client. The nurse calls the primary care provider to notify her of the error.
_____	Discipline	B. A nurse tries three different pouches before finding one that will contain the draining wound.
_____	Perseverance	C. A nurse uses a head-to-toe approach to conduct a physical assessment.
_____	Integrity	D. A nurse states that she has difficulties inserting IVs in clients who are dehydrated.
_____	Humility	E. A nurse offers to put an IV in a client who is dehydrated.

Chapter 8: Critical Thinking

Application Exercises Answer Key

Scenario: A nurse is caring for a 35-year-old man who is 24 hr postoperative for an inguinal hernia. The client is tolerating clear liquids well, has normal bowel sounds, and is expressing a desire for "real food." Preoperatively, he was cooperative and pleasant. Now, he is easily agitated. The nurse has explained the importance of coughing, deep breathing, and dangling. However, he refuses to comply for the most part. The client has pain medication ordered every 4 to 6 hr as needed. He has been accepting it every 6 to 7 hr. His vital signs taken prior to his last pain medication were heart rate 100/min, respiratory rate 16/min, temperature 37° C (98.6° F), and blood pressure 136/80 mm Hg. His surgical dressing is dry and intact.

1. The nurse tells the client that she will call the primary care provider to see whether or not he can have the ice cream and tomato soup that he is requesting. The provider gives her an order for a full liquid diet. This is an example of which level of critical thinking? Provide rationale.

   Basic critical thinking – Thinking is concrete and based on a set of rules (order for full liquids). Advanced experience and knowledge would allow the nurse to introduce full liquids based on normal bowel sounds and the client's tolerance of clear liquids.

2. The nurse suspects that the client is experiencing pain. Analyze the above situation and provide data to support or refute that judgment.

   Elevated blood pressure and pulse rate without elevated temperature, labored respirations, or signs of bleeding support that the client is in pain.

   Acceptance of pain medication only at or beyond the maximum time limit with atypical agitation also supports that the client is in pain.

   Refusal to comply with interventions that could increase his pain level (e.g., coughing, deep breathing) also supports that the client is in pain. Complex critical thinking would conclude that the client is experiencing unacceptable pain management.

3. Analyze the client's seeming noncompliance and provide alternative possibilities for the lack of cooperation.

The client is in pain and thus will not comply with potentially pain-inducing actions (e.g., coughing, deep breathing).

The client did not understand the nurse's explanation of the importance of coughing, deep breathing, and dangling. She needs to reflect on her presentation and readdress the educational issue.

The client is not able to retain instruction because of the pain he is experiencing; therefore, the pain must be managed appropriately and the education issue readdressed.

---

4. A client is experiencing hypertension, and the primary care provider orders a newly approved antihypertensive medication. Prior to administering the medication, the nurse gathers information about the medication using an electronic data base. The nurse is using which of the following components of critical thinking when reviewing the medication information?

    A. Knowledge
    B. Experience
    C. Intuition
    D. Competence

By using the electronic database, the nurse takes initiative to increase her knowledge base, which is the first component of critical thinking. The nurse has had no prior experience with the medication, and intuition requires experience. Competence involves making judgments, but judgments cannot be made about the safe administration of a medication until knowledge is obtained.

5. A nurse receives an order to administer an antibiotic to a 35-year-old man with cellulitis. The nurse checks the client's chart, discovers that the client is allergic to the antibiotic, and phones the primary care provider to obtain a different antibiotic. What critical thinking attitude did the nurse exhibit?

        A. Fairness

        B. Responsibility

        C. Risk taking

        D. Creativity

The nurse is responsible for administering medications in a safe manner according to standards of practice. Fairness is using a nonjudgmental, objective approach in looking at clients and situations. Risk taking is a calculated approach to solving a problem that is not responding to traditional methods. Creativity is an approach that uses imagination to find solutions to unique client problems.

6. Match the critical thinking attitude with the appropriate example.

E Confidence	A.	A nurse mistakenly gives the wrong dose of medication to a client. The nurse calls the primary care provider to notify her of the error.
C Discipline	B.	A nurse tries three different pouches before finding one that will contain the draining wound.
B Perseverance	C.	A nurse uses a head-to-toe approach to conduct a physical assessment.
A Integrity	D.	A nurse states that she has difficulties inserting IVs in clients who are dehydrated.
D Humility	E.	A nurse offers to put an IV in a client who is dehydrated.

Unit 1   **Foundations for Practice**

Section: Communication

Chapter 9:   Basic Communication
Contributor: Terri Astorino, EdD, MSN, RN

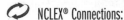 NCLEX® Connections:

> **Learning Objective**: Review and apply knowledge within **"Basic Communication"** in readiness for performance of the following nursing activities as outlined by the NCLEX® test plans:
>
> Δ   Assess/monitor the communication abilities and needs of clients and families.
>
> Δ   Use principles of communication theory to direct and/or provide nursing care to clients and families.

 Key Points

Δ   Communication is a complex process that incorporates a pattern of exchanging information and ideas with others.

Δ   It is a dynamic and ongoing process that creates a unique experience between the participants.

Δ   Effective communication is a skill that can be developed.

Δ   The nurse uses communication when providing care to establish relationships, collect information, influence behaviors, and demonstrate caring.

Δ   The helping relationship between the nurse and client occurs through the process of communication.

Key Factors

Δ **Three Primary Levels of Basic Communication**

- **Intrapersonal communication** – communication that occurs within an individual. Also identified as "self-talk." This occurs within one's self and is the internal discussion that takes place when an individual is thinking thoughts and not outwardly verbalizing them. In nursing, this allows the nurse to assess a client and/or situation and critically think about the client/situation before outwardly communicating.

- **Interpersonal communication** – communication that occurs between two or more people in a small group. This form of communication is the most common in nursing and requires an exchange of information with an individual or small group.

- **Public communication** – communication that occurs within large groups of people. In nursing, this commonly occurs during educational endeavors where the nurse is teaching a large group of individuals, such as in a community setting.

Δ Functional Components of Basic Communication

Referent	The incentive or motivation for communication to occur between one person and another
Sender	The person who initiates the message
Message	The verbal and/or nonverbal information that is expressed by the sender and intended for the receiver
Channel	The method of transmitting and receiving a message (received via sight, hearing, and/or touch)
Receiver	The person to whom the message is aimed
Environment	The emotional and physical climate in which the communication takes place
Feedback	• May be verbal and/or nonverbal, positive and/or negative • The message that is returned to the sender by the receiver that indicates that the message was received • An essential component for ongoing communication

Δ **Verbal Communication**

- **Vocabulary** – the words that are used to communicate. Limited vocabulary or speaking a language other than English may make it difficult for the nurse to communicate with the client. Use of medical jargon will make it difficult for the client to understand the nurse.

- **Denotative/connotative meaning** – when communicating, the meanings that are shared by participants. Shared words that have multiple meanings may cause miscommunication when interpreted differently.

- **Pacing** – The rate of speech can communicate a meaning to the receiver.

- **Intonation** – The tone of voice can communicate a variety of feelings.

- **Clarity/brevity** – The shortest, simplest types of communication are usually most effective.

- **Timing/relevance** – Knowing when to communicate allows the receiver to be more attentive to the message.

Δ **Nonverbal communication**

- Nurses should be aware of how they communicate nonverbally. The nurse should assess the client's nonverbal communications for the meaning being conveyed, remembering that culture impacts interpretation. Attention to the following behaviors is important, as it is compared to the verbal message being conveyed:

  ◊ Appearance.

  ◊ Posture.

  ◊ Gait.

  ◊ Facial expressions.

  ◊ Eye contact.

  ◊ Gestures.

  ◊ Sounds.

  ◊ Territoriality.

  ◊ Personal space.

Nursing Process

Δ **Assessment**

- Ability of the communicator to speak, hear, see, understand, and interpret

- Individual differences

- Cultural influences

- Values

- Emotions

- Knowledge level

- Health status

- Developmental level

NANDA Nursing Diagnoses

Δ   Impaired verbal communication

Δ   Readiness for enhanced communication

Δ   Impaired social interaction

Δ   **Planning**

- Identification of mutually agreed-upon client outcomes

- Setting priorities according to the client's needs

- Planning for adequate time for interventions

Δ   **Implementation**

Techniques that Enhance Communication	Techniques that Hinder Communication
• Active listening • Silence • Giving information • Sharing empathy, hope, humor, and feelings • Focusing • Reflecting and clarifying • Paraphrasing and restating	• Stereotyping • Challenging • Arguing • Giving unwarranted reassurance • Giving advice • Judgmental or defensive responses • Ignoring feelings • Not listening

Δ   **Evaluation**

- Determine if client outcomes were met.

- The nurse can also evaluate how effectively she communicated. Questions to ask include:

 ◊   Was openness encouraged?

 ◊   Were verbal and nonverbal cues identified?

 ◊   Did responses enhance or hinder communication?

 ◊   Were responses positive or judgmental?

 ◊   Were verbal and nonverbal communication congruent?

Primary Reference:

Potter, P. A., & Perry, A. G. (2005). *Fundamentals of nursing* (6th ed.). St. Louis, MO: Mosby.

Additional Resources:

NANDA International (2004). *NANDA nursing diagnoses: Definitions and classification 2005-2006*. Philadelphia: NANDA.

    Fundamentals for Nursing

Chapter 9: Basic Communication

Application Exercises

1. Give two examples of how a nurse can use intrapersonal communication to enhance communication with a client.

2. Match the element of verbal communication with the appropriate example that could cause miscommunication to occur.

_____ Pacing	A. Use of medical jargon such as "decubitus ulcer"
_____ Connotative meaning	B. Charting that is written "client complains of" vs "client reports"
_____ Vocabulary	C. A client not asking the nurse a question because the nurse is talking rapidly and seems very busy
_____ Clarity	D. A nurse attempting to teach a client about her medications while the client is waiting for a phone call from her granddaughter
_____ Timing	E. A nurse distractingly using the phrase "um" repetitively in her communication

Scenario: The following conversation occurs between a nurse and a client:
Nurse: "Do you have any pain from your knee incision this morning?"
Client: "No, but my back is really hurting. I think I want a pain pill for it."
Nurse: "Is the back pain a new problem or is this something you had before your surgery?"
Client: "Oh, I've had back problems for years."
Nurse: "I see you have a heating pad behind you. Does the heating pad help your back?"
Client: "Yes, it helps relax the muscles."

3. What is the referent for this conversation?

4. Who is the sender?

5. What were the channels for communication?

6. Who is the receiver?

7. What was the message?

8. What was the feedback?

9. A nurse who is bathing an older adult client tells the client to, "Turn to your side now, honey." The nurse believes she is demonstrating warmth and caring by calling the client "honey." However, the client finds the term offensive. What has caused this miscommunication to occur?

    A. The connotative meaning of the word is different to the client and the nurse.

    B. The client was unable to hear the nurse's message.

    C. The nurse's verbal communication was not congruent with her nonverbal communication.

    D. It is not the appropriate time for performing the client's bath.

Chapter 9: Basic Communication

Application Exercises Answer Key

1. Give two examples of how a nurse can use intrapersonal communication to enhance communication with a client.

   The nurse enters the client's room and sees that the client is crying. "Self-talk" asks, "I wonder why this client is so upset? Is he sad? Is he in pain? Does he have a social support system?" The nurse's assessment questions then stem from the intrapersonal communication. The nurse is using assessment skills to identify a potential problem, and she intervenes by asking the client pertinent questions to come to a more concrete answer.

   A client's condition is deteriorating and the nurse must phone the primary care provider. Intrapersonally, the nurse goes through a "self-talk" discussion about what is to be said to the primary care provider. This allows the nurse to be proactive and anticipate the provider's requests and/or questions. The nurse's intrapersonal communication enhances the interpersonal communication with the provider to best meet the needs of the client. The nurse is using "self-talk" to prepare for a future interpersonal communication encounter.

2. Match the element of verbal communication with the appropriate example that could cause miscommunication to occur.

   __C__ Pacing   A. Use of medical jargon such as "decubitus ulcer"

   __B__ Connotative meaning   B. Charting that is written "client complains of" vs "client reports"

   __A__ Vocabulary   C. A client not asking the nurse a question because the nurse is talking rapidly and seems very busy

   __E__ Clarity   D. A nurse attempting to teach a client about her medications while the client is waiting for a phone call from her granddaughter

   __D__ Timing   E. A nurse distractingly using the phrase "um" repetitively in her communication

Scenario: The following conversation occurs between a nurse and a client:

Nurse: "Do you have any pain from your knee incision this morning?"

Client: "No, but my back is really hurting. I think I want a pain pill for it."

Nurse: "Is the back pain a new problem or is this something you had before your surgery?"

Client: "Oh, I've had back problems for years."

Nurse: "I see you have a heating pad behind you. Does the heating pad help your back?"

Client: "Yes, it helps relax the muscles."

3. What is the referent for this conversation?

The nurse needed to assess the client's pain.

4. Who is the sender?

The nurse

5. What were the channels for communication?

Verbal communication, hearing

6. Who is the receiver?

The client

7. What was the message?

"Are you having pain and how are you experiencing it?"

8. What was the feedback?

"I have chronic pain in my back."

9. A nurse who is bathing an older adult client tells the client to, "Turn to your side now, honey." The nurse believes she is demonstrating warmth and caring by calling the client "honey." However, the client finds the term offensive. What has caused this miscommunication to occur?

> **A. The connotative meaning of the word is different to the client and the nurse.**
>
> B. The client was unable to hear the nurse's message.
>
> C. The nurse's verbal communication was not congruent with her nonverbal communication.
>
> D. It is not the appropriate time for performing the client's bath.

The nurse believes that the word "honey" communicates warmth and caring. The client interprets the word as being derogatory and perhaps unprofessional. The client did not have any difficulty hearing the message. There is no indication that verbal and nonverbal communication is not congruent, or that it is an inappropriate time for performing the bath.

Unit 1   Foundations for Practice
Section: Communication

Chapter 10:   **Therapeutic Communication**
               Contributor: Terri Astorino, EdD, MSN, RN

 NCLEX® Connections:

> **Learning Objective**: Review and apply knowledge within **"Therapeutic Communication"** in readiness for performance of the following nursing activities as outlined by the NCLEX® test plans:
>
> Δ   Use communication techniques to establish helping relationships with clients and families.
>
> Δ   Communicate the developmentally appropriate information to clients and families needed to achieve a high level of wellness.
>
> Δ   Encourage the client to verbalize feelings, needs, and beliefs.
>
> Δ   Plan and/or provide methods that compensate for impaired communication (e.g., translators, hearing aids, message boards).
>
> Δ   Use the nursing process to develop therapeutic relationships with clients of all ages.

 Key Points

Δ   Therapeutic communication is the **purposeful use of communication to build and maintain helping relationships** with clients, families, and significant others.

Δ   Therapeutic communication techniques **encourage the client to express feelings** and thoughts in a safe, nonjudgmental manner.

Δ   Children and older adults frequently require altered techniques to enhance communication.

Δ   Assessment, nursing diagnosis, planning, implementation, and evaluation of a client's care depend on therapeutic communication between the nurse, client/family/significant other, and the interdisciplinary health care team.

Key Factors

Δ **Characteristics**

- Client centered – not social or reciprocal

- **Purposeful, planned, and goal-directed**

- Has well-defined boundaries for the nurse and client

  ◊ **Orientation phase** – establishes the purpose of the relationship and the time frame available for work to be done. It is the initial contact.

  ◊ **Working phase** – sets goals and works toward meeting them.

  ◊ **Termination phase** – evaluates what has been accomplished and brings the relationship to a close.

Δ **Essential components**

- **Time** – Plan for and allow adequate time to communicate with others.

- **Active listening skills** – This is a nonverbal means of conveying interest in another.

  ◊ Face the client when engaging in communication.

  ◊ Lean forward toward the client and maintain an attentive, open posture.

  ◊ Maintain eye contact.

  ◊ Pay attention and maintain focus on the client's verbal and nonverbal cues.

- **Caring attitude** – Show concern and facilitate an emotional connection/ support between the nurse and the client/family/significant other.

- **Honesty** – Be open, direct, truthful, and sincere.

- **Trust** – Demonstrate to the client/family/significant other that they can rely on the nurse without doubt or question.

- **Empathy** – Convey an objective awareness and understanding of the feelings, emotions, and behaviors of the client/family/significant other, including trying to envision what it must be like to be in the client/family/ significant other's position.

- **Nonjudgmental attitude** – This is a display of tolerance/acceptance of the client/family/significant other that will encourage open, honest communication. Demonstrate respect for the client's unique approach and relate personal value beliefs.

Nursing Process

Δ **Assessment**

- Assess verbal and nonverbal communication needs.

- Consider the developmental level and how communication should be altered during the assessment phase.

  ◊ Children

    ° Use simple, straightforward language.

    ° Be aware of own nonverbal messages, as children are sensitive to nonverbal communication.

    ° Enhance communication by being at the child's eye level.

    ° Incorporate play in interactions.

  ◊ Older adult clients

    ° Recognize that the client may require amplification.

    ° Minimize distractions and face the client when speaking.

    ° Allow plenty of time for the client to respond.

    ° When impaired communication is assessed, ask for input from caregivers or family to determine the extent of the deficits and how best to communicate.

- Identify the client's cultural orientation and knowledge base during the assessment phase.

NANDA Nursing Diagnoses

Δ Health-seeking behaviors

Δ Interrupted family processes

Δ Risk for loneliness

Δ **Planning**

- Identify mutually agreed upon client outcomes.

- Set priorities according to the client's needs.

- Plan for adequate time for interventions.

Δ **Implementation**

- Establish a trusting nurse-client relationship. The client feels more at ease during the implementation phase when a helping relationship has been established.

  ◊ Provide empathetic responses and explanations to the client by using observations, hope, humor, and information.

- Encourage the client to verbalize feelings.

  ◊ Acknowledge the client's feelings.

  ◊ Use touch to communicate caring and comfort.

  ◊ Clarify whether or not the message received was accurate.

  ◊ Paraphrase the message to demonstrate understanding.

  ◊ Ask questions to seek additional information.

  ◊ Relevant self-disclosure by the nurse allows the client to see that his experience is shared by others and understood.

  ◊ Confrontation may be needed to help clients face emotions and behaviors that are contradictory, and to bring about greater self-awareness.

- Avoid mistakes that block therapeutic communication, which include:

  ◊ Asking irrelevant personal questions.

  ◊ Offering personal opinions as to how decisions should be made.

  ◊ Changing the topic.

  ◊ Responding without thinking.

  ◊ Asking judgmental "why" questions.

  ◊ Responding approvingly, disapprovingly, defensively, aggressively, or passively.

- Assist the client to communicate needs to health care staff.

- Therapeutic communication must continue to be used even though clients may have impaired communication ability (e.g., aphasia, decreased level of consciousness).

  ◊ Speak slowly and clearly, only amplifying the voice if indicated.

  ◊ Minimize distractions.

  ◊ Ensure that verbal and nonverbal communication is congruent.

  ◊ Include family member or caregiver if available.

  ◊ Listen actively.

  ◊ Maintain eye contact without staring.

Δ **Evaluation**

- Determine the client's responses to nursing actions.

- Evaluate the effectiveness of communications with client/family/significant others.

Primary Reference:

Potter, P. A., & Perry, A. G. (2005). *Fundamentals of nursing* (6th ed.). St. Louis, MO: Mosby.

Additional Resources:

NANDA International (2004). *NANDA nursing diagnoses: Definitions and classification 2005-2006*. Philadelphia: NANDA.

Chapter 10: Therapeutic Communication

Application Exercises

1. List the three phases of therapeutic communication. Indicate what occurs during each phase.

2. An adolescent client is admitted to the emergency department with a fever. None of the client's family members are present, and the client is tearful and withdrawn. Which of the following statements made by the nurse is an example of therapeutic communication?

   A. "I know you are frightened, but we will find out what is wrong with you soon."
   B. "Let me show you around so that you are less frightened."
   C. "Tell me why you are so frightened."
   D. "You look frightened. "

3. A nurse recognizes that a helping relationship is established with a client if the communication

   A. is equally reciprocal between the nurse and the client.
   B. encourages the client to express his thoughts and feelings.
   C. has no time limits.
   D. occurs spontaneously throughout the nurse-client relationship.

4. When communicating with a child who is seated, the nurse should

   A. touch the child.
   B. sit at eye level with the child.
   C. stand facing the child.
   D. stand with a relaxed posture.

5. Which of the following are behaviors of active listening? (Select all that apply.)

   _____ Maintaining an open posture
   _____ Writing down what the client says so that details are not forgotten
   _____ Establishing and maintaining eye contact
   _____ Nodding in agreement with the client throughout the conversation
   _____ Responding positively when giving feedback

6. For each pair of statements, select the one that does not block communication.

_____ "You have talked a lot about your symptoms of hypokalemia, but let's discuss the trouble you are having taking your potassium supplement."

_____ "Why are you not taking your potassium supplements?"

_____ "When did you last take your phenytoin?"

_____ "You should have taken your phenytoin this morning before breakfast. Did you?"

Chapter 10: Therapeutic Communication

Application Exercises Answer Key

1. List the three phases of therapeutic communication. Indicate what occurs during each phase.

   Orientation – Initiation of the relationship occurs within established time frames.

   Working – Develop and work toward the accomplishment of goals.

   Termination – Summarize and evaluate the work done and bring closure to the relationship.

2. An adolescent client is admitted to the emergency department with a fever. None of the client's family members are present, and the client is tearful and withdrawn. Which of the following statements made by the nurse is an example of therapeutic communication?

   A. "I know you are frightened, but we will find out what is wrong with you soon."

   B. "Let me show you around so that you are less frightened."

   C. "Tell me why you are so frightened."

   D. "You look frightened. "

   Option D demonstrates an empathetic and caring attitude where the nurse is addressing the nonverbal behavior in an open and honest manner. Option A diminishes the value of the client's feelings and is giving false reassurance that the fever will be diagnosed soon. In option B, the nurse is making the assumption that the client is tearful and withdrawn because he or she is in a strange environment. It actually may be viewed as changing the subject to an area that causes less anxiety and does not get to the root of the problem. Option C is incorrect because "why" questions may make the client defensive and may be hard for the client to answer.

3. A nurse recognizes that a helping relationship is established with a client if the communication

   A. is equally reciprocal between the nurse and the client.

   B. encourages the client to express his thoughts and feelings.

   C. has no time limits.

   D. occurs spontaneously throughout the nurse-client relationship.

   Therapeutic communication facilitates a helping relationship that maximizes the client's ability to openly express his or her thoughts and feelings. The communication is not reciprocal but client-focused. Therapeutic communication is limited to the boundaries of the therapeutic relationship. Therapeutic communication is well thought out and planned by a health care professional.

4. When communicating with a child who is seated, the nurse should

    A. touch the child.

    B. sit at eye level with the child.

    C. stand facing the child.

    D. stand with a relaxed posture.

The nurse should be at the same eye level as the child to facilitate communication. Touching may intimidate the child and block communication. Standing will prevent the nurse from being at eye level with the child.

5. Which of the following are behaviors of active listening? (Select all that apply.)

    __X__ Maintaining an open posture

    _____ Writing down what the client says so that details are not forgotten

    __X__ Establishing and maintaining eye contact

    _____ Nodding in agreement with the client throughout the conversation

    __X__ Responding positively when giving feedback

Having an open posture and leaning forward, establishing and maintaining eye contact, and responding positively when giving feedback are ways the nurse can demonstrate active listening. Writing down everything the client says will interfere with the nurse's ability to maintain eye contact and open posture. Nodding in agreement throughout the conversation may be interpreted as agreement with what the client is saying when it was only intended to indicate attending to what was being said.

6. For each pair of statements, select the one that does not block communication.

    __X__ "You have talked a lot about your symptoms of hypokalemia, but let's discuss the trouble you are having taking your potassium supplement."

    _____ "Why are you not taking your potassium supplements?"

The first option is nonjudgmental. Option two is a "why" question. It can be interpreted as judgmental and blocks communication.

    __X__ "When did you last take your phenytoin?"

    _____ "You should have taken your phenytoin this morning before breakfast. Did you?"

Option one is asking for more information and is appropriate for performing assessments. Option two is opinionated and could impact future answers given by a client wishing to avoid the nurse's disapproval.

Unit 1   Foundations for Practice
Section: Communication

Chapter 11:   Client Education
Contributor: LaToya T. Marsh, MSN, RN

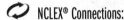 NCLEX® Connections:

> **Learning Objective**: Review and apply knowledge within **"Client Education"** in readiness for performance of the following nursing activities as outlined by the NCLEX® test plans:
>
> Δ   Assess/monitor the client's learning needs and readiness to learn.
>
> Δ   Consider the developmental stage of the client when planning content and interventions.
>
> Δ   Plan and/or provide appropriate instruction to the client to meet learning needs using a variety of teaching tools.
>
> Δ   Use information technology to enhance/augment client education resources.
>
> Δ   Teach/reinforce identified content areas.
>
> Δ   Evaluate achievement of client learning outcomes.

 Key Points

Δ   **Client education** assists individuals, families, and communities in achieving optimal health.

Δ   Client education is a basic standard of professional nursing care.

Δ   **Teaching** is interactive, promotes learning, and leads to a change in behavior.

Δ   **Learning** is an intentional gain of new information.

Δ   Information technology can be used to enhance access to and delivery of knowledge.

Key Factors

Δ   Purposes of client teaching include:

- Health maintenance and promotion and illness prevention (e.g., immunizations, lifestyle changes, prenatal care).

- Health restoration (e.g., teaching a client how to administer insulin).

- Coping with impaired function (e.g., ostomy care, learning swallowing techniques, speech therapy).

Δ   Domains of learning include:

- Cognitive learning, which includes all intellectual activities. For example, cognitive learning takes place when a client is taught and then can list the signs and symptoms of hypoglycemia.

- Affective learning, which includes feelings, opinions, and values. For example, affective learning takes place when the client is attentive and willing to listen to the nurse discuss new-onset diabetes.

- Psychomotor learning, which is learning how to complete a physical activity. For example, psychomotor learning takes place when a client practices preparing insulin injections.

Δ   Factors Affecting Learning

Factors that Enhance Learning	Barriers to Learning
• Perceived benefit	• Fear, anxiety, depression
• Cognitive and physical ability	• Physical discomfort, pain, fatigue
• Health and cultural beliefs	• Environmental distractions
• Active participation	• Health and cultural beliefs
• Age/educational level-appropriate methods	• Sensory and perceptual deficits
	• Psychomotor deficits

Nursing Process

Δ   **Assessment**

- Assess/monitor the **client's learning needs.**

- Assess/monitor the client's learning style (e.g., auditory, visual, kinesthetic).

- Identify areas of concern.

- Assess/monitor available resources (e.g., financial, social, community).

- Identify the client's developmental stage.

- Determine the client's physical and cognitive ability.

- Identify special needs (e.g., visual impairment, decreased manual dexterity).

- Determine the client's motivation and readiness to learn.

NANDA Nursing Diagnoses

- Deficient knowledge

- Noncompliance

- Ineffective health maintenance

- Health-seeking behaviors

Δ **Planning**

- Identify **mutually agreed upon client outcomes.**

- Prioritize the learning objectives with the client's needs in mind.

- Use methods that emphasize the **client's learning style**.

- Select age-appropriate teaching methods/material.

- Provide electronic educational resources as appropriate (e.g., CDs, DVDs, computer/PDA software programs).

- Demonstrate use of Internet in regard to acessing information and support services.

- Organize learning activities to move from **simple to more complex** tasks.

- Incorporate active participation in the learning process.

- Schedule teaching sessions to coincide with the client's daily activities.

Δ **Implementation**

- Create an environment conducive to learning (e.g., minimize distractions and interruptions, provide for privacy).

- Use therapeutic communication to develop a trusting relationship that allows the client to express areas of concern (e.g., active listening, empathy).

- Review previous knowledge and experiences.

- Explain the therapeutic regimen or procedure.

- Present steps building to more complex tasks.

- Demonstrate psychomotor skills.

- Allow time for return demonstrations.

- Provide positive reinforcement.

Δ   Evaluation

- Observe the client demonstrating the learned activity (best for evaluation of psychomotor learning).

- Ask questions.

- Listen to the client explain the information learned.

- Use written tools to measure accuracy of information.

- Request the client's self-evaluation of progress.

- Observe verbal and nonverbal communication.

- Revise the care plan as needed.

Primary Reference:

Potter, P. A., & Perry, A. G. (2005). *Fundamentals of nursing* (6th ed.). St. Louis, MO: Mosby.

Additional Resources:

NANDA International (2004). *NANDA nursing diagnoses: Definitions and classification 2005-2006*. Philadelphia: NANDA.

Chapter 11: Client Education

Application Exercises

1. When teaching a client how to draw up and mix insulin injections, which of the following is the best evaluation method to know that psychomotor learning has taken place?

   A. The client is able to discuss the appropriate technique.

   B. The client is able to demonstrate the appropriate technique.

   C. The client states that he understands.

   D. The client is able to write the steps down on a piece of paper.

2. Teaching a group of college students how to avoid sexually transmitted diseases is referred to as

   A. planning.

   B. health restoration.

   C. illness prevention.

   D. coping with impaired function.

3. A nurse is working with a client that believes all children should be toilet trained by age 1. Following an educational session by the nurse, the client now states that her earlier ideas have changed. She is now willing to postpone toilet training until the child is older. Learning has occurred in which domain of learning?

   A. Cognitive

   B. Affective

   C. Psychomotor

   D. Coping

Scenario: A nurse is responsible for reviewing the preoperative and postoperative teaching for a client who is newly diagnosed with breast cancer. The client is scheduled for a mastectomy. The client is tearful when the nurse enters her room.

---

4. Before starting client education, the nurse must identify possible barriers to learning. What possible barriers are present for this client?

5. What nursing interventions could be implemented to overcome these barriers to learning?

6. What are some possible statements by the client that would indicate she is ready to learn?

7. Which of the following may enhance client learning? (Select all that apply.)

      _____ Fear

      _____ Fatigue

      _____ Active participation

      _____ Sensory deficits

      _____ Perceived benefit

Chapter 11: Client Education

Application Exercises Answer Key

1. When teaching a client how to draw up and mix insulin injections, which of the following is the best evaluation method to know that psychomotor learning has taken place?

    A. The client is able to discuss the appropriate technique.

    B. The client is able to demonstrate the appropriate technique.

    C. The client states that he understands.

    D. The client is able to write the steps down on a piece of paper.

    Having the client perform a return demonstration is the best method to evaluate a learning objective from the psychomotor domain. Discussing the appropriate technique, stating understanding, and writing down steps will demonstrate learning, but only actual demonstration by the client will evaluate psychomotor learning.

2. Teaching a group of college students how to avoid sexually transmitted diseases is referred to as

    A. planning.

    B. health restoration.

    C. illness prevention.

    D. coping with impaired function.

    Teaching clients how to avoid sexually transmitted diseases is teaching them how to prevent illness. Planning is a step of the nursing process and is not a category of client teaching. Teaching a client how to manage his blood pressure medication assists him with health restoration. Teaching a client how to use a front-wheeled walker when ambulating is assisting a client to learn how to cope with impaired function.

3. A nurse is working with a client that believes all children should be toilet trained by age 1. Following an educational session by the nurse, the client now states that her earlier ideas have changed. She is now willing to postpone toilet training until the child is older. Learning has occurred in which domain of learning?

> A. Cognitive
>
> **B. Affective**
>
> C. Psychomotor
>
> D. Coping

Affective learning has taken place as evidenced by the client's changed ideas regarding toilet training. Cognitive learning would be demonstrated if the client could state the behaviors that her child will demonstrate when ready to toilet train. Psychomotor learning would be demonstrated if the client performed the proper techniques for introducing her child to toilet training. Coping is not a domain of learning.

Scenario: A nurse is responsible for reviewing the preoperative and postoperative teaching for a client who is newly diagnosed with breast cancer. The client is scheduled for a mastectomy. The client is tearful when the nurse enters her room.

---

4. Before starting client education, the nurse must identify possible barriers to learning. What possible barriers are present for this client?

The client's new diagnosis of cancer may cause anxiety, fear, or depression, all of which can interfere with the learning process.

5. What nursing interventions could be implemented to overcome these barriers to learning?

Use therapeutic communication (e.g., active listening, demonstration of empathy) to develop a trusting relationship that will encourage the client to talk about areas of concern.

Use short sessions to prevent the client from feeling overwhelmed with new information.

6. What are some possible statements by the client that would indicate she is ready to learn?

"How long does the surgery take?"

"Will I receive breast reconstruction surgery at a later date?"

7. Which of the following may enhance client learning? (Select all that apply.)

_____ Fear

_____ Fatigue

_X_ Active participation

_____ Sensory deficits

_X_ Perceived benefit

Active participation and perceived benefit may enhance learning. Fear, fatigue, and sensory deficits can all impair client learning.

Unit 1   Foundations for Practice
Section: Communication

Chapter 12:   Documentation and Reporting
                Contributor: LaToya T. Marsh, MSN, RN

 NCLEX® Connections:

Learning Objective: Review and apply knowledge within **"Documentation and Reporting"** in readiness for performance of the following nursing activities as outlined by the NCLEX® test plans:

Δ   Document client information in a legally responsible manner in the medical record.

Δ   Promote continuity of care by documenting pertinent information about the client according to facility/agency policy.

Δ   Manage aspects of the client's care by collaborating with other health care team members as appropriate.

Δ   Provide accurate and relevant information during reports.

Δ   Reduce potential health risks to the client by promptly interpreting assessments and reporting status changes to the primary care provider.

Δ   Maintain computer-based client care records using electronic resources.

Δ   Maintain confidentiality of all client medical information.

 Key Points

Δ   The client's chart or medical record is the **legal** record of care.

Δ   The nursing care provided is recorded as **documentation** or **charting** and should reflect the nursing process.

Δ   The client's chart is a **confidential, permanent,** and **legal document** that is admissible in court. The nurse is legally and ethically responsible for ensuring that confidentiality is maintained. Access to the client's medical record should be restricted to only those health care providers who are involved directly in the client's care.

Δ   There is a rapidly growing trend for the client's records to be electronically maintained.

△ Nursing documentation must be **accurate** to correctly record information regarding the client's care.

△ Information to be charted includes:

- Assessments.

- Medication administration.

- Treatments given and client responses.

- Client education.

△ Documentation is a standard for many accrediting agencies including The Joint Commission (formerly JCAHO) Purposes for medical records include communication, legal documentation, financial billing, education, research, and auditing.

△ The purpose of reporting is to provide continuity of care for clients when several nurses provide care.

△ Reporting should be conducted in a confidential manner.

Key Factors

△ **Factual** – Subjective or objective data can be documented.

- Subjective data can be documented as direct quotes, within quotation marks, or summarized and identified as the client's statement.

- Objective data should be descriptive and should include things that the nurse sees, hears, feels, and smells. Document without use of derogatory words, judgment, or stating opinion. Document client behavior accurately. Instead of writing "client is agitated," write "client pacing back and forth in his room, yelling loudly."

△ **Accurate and concise** – Information that is documented must be precise. Avoid the use of unnecessary words and irrelevant details. Use only institutionally accepted abbreviations and correct spelling to prevent errors. If facility/agency policy allows, use monitor strips when appropriate.

△ **Complete and current** – Information that is documented should be comprehensive and documented at the time of the occurrence. Never prechart an assessment, intervention, or evaluation.

△ **Legal Guidelines**

- Begin each entry with the date and time.

- Record entries legibly, in black ink, and do not leave blank spaces in the nurse's note.

- Do not use correction fluid or blacken out errors that are made while documenting in the client record. Make corrections per facility/agency protocol.

- Information that was inadvertently omitted may be added in the form of a "late entry." A late entry must include the time the charting actually occurred and the specific time the charting reflects.

- All documentation must be signed with the signature and the title of the individual making the entry.

- Documentation should reflect assessments, interventions, and evaluations performed by the person signing the entry.

- Guidelines may vary for electronic charting.

Δ   Documentation Formats

- **Flow charts** can be used to record vital signs, blood glucose levels, pain level, and other assessments that are performed frequently and in order to show trends.

- **Narrative** documentation records information as a sequence of events.

- **Charting by exception** makes use of standardized forms that identify normal findings/values and allows for selective documentation of abnormal findings.

- **Problem-oriented medical records** consist of a database, problem list, care plan, and progress notes. Various formats can be used to complete a progress note.

    ◊   **SOAPE**:

    - **S** – Subjective data

    - **O** – Objective data

    - **A** – Assessment (includes a nursing diagnosis based on the assessment)

    - **P** – Plan

    - **E** – Evaluation

    ◊   **PIE**:

    - **P** – Problem

    - **I** – Intervention

    - **E** - Evaluation

    ◊   **DAR**:

    - **D** – Data

    - **A** – Action

    - **R** – Response

- **Computerized documentation** has been developed to include a computer-based client care record (CBPCR).

  ◊ Advantages include standardization, accuracy, confidentiality, and easy access for multiple users. In addition, acquisition and transfer of client information is expediated.

  ◊ Challenges include learning the computerized system, knowing how to correct errors, and maintaining security.

  ◊ Documentation rules and formats are the same as paper charting.

Δ Reporting Formats

- **Change-of-shift reports**

  ◊ This report is given at the conclusion of each shift by the nurse leaving to the nurse assuming responsibility for the client.

  ◊ Ways in which the report can be given include face-to-face, audiotape, or during walking rounds in the client's room.

  ◊ An effective report should:

    ° Include significant objective information about the client and her health problems.

    ° Be given in a logical order.

    ° Be free of gossip and personal opinion.

    ° Relate recent changes in medications, treatments, procedures, or the discharge plan.

- **Telephone reports** are useful when contacting the primary care provider or other members of the interdisciplinary team.

  ◊ It is important to:

    ° Have all the data prepared prior to contacting any member of the interdisciplinary team.

    ° Use professional nurse demeanor.

    ° Use exact, relevant, and accurate information.

    ° Document the name of the person called, the time, content of the message, and what instructions or information was received following the report.

- **Telephone orders (TO) or verbal orders (VO)**

  ◊ These types of orders should be avoided but may be necessary during emergencies and unusual hours.

Δ **Transcribing Medical Orders**

- Use strategies to prevent errors when taking a medical order that is given verbally or over the phone by the primary care provider.

◊ Have a second RN/LPN listen on a phone order.

◊ Repeat back the order given, making sure to include medication name (spell if necessary), dosage, time, and route.

◊ Document reading back the order and the presence of the second nurse on the phone extension.

◊ Question any order that may seem contraindicated due to a previous order or client condition.

- **Transfer reports** should include:

  ◊ Client demographic information.

  ◊ Summary of progress up to transfer.

  ◊ Current health status, both physical and psychosocial.

  ◊ Critical assessments or interventions to be completed.

  ◊ Current nursing diagnoses, care plan, and any problems that may have occurred.

  ◊ Medications currently taken and last dose administered.

  ◊ Allergies.

  ◊ Diet and activity orders.

  ◊ Advance directives.

  ◊ Family support.

  ◊ Special equipment needed (e.g., oxygen, suction, wheelchair).

- **Incident reports (unusual occurrences)**

  ◊ Incident reports are an important part of a facility/agency's quality improvement plan.

  ◊ Any occurrence that is inconsistent with the routine care of the client is considered an incident. Examples of incidents include: medication errors, falls, and needle sticks.

  ◊ The facts should be documented without judgment or opinion.

  ◊ The incident report should not be referred to in the client's medical record.

  ◊ Incident reports help improve health care quality by contributing to changes designed to make improvements.

Primary Reference:

Potter, P. A., & Perry, A. G. (2005). *Fundamentals of nursing* (6th ed.). St. Louis, MO: Mosby.

Additional Resources:

NANDA International (2004). *NANDA nursing diagnoses: Definitions and classification 2005-2006*. Philadelphia: NANDA.

Chapter 12: Documentation and Reporting

Application Exercises

Scenario: A nurse is caring for a 79-year-old man who will be transferred from the acute care facility to a long-term care facility in a city close to his family. Before the transfer, the nurse needs to prepare the transfer forms, remembering the principles of documentation.

1. What information should be reported in the transfer paper work?

2. Prior to the client being transferred, his neighbor calls to receive information about the location of the city and the facility where the client will be transferred. How should the nurse respond to the neighbor?

3. The night shift nurse is preparing information for change-of-shift report. Which of the following is the most important piece of information that the nurse should include in the report?

   A. The client's input and output for the shift

   B. The client's blood pressure from yesterday

   C. A bone scan that is scheduled for today

   D. The medication routine from the medication administration record

4. A nurse enters a client's room and finds the client sitting in his chair. He states, "I fell in the shower but I got myself back up and into my chair." How should the nurse document this in the client's chart?

   A. The client fell in the shower.

   B. The client states he fell in the shower and was able to get himself back into his chair.

   C. This information should not be documented in the chart because the nurse did not witness the fall.

   D. The client fell in the shower but is now resting comfortably.

5. A nurse on the medical unit notices a client has just developed a temperature and does not have an order for acetaminophen (Tylenol). Which of the following is the most appropriate action to take?

> A. Call the primary care provider immediately and then review the client's chart.
> B. Review the client's chart and have all information ready prior to calling the primary care provider.
> C. Talk with the charge nurse, give the client Tylenol, and then call the primary care provider.
> D. Give Tylenol because an order for over-the-counter medications is not needed.

6. A client is given the nursing diagnosis of *impaired mobility* because the skin barrier covering her intestinal fistula keeps falling off when she stands up to ambulate. The skin barrier has been applied twice during shift and remains intact only when the client is supine in bed. The nurse telephoned the physical therapist to tell her about the difficulties containing the drainage from the fistula, so the therapist did not work with the client today. The client sat in a chair during lunch with an absorbent pad over the fistula. A wound care nurse was called and states she will be coming in later today to see the client. The client states she is getting frustrated at not being able to work with her physical therapist. List the information that should be included in the end-of-shift report.

7. Which of the following legal guidelines should the nurse follow when documenting in the client's record? (Select all that apply.)

_____ If an error is made, cover it with correction fluid and write in the correct information.

_____ All entries should be dated and timed.

_____ Document objective data, leaving out personal bias.

_____ Use as many abbreviations as possible.

_____ To save time, wait until the end of the shift to document any information.

Chapter 12: Documentation and Reporting

Application Exercises Answer Key

Scenario: A nurse is caring for a 79-year-old man who will be transferred from the acute care facility to a long-term care facility in a city close to his family. Before the transfer, the nurse needs to prepare the transfer forms, remembering the principles of documentation.

1. What information should be reported in the transfer paper work?

   State the client's name, age, medical diagnosis, nursing care plan, diet and activity parameters, family, support system, allergies, current medications, and advance directives.

2. Prior to the client being transferred, his neighbor calls to receive information about the location of the city and the facility where the client will be transferred. How should the nurse respond to the neighbor?

   Explain to the neighbor that the information is confidential and that he must contact the client's family.

3. The night shift nurse is preparing information for change-of-shift report. Which of the following is the most important piece of information that the nurse should include in the report?

   A. The client's input and output for the shift

   B. The client's blood pressure from yesterday

   C. A bone scan that is scheduled for today

   D. The medication routine from the medication administration record

   The bone scan is the most important because the client's care may need to be modified to accommodate leaving the unit. Unless there is something significant concerning the client's intake and output (I&O), blood pressure, and medication routine, the day shift nurse can read that information in the chart.

4. A nurse enters a client's room and finds the client sitting in his chair. He states, "I fell in the shower but I got myself back up and into my chair." How should the nurse document this in the client's chart?

> A. The client fell in the shower.
>
> **B. The client states he fell in the shower and was able to get himself back into his chair.**
>
> C. This information should not be documented in the chart because the nurse did not witness the fall.
>
> D. The client fell in the shower but is now resting comfortably.

The nurse did not witness the fall, but it is important to include in the chart. Because the nurse did not witness the fall, it cannot be documented as objective data. By writing what the client states, the information is considered subjective data. The nurse should also complete an incident report per facility/agency protocol.

5. A nurse on the medical unit notices a client has just developed a temperature and does not have an order for acetaminophen (Tylenol). Which of the following is the most appropriate action to take?

> A. Call the primary care provider immediately and then review the client's chart.
>
> **B. Review the client's chart and have all information ready prior to calling the primary care provider.**
>
> C. Talk with the charge nurse, give the client Tylenol, and then call the primary care provider.
>
> D. Give Tylenol because an order for over-the-counter medications is not needed.

By reviewing the chart, the nurse will have the opportunity to note whether an order for Tylenol was missed or if the client has an allergy that would contraindicate the medication. The nurse should be prepared prior to calling the primary care provider. Any medication given to a client in a health care facility/agency must have a primary care provider's order.

6. A client is given the nursing diagnosis of *impaired mobility* because the skin barrier covering her intestinal fistula keeps falling off when she stands up to ambulate. The skin barrier has been applied twice during shift and remains intact only when the client is supine in bed. The nurse telephoned the physical therapist to tell her about the difficulties containing the drainage from the fistula, so the therapist did not work with the client today. The client sat in a chair during lunch with an absorbent pad over the fistula. A wound care nurse was called and states she will be coming in later today to see the client. The client states she is getting frustrated at not being able to work with her physical therapist. List the information that should be included in the end-of-shift report.

Client has an intestinal fistula.

Skin barrier stays intact when the client is supine, but the seal loosens when the client stands.

Physical therapy did not ambulate the client today.

Client sat in the chair during lunch.

Client states she is frustrated with not being able to work on improving mobility.

Wound care nurse was called and will see the client later today.

7. Which of the following legal guidelines should the nurse follow when documenting in the client's record? (Select all that apply.)

_____ If an error is made, cover it with correction fluid and write in the correct information.

__X__ **All entries should be dated and timed.**

__X__ **Document objective data, leaving out personal bias.**

_____ Use as many abbreviations as possible.

_____ To save time, wait until the end of the shift to document any information.

All entries must be dated and timed. Documentation should be objective without personal bias. Correction fluid should never be used in a permanent record. The nurse should follow facility/agency protocol for making corrections. Too many abbreviations may make the entry difficult to understand, and only institutionally accepted abbreviations should be used. Documentation should be kept current. Waiting until the end of the shift may lead to omitted documentation.

Unit 1   Foundations for Practice
Section: Professional Standards

Chapter 13:   Ethics and Values
                Contributor: Linda Turchin, MSN, RN

 NCLEX® Connections:

Learning Objective: Review and apply knowledge within **"Ethics and Values"** in readiness for performance of the following nursing activities as outlined by the NCLEX® test plans:

Δ   Protect client's confidentiality and privacy.

Δ   Discuss the Nursing Code of Ethics and its impact on nursing care.

Δ   Identify and describe ethical issues affecting nurses and client care.

Δ   Participate in reasoning ethical solutions for practice and client problems.

Δ   Identify and respect the unique characteristics and values of clients.

Δ   Advocate for the client to assist with meeting the client's needs.

 Key Points

Δ   **Ethics** refers to a method of inquiry concerning the rightness/wrongness of human behavior, as well as the standards of man's behavior described in his formal **code of ethics.**

Δ   **Bioethics** refers specifically to issues that affect health and the delivery of health care.

Δ   **Nursing ethics** refers to issues or questions that nurses must address resulting from their professional practice.

Δ   **Values** are freely chosen, long-lasting beliefs about the correctness of certain items, ideas, attitudes, or customs that influence the behavior of an individual or group.

•   Values reflect cultural and social influences, relationships, and personal needs.

•   Values develop and change over time.

Δ   Ethical nursing dilemmas arise from differences in personal **values**, changing professional roles, technological advances, and social issues that impact the quality of life.

Δ A standard process for thinking through ethical problems (**ethical reasoning**), which is based on critical thinking, helps professional nurses resolve ethical dilemmas arising from their practice.

Δ The goal of ethical reasoning is to reach a mutual, peaceful agreement that is in the best interest of the client while upholding the nurse's individual and professional values.

Key Factors

Δ **Ethical principles** are standards of what is right or wrong with regard to important social values and norms. Ethical principles pertaining to the treatment of the client include:

- **Autonomy** – the ability of the client to make personal decisions, even when those decisions may not be in the client's own best interest.

- **Beneficence** – the care given is in the best interest of the client.

- **Nonmaleficence** – to be spared from harm or pain as much as possible when receiving treatments.

- **Justice** – to be treated fairly in matters related to physical and psychosocial care and use of resources.

- **Fidelity** – to keep one's promise to the client about care that was offered.

Δ **Code of Ethics** – a formal statement of the ethical values and principles that are shared by members of a group. This code serves as a standard for professional actions. The code should be compatible with the individual's personal values.

- The code of ethics demonstrates the profession's commitment to the public, provides a context for making judgments in difficult nursing situations, and offers general guidelines for professional conduct.

- The *American Nurses Association Code of Ethics for Nurses* (2001) and the *International Council of Nurses' Code of Ethics for Nurses* (2000) are documents commonly accepted by professional nurses.

- Professional conduct is demonstrated by:

  ◊ **Accountability** – to be answerable for one's own actions.

  ◊ **Responsibility** – to be trustworthy and dependable.

  ◊ **Advocacy** – to support or defend the client, looking out for the well-being of the client.

  ◊ **Confidentiality** – providing privacy in all matters of health care delivery without diminishing access to quality care.

  ◊ **Veracity** – to tell the truth with no information being withheld.

Δ **Values**

- Understanding one's personal value system and assessing the value systems of others helps to facilitate decision making while ensuring respect for client autonomy.

- Nurses acquire professional values from:

  ◊ Interactions with other nurses.

  ◊ Professional codes of ethics.

  ◊ Nursing experiences.

- Professional values include:

  ◊ Aesthetics (e.g., creativity, sensitivity).

  ◊ Altruism (e.g., caring, commitment, loyalty).

  ◊ Equality/impartiality.

  ◊ Dignity/poise.

  ◊ Justice/fairness.

  ◊ Truthfulness/honesty.

Δ **Ethical reasoning**

- Ethical reasoning is similar to the nursing process because it requires deliberate, systematic, and critical thinking.

- It differs from the nursing process because it requires negotiation of differences, incorporation of conflicting ideas, and an effort to respect differences of opinion.

- The problem is an ethical dilemma if:

  ◊ It cannot be solved solely by a review of scientific data.

  ◊ It is perplexing – not easily solved.

  ◊ The answer will have profound effect on the situation/client.

- The seven steps of ethical reasoning include:
  1. Ask, "Is this an ethical question?"

  2. Review all pertinent information.

  3. Examine and determine personal values related to the issue (values clarification).

  4. Verbalize the problem – produce a clear, simple statement describing the dilemma.

  5. Formulate possible courses of action. This is especially important when there are conflicting opinions.

  6. Negotiate the outcome. This requires a confidence in one's own point of view while having a deep respect for the opinions of others.

  7. Evaluate the action and the outcome.

Primary Reference:

Potter, P. A., & Perry, A. G. (2005). *Fundamentals of nursing* (6th ed.). St. Louis, MO: Mosby.

Additional Resources:

NANDA International (2004). *NANDA nursing diagnoses: Definitions and classification 2005-2006*. Philadelphia: NANDA.

Chapter 13: Ethics and Values

Application Exercises

Scenario: A 72-year-old woman is admitted to the coronary intensive care unit with a diagnosis of acute myocardial infarction. She has a history of cardiac problems stemming from a myocardial infarction 5 years ago. She has expressed a desire to be "spared all the fuss" if she experiences another heart attack. She states she wants to "die with dignity," which means no tubes or machines. She has signed an advance directive expressing these wishes and has given a copy of this directive to her primary care provider and her son.

A postman delivering mail finds the woman unconscious on her doorstep. He immediately dials 911 and initiates CPR. She is transported by ambulance to the emergency department and is placed on life support.

When the son arrives at the hospital, he presents a copy of the client's directive to the attending provider. With this document and her current status, the decision is made to remove her from life support while maintaining palliative care. The client dies the following day.

1. Apply the seven steps of ethical reasoning to this situation.

2. Match the ethical principle with the correct example.

_____ Justice

_____ Autonomy

_____ Beneficence

_____ Nonmaleficence

_____ Fidelity

A. A client decides not to have open heart surgery despite significant blockages.

B. A nurse offers pain medication to a client who is postoperative prior to ambulation.

C. A nurse takes the client outdoors in a wheelchair after lunch as promised.

D. All clients waiting for a kidney transplant have to meet the same qualifications.

E. A nurse questions a medication order as being too extreme in light of the client's advanced age and unstable condition.

3. An ethical dilemma exists due to the difference of opinions regarding performing surgery for a premature infant. The facility/agency's ethics committee has met and all members were given the information required to make a decision. What is the next step in the reasoning process?

    A. Everyone examines his/her own values.

    B. A statement is developed describing the dilemma.

    C. All possible solutions are listed.

    D. A solution is negotiated.

4. A nurse has determined that a client does not understand the implications of a surgical procedure scheduled for the next day. The nurse will not ask the client to sign the informed consent form until the surgeon provides further explanations, and the client verbalizes understanding. The professional nursing ethical principle applicable in this situation is

    A. autonomy.

    B. confidentiality.

    C. fidelity.

    D. veracity.

5. State three ways nurses obtain their professional values.

6. The ANA code of ethics serves which of the following purposes?

    A. Establishes standardized curricula for nursing educational programs

    B. Sets formal guidelines and standards for professional nursing conduct

    C. Ensures that nurses provide client care based on scientific principles

    D. Determines qualifications for advanced practice nurses

Chapter 13: Ethics and Values

Application Exercises Answer Key

Scenario: A 72-year-old woman is admitted to the coronary intensive care unit with a diagnosis of acute myocardial infarction. She has a history of cardiac problems stemming from a myocardial infarction 5 years ago. She has expressed a desire to be "spared all the fuss" if she experiences another heart attack. She states she wants to "die with dignity," which means no tubes or machines. She has signed an advance directive expressing these wishes and has given a copy of this directive to her primary care provider and her son.

A postman delivering mail finds the woman unconscious on her doorstep. He immediately dials 911 and initiates CPR. She is transported by ambulance to the emergency department and is placed on life support.

When the son arrives at the hospital, he presents a copy of the client's directive to the attending provider. With this document and her current status, the decision is made to remove her from life support while maintaining palliative care. The client dies the following day.

1. Apply the seven steps of ethical reasoning to this situation.

Step 1
Is this an ethical question?
Yes, the question is profound. The client's life is the concern.

Step 2
Review all pertinent information.
The postman and the emergency personnel were not aware of her advanced directive, and therefore CPR was initiated and she was placed on life support.

Step 3
Examine and determine personal values related to the issue.
Personal values regarding withholding of medical treatment and an individual's right to make such decisions will influence personal feelings.

Step 4
Verbalize the problem.
The client was resuscitated and is being kept alive despite expressing desires to the contrary in an advance directive.

Step 5
Formulate possible courses of action.
Possible courses of action are removal of all forms of life support, continuation of all forms of life support, and removal of medication support while continuing mechanical support.

Step 6
Negotiate the outcome.
Discuss problems that might arise if a family member was resistant to the termination of life support.

Step 7:
Evaluate the action and the outcome.
State how the problem was resolved.

2. Match the ethical principle with the correct example.

__D__	Justice	A. A client decides not to have open heart surgery despite significant blockages.
__A__	Autonomy	B. A nurse offers pain medication to a client who is postoperative prior to ambulation.
__B__	Beneficence	C. A nurse takes the client outdoors in a wheelchair after lunch as promised.
__E__	Nonmaleficence	D. All clients waiting for a kidney transplant have to meet the same qualifications.
__C__	Fidelity	E. A nurse questions a medication order as being too extreme in light of the client's advanced age and unstable condition.

3. An ethical dilemma exists due to the difference of opinions regarding performing surgery for a premature infant. The facility/agency's ethics committee has met and all members were given the information required to make a decision. What is the next step in the reasoning process?

A. Everyone examines his/her own values.

B. A statement is developed describing the dilemma.

C. All possible solutions are listed.

D. A solution is negotiated.

Values clarification is the third step in solving an ethical dilemma. Developing a statement describing the dilemma is the fourth step, listing all possible solutions is the fifth step, and negotiating a solution is the sixth step.

4. A nurse has determined that a client does not understand the implications of a surgical procedure scheduled for the next day. The nurse will not ask the client to sign the informed consent form until the surgeon provides further explanations, and the client verbalizes understanding. The professional nursing ethical principle applicable in this situation is

>   A. autonomy.
>
>   B. confidentiality.
>
>   C. fidelity.
>
>   **D. veracity.**

Veracity means that the client has a right to be told the truth with no information being withheld. Autonomy and confidentiality are general ethical principles, not professional nursing ethical principles. Confidentiality refers to the client's right to privacy that is not in question in the given situation.

5. State three ways nurses obtain their professional values.

Interactions with other nurses

Professional codes of ethics

Nursing experiences

6. The ANA code of ethics serves which of the following purposes?

>   A. Establishes standardized curricula for nursing educational programs
>
>   **B. Sets formal guidelines and standards for professional nursing conduct**
>
>   C. Ensures that nurses provide client care based on scientific principles
>
>   D. Determines qualifications for advanced practice nurses

The ANA code of ethics offers general guidelines for professional conduct. State boards of nursing are responsible for setting nursing educational curricula and determining qualifications of professional nurses. Providing care based on scientific principles is a component of the ANA Standards of Professional Performance.

Unit 1   Foundations for Practice
Section: Professional Standards

Chapter 14:   **Legal Responsibilities**
Contributor: Linda Turchin, MSN, RN

 NCLEX® Connections:

Learning Objective: Review and apply knowledge within **"Legal Responsibilities"** in readiness for performance of the following nursing activities as outlined by the NCLEX® test plans:

- Δ   Discuss the legal regulation of nursing practice.

- Δ   Assess the client's understanding of his/her rights and offer explanations when necessary (e.g., advance directives, refusal of treatment, privacy).

- Δ   Recognize and respect the client's right to treatment.

- Δ   Assist in obtaining informed consent by evaluating whether or not the client is appropriate to give consent (e.g., is of legal age, cognitively aware, has understanding of the treatment or procedure to be performed) before the form is signed.

- Δ   Perform nursing care within the scope of practice.

- Δ   Report client neglect or abuse when identified.

- Δ   Report incidences or variances in accordance with facility guidelines when identified.

 Key Points

- Δ   Nurses are legally responsible for the care they provide and are required to critically think to understand and observe the legal guidelines whereby a nurse must function.

- Δ   Knowledge of the law helps to maintain standards of nursing practice and protects the nurse from liability.

- Δ   The legal guidelines for practice are established and enforced through a state board of nursing or other government agency and state **nurse practice acts**.

- Δ   **Standards of care** are legal guidelines for practice described in the nurse practice acts of each state, professional nursing organizations (nursing specialties), and healthcare facility/agency polices and procedures.

Δ Protecting a client's right to appropriate, **consensual,** confidential health care, and freedom from unauthorized release of any related information is a legal and ethical responsibility of nursing.

Δ Federal statutes offering the client protection include Americans with Disabilities Act, Emergency Medical Treatment and Active Labor Act, Mental Health Parity Act, Patient Self-Determination Act (advance directives), Uniform Anatomical Gift Act, Health Insurance Portability and Accountability Act, and Uniform Determination of Death Act.

Δ All professional nurses must be **licensed** by the state in which they are practicing.

Δ As determined by a nurse's behavior, he/she may be held **liable** for either **intentional** or **unintentional torts.**

Δ Nurses are client advocates and play a role in ensuring quality of care through risk management and legislative lobbying.

Key Factors

Δ **Nurse practice acts** are statutes created and enacted by the legislature of each state to ensure public safety. Rules and regulations created by state boards of nursing impose regulatory law on nursing practice.

- **The nurse practice act** defines

  ◊ The general scope of professional nursing practice (**standard of care**). Guidelines in each act are used to measure nursing conduct and determine whether or not the nurse acted as any reasonable prudent nurse would act under the same or similar circumstances.

  ◊ Educational requirements (basic and continuing) for nurses.

  ◊ Makeup of the board of nursing and what authority it holds.

  ◊ **Licensure** – permits a nurse to provide special skilled services to the public while providing the public with certain assurances concerning the quality of those services.

    ° Requirements for this licensure may vary, but all states demand educational requirements and the successful passing of the National Council Licensure Examination (NCLEX®).

    ° The license may be suspended or revoked for improper conduct.

  ◊ The appropriate tasks that can be delegated to assistive personnel based on the delegate's knowledge and experience and the client's condition.

Δ **Client Rights**

- **The Patient Care Partnership**

  ◊ The American Hospital Association (AHA) Patients' Bill of Rights specifies the rights of individuals in health care settings.

◊ The wording of these rights has recently been revised to a plain language, multilingual document called The Patient Care Partnership. For information about this document, go to http://www.aha.org/aha/issues/Communicating-With-Patients/pt-care-partnership.html.

◊ The nurse should use these documents to advocate for the client.

- **Patient Self-Determination Act (advance directives)** requires that a client be given written information explaining his right to refuse treatment and establish advance directives. Documentation in the client's medical record must show whether or not a client has an advance directive in effect.

  ◊ **Advance directives** include:

    ° A living will, which is a written declaration of the client's directions for health care in the event the client is not able to communicate.

    ° A durable power of attorney for health care, which is a written declaration stating that another person may act on behalf of the client in health care decisions when the client becomes unable to express his own desires.

- **Uniform Anatomical Gift Act** allows a competent client to make an informed decision to donate all or part of her body for organ donation or medical research after death.

  ◊ The nurse may act as a witness to this decision.

  ◊ The nurse must be familiar and comply with facility/agency policies and procedures regarding organ donation.

- **Health Insurance Portability and Accountability Act (HIPAA)** prohibits health insurance companies from discriminating based on health status and sets standards regarding the exchange of private and sensitive health information. Nurses are legally responsible for being informed, aware, and in compliance with the HIPAA policies and procedures of their facility/agency.

- **Uniform Determination of Death Act** provides a consistent definition of death in each state based on a whole-brain or a cardiopulmonary definition. Nursing responsibilities include:

  ◊ Being aware of the legal definitions of death in order to produce appropriate and accurate documentation regarding the client's death.

  ◊ Treating the deceased with dignity.

  ◊ Obtaining permission for an autopsy from one of the following:

    ° The client prior to death.

    ° A close family member after death.

Δ   **Civil and Common Law**

- The nurse is responsible for knowing and following the legal guidelines concerning client rights and the importance of consent.

- **Torts** are civil wrongs against a person or property and are potential areas of nursing liability. There are two forms of torts:

  ◊   **Intentional** – willful act that violates another's rights.

Intentional Tort	Description	Example
Assault	A threat to cause harm	"If you don't eat your breakfast, I'll make you stay in the chair all day."
Battery	• Purposeful, wrongful (inappropriate) touching without consent • Relies on implied consent as an agreement inferred by the client's cooperative behavior	• A client who presents his hand when told it is time to test his blood glucose implies consent. • Continuing to give the client an enema even when she says "Stop" is battery.
Invasion of privacy	The unwanted intrusion of others in a client's private affairs	Sharing a client's condition over the phone with someone who identifies himself as a "friend" of the client is considered an invasion of privacy.
Defamation of character	Knowingly or unknowingly presenting a false statement, either written (libel) or oral (slander) that results in harm to a client's reputation	Stating, "The client in exam room A has to be selling his pain medication, since he always wants the prescription renewed," can be construed as defamation of the client's character.
False imprisonment	Restraining or detaining a competent client against his or her will	A nurse refusing to give a client his clothing when he decides to leave the hospital against medical advice is considered false imprisonment.

  ◊   **Unintentional torts or negligence** is nursing conduct that fails to meet the standard of care and thus places the client at risk for injury. One type of an unintentional tort is **malpractice.** Malpractice occurs when a nurse fails to meet standards of care, and the following elements are present:

    °   There is an established relationship between the nurse and the client (e.g., the nurse is assigned the care of the client).

    °   The nurse ignores a standard of care that is expected in a specific situation (e.g., not checking the client's identification bracelet prior to the administration of whole blood).

    °   The client sustains harm, injury, or damage as a result of the nurse's omission (e.g., the client suffers a blood transfusion reaction due to receiving blood of the wrong type).

       ° The harm occurs as a result of the nurse not performing in a reasonable manner.

- Other areas of potential liability include:

  ◊ Unprofessional conduct (e.g., reporting to work under the influence of alcohol or drugs).

  ◊ Failure to carry out a primary care provider's order, with exceptions being:

      ° A nurse is obligated to carry out such an order unless the correctness of the order is in doubt or certainly detrimental to the client (e.g., "Meperidine [Demerol] 100 mg IV q 3 to 4 hr PRN" for a client with a documented hypersensitivity to meperidine).

      ° A nurse is obligated to make a serious attempt to clarify any order that is illegible, unclear, or incomplete (e.g., "Meperidine [Demerol] 50 mg PRN" – incomplete prescription [no route] for safe administration).

  ◊ Abandonment: termination of the nurse-client relationship by the nurse without adequate notice or appropriate transfer of care (e.g., 7 a.m. – 7 p.m. nurse leaves her clients unattended when her 7 p.m. – 7 a.m. shift replacement calls in sick).

Δ Consent

- Consent is required for all treatment that is given to the client in a health care facility.

- State laws prescribe who is able to give informed consent. Laws will vary regarding age limitations and emergencies. The nurse is responsible for knowing the laws in the state of practice.

Δ Informed Consent

- Consent is required for all treatment that is given to the client in a health care facility.

- State laws prescribe who is able to give informed consent. Laws will vary regarding age limitations and emergencies. The nurse is responsible for knowing the laws in the state of practice.

- People authorized to grant consent for another person include:

  ◊ Parent of a minor.

  ◊ Legal guardian.

  ◊ Court-specified representative by a court order.

  ◊ Spouse or closest available relative who has durable power of attorney for health care.

Responsibilities for Informed Consent		
The Provider	**The Client**	**The Nurse**
Obtains informed consent. To do so, the provider must give the client:	**Gives informed consent.** To give informed consent, the client must:	**Witnesses informed consent.** This means the nurse is responsible for:
• A complete description of the treatment/procedure. • A description of the professionals who will be performing and participating in the treatment. • A description of the potential harm, pain, and/or discomfort that might occur. • Options for other treatments. • The right to refuse treatment.	• Give it voluntarily (no coercion involved). • Be competent and of legal age (otherwise an authorized person must give consent). • Receive enough information to make a decision based on an understanding of what is expected.	• Ensuring that the provider gave the client the necessary information. • Ensuring that the client understood the information and is competent to give informed consent. • Having the client sign the informed consent document. • Notifying the provider if the client has more questions or appears not to understand any of the information provided. (The provider is then responsible for giving clarification.)

- Informed consent must be obtained by the provider performing the procedure.

- Informed consent is the giving of permission for a procedure to be performed with the assumption that:

  ◊ Consent was voluntary (no coercion was involved).

  ◊ The client was competent and of legal age.

  ◊ The client had enough information to make a decision based on an understanding of what is expected. This should include:

     ° Complete description of treatment/procedure.

     ° Professionals who will be performing and participating in the treatment/procedure.

     ° Potential harm, pain, and/or discomfort that may occur.

     ° Options for other treatments.

     ° The right to refuse treatment.

- A nurse is responsible for confirming that informed consent has been obtained. Witnessing the client's signature implies that the requirements for giving informed consent have been met.

- If the nurse believes the client is not adequately informed the primary care provider must be notified.

Δ   **Reporting and Documentation**

- Nurses should follow all laws and facility policies regarding reporting and documenting.

- Depending on state law, professional nurses are legally bound to report possible criminal behaviors such as child and/or older adult abuse, domestic violence, rape, and certain communicable diseases.

- Incident/unusual occurrence reports can be used to record actions that cause or have the potential to cause harm.

- Documentation of incidents should follow good charting guidelines (e.g., timely, accurate, complete, concise).

Primary Reference:

Potter, P. A., & Perry, A. G. (2005). *Fundamentals of nursing* (6th ed.). St. Louis, MO: Mosby.

Additional Resources:

NANDA International (2004). *NANDA nursing diagnoses: Definitions and classification 2005-2006.* Philadelphia: NANDA.

Chapter 14: Legal Responsibilities

Application Exercises

Scenario: A nurse enters a client's room to reassess him after administration of an IV pain medication. The nurse finds the client sleeping with normal respirations and no signs of pain. The phone rings, and the nurse answers it to prevent the client from being disturbed. The caller identifies himself as the client's son and asks, "How is dad doing?" The nurse tells the caller that his father is resting comfortably now after receiving "a shot" but that earlier he was "cranky and difficult to deal with." The nurse also tells the caller that the client's "x-rays were not good, but you'll need to discuss that with his doctor."

1. Has the nurse breached any client rights? Defend your conclusion.

2. Is the nurse guilty of any tort? Defend your answer.

3. List several ways that a nurse can manage questions posed by the client's family?

4. Identify the reasons a nursing license may be suspended or revoked by the state board of nursing.

5. HIPPA provides which client right?

    A. The right to a consistent determination of death

    B. The right to donate all or part of the body for organ donation or medical research after death

    C. The right to refuse treatment and establish advance directives

    D. The right for sensitive health information to be kept confidential

6. Which of the following are functions that are most likely to be performed by a state board of nursing? (Select all that apply.)

_____ Determining qualifications of applicants for licensure

_____ Approving nursing education curricula

_____ Settling ethical dilemmas within a health care setting

_____ Setting minimum standards for practice

_____ Determining hospital hiring policies

7. A client tells the nurse she does not understand why she has to have surgery for her problems when her best friend, who has similar symptoms, is able to take medications for her problems. Which of the following is the most appropriate communication by the nurse?

    A. Reassure the client that the surgeon is the most competent physician on staff.

    B. Notify the surgeon regarding the client's concerns.

    C. Tell the client that she should not be concerned with her friend's health.

    D. Change the subject so that the client will not focus on her concerns.

Chapter 14: Legal Responsibilities

Application Exercises Answer Key

Scenario: A nurse enters a client's room to reassess him after administration of an IV pain medication. The nurse finds the client sleeping with normal respirations and no signs of pain. The phone rings, and the nurse answers it to prevent the client from being disturbed. The caller identifies himself as the client's son and asks, "How is dad doing?" The nurse tells the caller that his father is resting comfortably now after receiving "a shot" but that earlier he was "cranky and difficult to deal with." The nurse also tells the caller that the client's "x-rays were not good, but you'll need to discuss that with his doctor."

1. Has the nurse breached any client rights? Defend your conclusion.

   Yes – confidential care. Information relating to both his present condition and the results of his x-rays were shared inappropriately.

2. Is the nurse guilty of any tort? Defend your answer.

   Yes – Breach of confidentiality and defamation of character ("cranky and difficult")

3. List several ways that a nurse can manage questions posed by the client's family?

   Unplugging the phone so the phone doesn't ring in the client's room

   Suggesting to the family member that he/she contact the primary care provider regarding the status of the client

   Telling the family member that the nurse will inform the client that he received a phone call from a family member and suggesting that he call the family member back

4. Identify the reasons a nursing license may be suspended or revoked by the state board of nursing.

   These will vary by state, but some common reasons include: stealing/selling controlled substances, substance abuse, sexual misconduct with a client, and abuse and/or neglect of clients.

5. HIPPA provides which client right?

> A. The right to a consistent determination of death
>
> B. The right to donate all or part of the body for organ donation or medical research after death
>
> C. The right to refuse treatment and establish advance directives
>
> **D. The right for sensitive health information to be kept confidential**

The right to confidentiality is protected by the Health Insurance Portability and Accountability Act (HIPAA). The accurate determination of death is a right protected by the Uniform Determination of Death Act. The right to donate body organs is protected by the Uniform Anatomical Gift Act. The right to refuse treatment is the right protected by the Patient Self-Determination Act.

6. Which of the following are functions that are most likely to be performed by a state board of nursing? (Select all that apply.)

> __X__ **Determining qualifications of applicants for licensure**
>
> __X__ **Approving nursing education curricula**
>
> _____ Settling ethical dilemmas within a health care setting
>
> __X__ **Setting minimum standards for practice**
>
> _____ Determining hospital hiring policies

Through state nurse practice acts, the state board of nursing is usually responsible for determining qualifications of applicants for licensure, approving curricula for nursing education programs, and setting minimum standards for practice. State nurse practice acts do not settle ethical dilemmas, nor do they determine hiring policies of hospitals.

7. A client tells the nurse she does not understand why she has to have surgery for her problems when her best friend, who has similar symptoms, is able to take medications for her problems. Which of the following is the most appropriate communication by the nurse?

> A. Reassure the client that the surgeon is the most competent physician on staff.
>
> **B. Notify the surgeon regarding the client's concerns.**
>
> C. Tell the client that she should not be concerned with her friend's health.
>
> D. Change the subject so that the client will not focus on her concerns.

It is within the nurse's scope of practice to determine that the client will not be able to give informed consent based on her comments. Therefore, the nurse must notify the surgeon and inform him that the client has questions. Reassuring the client, telling her not to worry about her friend, and changing the subject are all nontherapeutic responses.

Unit 1   Foundations for Practice

Section: Nursing Throughout the Lifespan

Chapter 15:   Infant (Birth to 1 year)

Contributor: Sally Swenson, MA, RN

 NCLEX® Connections

> **Learning Objective**: Review and apply knowledge within "**Infant (Birth to 1 year)**" in readiness for performance of the following nursing activities as outlined by the NCLEX® test plans:
>
> Δ   Assess/monitor an infant's physical, cognitive, and psychosocial development and compare to expected growth and development for age.
>
> Δ   Identify and report variances from expected growth and development.
>
> Δ   Plan and/or provide care to assist the infant to achieve expected growth and development outcomes.
>
> Δ   Plan and/or provide care appropriate to the infant's developmental level, inclusive of age-appropriate recreational/diversional activities.
>
> Δ   Teach children/family expected normal growth and development and age-appropriate health maintenance recommendations for the infant.
>
> Δ   Teach/reinforce accident prevention and health promotion activities for the infant.

 Key Points

Δ   **Stages of Development** – The infant (birth to 1 year)

Theorist	Type of Development	Stage
Erikson	Psychosocial	Trust vs mistrust
Freud	Psychosocial	Oral
Piaget	Cognitive	Sensorimotor

Expected Growth and Development

Δ   **Physical Development**

•   The infant's **posterior fontanel** close at 2 to 3 months of age.

- The infant's **size** is tracked by weight, height, and head circumference.

  ◊ **Weight**: The infant gains 0.7 kg (1.5 lb) per month the first 6 months, and 0.3 kg (0.75 lb) per month the last 6 months. The infant triples birth weight by end of the first year.

  ◊ **Height**: The infant grows 2.5 cm (1 in) per month the first 6 months, and then 1.25 cm (0.5 in) per month the last 6 months.

  ◊ **Head circumference**: The circumference of the infant's head increases 1.25 cm (0.5 in) per month for the first 6 months.

- Following size, the infant develops **gross motor skills**.

  ◊ Holds head up (3 months)

  ◊ Rolls over (5 to 6 months)

  ◊ Holds head steady when sitting (6 months)

  ◊ Gets to sitting position alone and can pull up to standing position (9 months)

  ◊ Stands holding on (12 months)

  ◊ Stands alone (12 months)

- **Fine motor** development follows next in the sequence.

  ◊ Brings hands together

  ◊ Grasps rattle

  ◊ Looks for items that are dropped from view

  ◊ Transfers an object from one hand to the other (6 months)

  ◊ Rakes finger foods with hand (6 months)

  ◊ Uses thumb-finger to grasp items (9 months)

  ◊ Bangs two toys together (9 months)

  ◊ Can nest one object inside another (12 months)

Δ **Cognitive Development**

- **The sensorimotor** period for an infant (Piaget) is characterized by:

  ◊ Initial reflexes replaced by voluntary movements that are self-centered on having needs met.

    ° Object permanence – The infant realizes that an object still exists even when it is no longer in view (occurs between 6 to 12 months).

    ° The infant's discrimination between persons.

    ° The infant comprehends word meanings.

- **Language** development follows the sensorimotor period.
  - ◊ Responds to noises
  - ◊ Vocalizes with "ooos" and "aahs"
  - ◊ Laughs and squeals
  - ◊ Turns head to the sound of a rattle
  - ◊ Pronounces single-syllable words
  - ◊ Begins speaking two and then three-word phrases

Δ **Psychosocial Development**

- **Personal-social** development occurs next in the sequence.
  - ◊ Regards faces
  - ◊ Smiles in response to others
  - ◊ Regards own hands
  - ◊ Works to reach toys
  - ◊ Feeds self by eating finger foods
  - ◊ Waves goodbye
  - ◊ Plays pat-a-cake
  - ◊ Drinks from a cup with handles

- **The infant begins to bond with its parents** within the first month. The process is enhanced when both the infant and parents are in good health, have positive feeding experiences, and receive adequate rest.

- **Separation** recognition occurs during the first year as the infant learns his physical boundaries from that of other people. Learning how to respond to people in his environment is the next phase of development. Positive interactions with parents, siblings, and other caregivers help to establish trust (Erikson).

- **Separation anxiety** develops the latter half of the first year. Therefore, parents should be encouraged not to leave the infant for long periods of time.

Δ **Self-concept Development**

- By the end of the first year, infants will be able to distinguish themselves as being separate from their parents.

Δ **Body-image Changes**

- The infant discovers that his mouth is a pleasure producer (Freud: oral stage).

- Hands and feet are seen as objects of play.

- The infant discovers that smiling causes others to react.

Δ   **Age-appropriate Activities**

- Infants have short attention spans and do not interact with other children during play (solitary play). Appropriate toys include those that stimulate the senses and encourage development. These toys include:

  ◊   Rattles.

  ◊   Mobiles.

  ◊   Teething toys.

  ◊   Nesting toys.

  ◊   Playing pat-a-cake.

  ◊   Playing with balls.

  ◊   Reading books.

Δ   **Nutrition**

- **Feeding alternatives** for an infant include:

  ◊   Breastfeeding (recommended).

  ◊   Iron-fortified formula (acceptable alternative to breast milk).

  ◊   Cow's milk (not recommended).

- **Solids** can be introduced around the time the infant doubles his birth weight (5 to 6 months).

  ◊   First, give the infant cereals.

  ◊   Next, give the infant puréed or strained foods one at a time to assess for food allergies.

  ◊   Finally, breast milk/formula should be decreased as intake of solid foods increases.

- **Weaning** can be accomplished when the infant is able to drink from a cup with handles (sometime after 6 months).

  ◊   One of the infant's feedings is switched to a cup with handles.

  ◊   The infant's bedtime feeding is the last one to be replaced.

Δ   **Health Promotion and Prevention**

- **Hyperbilirubinemia** (newborns) is commonly caused by immaturity of the liver and is observed as jaundice. Bilirubin levels are assessed, and if elevated, are treated with phototherapy. If left untreated, hyperbilirubinemia can cause brain damage.

- **Child abuse** is a potential risk and may be **manifested as:**

  ◊   **Physical neglect**: poor hygiene, failure to demonstrate adequate growth and development, injuries related to insufficient safeguards.

◊ **Emotional abuse and neglect**: failure to demonstrate adequate growth and development, poor social interactions, and fear of strangers.

◊ **Physical abuse**: bruising, welts, lacerations, burns, fractures, bite marks, fear of a parent(s) or lack of reactions, abdominal distension, vomiting, or missing hair.

◊ **Sexual abuse**: bruising; bleeding; abrasions around external genitalia, rectum, or mouth; STDs; and urinary tract infections.

• **Dentition** – 6 to 8 teeth erupt in the infant's mouth by the end of the first year.

◊ Teething pain can be eased using cold teething rings, over-the-counter teething gels, or acetaminophen (Tylenol) and/or ibuprofen.

◊ Clean the infant's teeth using a wet washcloth.

◊ Bottles should not be given to infants when they are falling asleep. This will help to avoid prolonged exposure to milk or juice that can cause dental caries (bottle mouth syndrome).

• 2007 Centers for Disease Control and Prevention (CDC) **immunization recommendations** for healthy infants **less than 12 months** include:

◊ **Birth** – hepatitis B (Hep B).

◊ **2 months** – Hep B; rotavirus vaccine (Rota); diphtheria and tetanus toxoids and pertussis (DTaP); *Haemophilus influenzae* type B (Hib); pneumococcal vaccine (PCV); inactivated poliovirus (IPV).

◊ **4 months** – Rota, DTaP, Hib, PCV, IPV.

◊ **6 months** – Hep B (6 to 12 months), Rota, DTaP, PCV, IPV (6 to 18 months).

◊ Infants 6 to 12 months should receive a yearly **influenza** vaccination. The trivalent inactivated influenza vaccine (TIV) is available as an intramuscular injection, or the live, attenuated influenza vaccine (LAIV) is available as an intranasal spray.

• **Diaper rash treatment and prevention includes:**

◊ Changing the infant's diapers frequently.

◊ Cleansing the infant's skin with water and drying thoroughly at each change.

◊ Applying either A&D or zinc oxide ointment to the infant's rash before replacing the diaper.

◊ Exposing the infant's reddened skin to air during the day when possible.

• Injury prevention includes:

◊ Suffocation.

° Plastic bags should be avoided.

- A firm crib mattress should fit tight.

- Crib slats should be no further apart than 6 cm (2.4 in).

- No pillows should be allowed in the infant's crib.

- The infant should be placed on the back for sleep.

- The infant should never be left alone in the bath.

◊ Falls.

- Rails should be up on the crib.

- Use restraints in infant seats.

- Place the seat on the ground or floor if used outside of the car, and do not leave it unattended or on elevated surfaces.

- Use safety gates across stairs.

◊ Poisoning.

- Avoid exposing the infant to lead paint.

- Keep toxins and plants out of the infant's reach.

- Keep safety locks on cabinets with cleaners and other household chemicals.

- Keep poison control number near the phone.

- Keep medications in childproof containers.

◊ Burns.

- Check temperature of bath water.

- Turn down the thermostat on hot water heater.

- Make sure smoke detectors are working at all times.

- Elevate hot objects.

- Use sunscreen during the infant's exposure to the sun.

- Cover electrical outlets.

◊ Motor vehicles.

- Use an approved rear-facing car seat in the back seat (away from air bags) to transport the infant. Infants should be in rear-facing car seats for the first year of life and until they weigh 9.1 kg (20 lb). It is recommended to have the infant ride rear-facing until he has reached the height and weight limit allowed by the manufacturer of the car seat.

◊ Bodily damage.

- Keep sharp objects out of the infant's reach, and turn diaper pins away from the infant.

Primary Reference:

Potter, P. A., & Perry, A. G. (2005). *Fundamentals of nursing* (6th ed.). St. Louis, MO: Mosby.

Additional Resources:

American Academy of Pediatrics. (2007, February). *Car safety seats: A guide for families 2007*. Retrieved March 15, 2007, from http://www.aap.org/family/carseatguide.htm

Centers for Disease Control and Prevention. (2007). *Recommended childhood and adolescent immunization schedule*. Retrieved January 17, 2007, from *www.cdc.gov/*

Hockenberry, M. (2005). *Wong's essentials of pediatric nursing*. (7th ed.). St. Louis, MO: Mosby.

NANDA International (2004). *NANDA nursing diagnoses: Definitions and classification 2005-2006*. Philadelphia: NANDA.

Chapter 15: Infant (Birth to 1 year)

Application Exercises

Scenario: A 6-month-old infant weighed 3.2 kg (7 lb) at birth. Currently, at his well-infant check-up he weighs 7.7 kg (17 lb).

1. Is the infant's weight normal for this age?

2. The infant's mother states that her infant just started sitting with support. List several gross motor skills that the nurse would expect the infant to develop over the next few months?

3. One of the personal-social skills the infant demonstrates is reaching to get toys. What activities should the nurse suggest to the infant's mother to promote personal and social development over the next few months?

4. The infant says "Dada" and turns to see where various sounds are coming from. What language skills will the infant develop over the next several months?

5. What immunizations should the infant receive at this visit if his previous immunizations are current?

6. During a well-infant check, the mother of a 9-month-old infant states that her infant is easily distracted from breastfeeding and does not seem that interested. What teaching can the nurse provide?

7. What information can a nurse provide to assist a mother to wean her infant?

8. When assessing an infant for abuse, a nurse should look for which of the following signs and symptoms? (Select all that apply.)

_____ Altered growth and development

_____ Bruising, welts, and lacerations

_____ Poor hygiene

_____ Poor social interactions

_____ Comfort with strangers

9. Cognitive development of the infant includes development of object permanence. This means the infant

A. has long-term memory capabilities.

B. realizes that an object continues to exist even though it is no longer in view.

C. recognizes that she is a separate object from her parents.

D. tries to respond voluntarily versus reflexively to stimuli.

Chapter 15: Infant (Birth to 1 year)

Application Exercises Answer Key

Scenario: A 6-month-old infant weighed 3.2 kg (7 lb) at birth. Currently, at his well-infant check-up he weighs 7.7 kg (17 lb).

1. Is the infant's weight normal for this age?

   Yes. The infant has doubled his birth weight by 5 to 6 months of age.

2. The infant's mother states that her infant just started sitting with support. List several gross motor skills that the nurse would expect the infant to develop over the next few months?

   Rolling over

   Standing holding on, standing alone

   Getting to sitting position and sitting alone

3. One of the personal-social skills the infant demonstrates is reaching to get toys. What activities should the nurse suggest to the infant's mother to promote personal and social development over the next few months?

   Feeding self with finger foods

   Waving goodbye

   Playing pat-a-cake

   Drinking from a cup with handles

4. The infant says "Dada" and turns to see where various sounds are coming from. What language skills will the infant develop over the next several months?

   Pronouncing other single-syllable words

   Speaking two-and then three-word phrases

5. What immunizations should the infant receive at this visit if his previous immunizations are current?

6 months – hepatitis B, Rota, DTaP, IPV, PCV, and TIV. In addition, infants 6 to 12 months should receive a yearly influenza vaccination.

6. During a well-infant check, the mother of a 9-month-old infant states that her infant is easily distracted from breastfeeding and does not seem that interested. What teaching can the nurse provide?

This infant may be ready to drink from a cup with handles. Solids can also be started by offering cereals first, followed by puréed or strained foods one at a time to assess for food allergies.

7. What information can a nurse provide to assist a mother to wean her infant?

One of the infant's feedings is switched to a cup with handles.

The infant's bedtime feeding is the last one to be replaced.

8. When assessing an infant for abuse, a nurse should look for which of the following signs and symptoms? (Select all that apply.)

   __X__ **Altered growth and development**
   __X__ **Bruising, welts, and lacerations**
   __X__ **Poor hygiene**
   __X__ **Poor social interactions**
   _____ Comfort with strangers

Signs of altered growth and development, physical injury, poor hygiene, and social interactions, as well as fear of strangers, are all signs and symptoms of infant abuse. Abuse will interfere with adequate growth and development.

9. Cognitive development of the infant includes development of object permanence. This means the infant

    A. has long-term memory capabilities.

    B. realizes that an object continues to exist even though it is no longer in view.

    C. recognizes that she is a separate object from her parents.

    D. tries to respond voluntarily versus reflexively to stimuli.

Object permanence is realizing that an object still exists even when it is no longer in view. The infant develops this skill during the last 6 months of the first year.

Unit 1 Foundations for Practice
Section: Nursing Throughout the Lifespan

Chapter 16: Toddler (12 months to 3 years)
Contributor: Sally Swenson, MA, RN

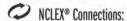 NCLEX® Connections:

Learning Objective: Review and apply knowledge within "**Toddler (12 months to 3 years)**" in readiness for performance of the following nursing activities as outlined by the NCLEX ® test plans:

Δ   Assess/compare the toddler's physical, cognitive, and psychosocial development to expected growth and development for age.

Δ   Identify and report variances from expected growth and development.

Δ   Plan and/or provide care to assist the toddler to achieve expected growth and development outcomes.

Δ   Plan and/or provide care appropriate to the toddler's developmental level, inclusive of age-appropriate recreational/diversional activities.

Δ   Teach children/family expected normal growth and development and age-appropriate health maintenance recommendations for the toddler.

Δ   Teach/reinforce accident prevention and health promotion activities for the toddler.

 Key Points

Δ   **Stages of development** – The toddler (12 months to 3 years)

Theorist	Type of Development	Stage
Erikson	Psychosocial	Autonomy vs shame
Freud	Psychosocial	Anal
Piaget	Cognitive	Sensorimotor transitions to preoperational

Expected Growth and Development

Δ **Physical Development**

- **The toddler's anterior fontanel** closes by 18 months of age.

- **Weigh**t: At 30 months the toddler should weigh 4 times his birth weight

- **Height**: The toddler grows by 7.5 cm (3 in) per year.

Δ **Developmental skills** achieved by the toddler include:

- Development of steady gait.

- Climbing stairs.

- Jumping and standing on one foot for short periods.

- Stacking blocks in increasingly higher numbers.

- Drawing stick figures.

- Undressing and feeding self.

- Toilet training.

Δ **Cognitive Development**

- The concept of **object permanence** is fully developed.

- Toddlers demonstrate **memory** of events that relate to them.

- **Language** increases to about 400 words with the toddler speaking in 2- to 3-word phrases.

- **Preoperational thought** does not allow for the toddler to understand other viewpoints, but it does allow toddlers to symbolize objects and people in order to imitate activities they have seen previously.

Δ **Psychosocial Development**

- **Independence** is paramount for the toddler who is attempting to do everything for himself.

- **Separation anxiety** continues to occur when a parent leaves the child.

Δ **Moral Development**

- Moral development is closely associated with cognitive development.

- Egocentric – Toddlers are unable to see another's perspective; they can only view things from their point of view.

- The toddler's punishment and obedience orientation begins with a sense that good behavior is rewarded and bad behavior is punished.

Δ   **Self-concept Development**

- Toddlers progressively see themselves as separate from their parents and increase their explorations away from them.

Δ   **Body-image Changes**

- The toddler appreciates the usefulness of various body parts.

- Toddlers develop gender identify by age 3.

Δ   **Age-appropriate Activities**

- Solitary play evolves into parallel play where the toddler observes other children and then may engage in activities nearby.

    ◊   Filling and emptying containers

    ◊   Playing with blocks

    ◊   Reading books

    ◊   Playing with toys that can be pushed and pulled

        °   Tossing a ball

Δ   **Nutrition**

- Toddlers are picky eaters with repeated requests for favorite foods.

- The toddler should be switched to 3 or 4 glasses of cow's milk a day, and serving sizes should be kept small to avoid overwhelming the toddler.

Δ   **Health Promotion and Prevention**

- **Child abuse** is a potential risk and may be **manifested as**

    ◊   **Physical neglect**: poor hygiene, failure to demonstrate adequate growth and development, injuries related to insufficient safe guards.

    ◊   **Emotional abuse and neglect**: failure to demonstrate adequate growth and development, poor social interactions, and fear of strangers.

    ◊   **Physical abuse**: bruising, welts, lacerations, burns, fractures, bite marks, fear of a parent(s) or lack of reactions, abdominal distension, vomiting, or missing hair

    ◊   **Sexual abuse**: bruising; bleeding; abrasions around external genitalia, rectum, or mouth; STDs; and urinary tract infections.

- **Upper respiratory tract infections and otitis media**: Acetaminophen (Tylenol) and cool mist vaporizers may be useful. Antibiotics or decongestants may be prescribed by a primary care provider.

- **Temper tantrums** result when the toddler is frustrated with restrictions on his independence. Providing consistent, age-appropriate expectations helps the toddler work through his frustration.

- **Toilet training** can begin when it is recognized that the child has the sensation of needing to urinate or defecate. Parents should demonstrate patience and consistency in toilet training their child. Nighttime control may develop last of all.

- **Discipline** should be consistent with well-defined boundaries that are established to develop appropriate social behavior.

Δ   2007 Centers for Disease Control and Prevention (CDC) **immunization recommendations** for healthy toddlers **12 months to 3 years** of age include:

- **12 to 15 months** – *Haemophilus influenzae* type B (Hib); pneumococcal vaccine (PCV); IPV(6 to 18 months); measles, mumps, and rubella (MMR); and varicella.

- **12 to 23 months** – Hepatitis A (Hep A), given in two doses, at least 6 months apart.

- **15 to 18 months** – Diphtheria and tetanus toxoids and pertussis (DTaP).

- **12 to 36 months** – Yearly trivalent inactivated influenza vaccine (TIV).

Δ   **Injury Prevention**

- **Drowning** – Do not leave the toddler unattended in the bathtub. Keep toilet lids closed. Closely supervise the child at the pool or any other body of water.

- **Falls** – Keep doors and windows locked. Keep crib mattress in the lowest position with the rails all the way up. Use safety gates across stairs.

- **Suffocation** – Keep toys with small parts out of reach. Make sure food items are cut into small pieces and are without seeds, small bones, nuts, or popcorn. Remove drawstrings from jackets and other clothing.

- **Poisoning** – Avoid exposing the toddler to lead paint, elevate toxins and plants, place safety locks on cabinets with cleaners and other chemicals. Keep poison control number near the phone. Keep medications in childproof containers.

- **Burns** – Check temperature of bath water, turn down thermostat on hot water heater, have working smoke detectors at all times, turn pot handles toward the back of the stove, cover electrical outlets, use sunscreen when outside.

- **Motor vehicles** – Use an approved car seat in the back seat (away from air bags). Toddlers should be in rear-facing car seats for the first year of life and until they weigh 9.1 kg (20 lb). It is recommended to have the toddler ride rear-facing until he has reached the height and weight limit allowed by the manufacturer of the car seat.

- Supervise children when playing outside.

- **Bodily damage** – Keep sharp objects out of the toddler's reach.

    ◊   Educate the toddler regarding what to do when he is approached by a stranger.

    ◊   Teach toddlers to avoid unknown animals.

Primary Reference:

Potter, P. A., & Perry, A. G. (2005). *Fundamentals of nursing* (6th ed.). St. Louis, MO: Mosby.

Additional Resources:

American Academy of Pediatrics. (2007, February). *Car safety seats: A guide for families 2007*. Retrieved March 15, 2007, from http://www.aap.org/family/carseatguide.htm

Centers for Disease Control and Prevention. (2007). *Recommended childhood and adolescent immunization schedule*. Retrieved January 17, 2007, from *www.cdc.gov/*

Hockenberry, M. (2005). *Wong's essentials of pediatric nursing*. (7th ed.). St. Louis, MO: Mosby.

NANDA International (2004). *NANDA nursing diagnoses: Definitions and classification 2005-2006*. Philadelphia: NANDA.

Chapter 16: Toddler (12 months to 3 years)

Application Exercises

1. A nurse is teaching a class on accident prevention to a group of parents with toddlers. Which of the following strategies should the nurse teach the parents to implement to prevent accidents? (Select all that apply.)

   _____ Keep toxic agents out of reach.

   _____ Keep sharp objects out of reach.

   _____ Keep toilet seats up.

   _____ Turn pot handles toward the back of the stove.

   _____ Place safety gates across stairways.

   _____ Raise setting on hot water heater.

   _____ Place fences around swimming pools.

2. What immunizations should a toddler receive between the ages of 12 months and 3 years?

3. Describe what a nurse should expect to observe when watching 18-month-old children play in a daycare facility?

4. What developmental accomplishments make accidents prevalent among toddlers?

5. Effective discipline of a toddler includes

   A. consistent enforcement of well-defined boundaries or limits.

   B. punishment for poor behavior.

   C. allowing the child to learn the majority of the time by trial and error.

   D. consistently rewarding only good behavior.

6. A 20-month-old child is being discharged from the hospital. Which of the following potential health risks should be addressed with the parents? (Select all that apply.)

   _____ Cholesterol screening for cardiovascular disease

   _____ Poisoning

   _____ Peer pressure

   _____ Burns

   _____ Falls

7. A mother of a 2-year-old child states that her child has temper tantrums. The child says "No" every time the mother tries to help her. The nurse explains that developmentally, the toddler is

    A. trying to increase her independence.

    B. developing a sense of trust.

    C. manifesting an anger management problem.

    D. attempting to finish a project she set out to do.

Chapter 16: Toddler (12 months to 3 years)

Application Exercises Answer Key

1. A nurse is teaching a class on accident prevention to a group of parents with toddlers. Which of the following strategies should the nurse teach the parents to implement to prevent accidents? (Select all that apply.)

   __X__ **Keep toxic agents out of reach.**

   __X__ **Keep sharp objects out of reach.**

   _____ Keep toilet seats up.

   __X__ **Turn pot handles toward the back of the stove.**

   __X__ **Place safety gates across stairways.**

   _____ Raise setting on hot water heater.

   __X__ **Place fences around swimming pools.**

   Keeping toxic agents and sharp objects out of reach, turning pot handles to the back of the stove, placing safety gates across stairways and fences around pools are ways to prevent accidents. Toilet seats should be kept down and the temperature on the hot water heater should be lowered.

2. What immunizations should a toddler receive between the ages of 12 months and 3 years?

   DTaP, Hib, PVC, IPV, MMR, varicella, Hep A, yearly influenza

3. Describe what a nurse should expect to observe when watching 18-month-old children play in a daycare facility?

   The children will engage in solitary play initially that will eventually evolve into parallel play. The toddler will observe other children and engage in activities nearby.

4. What developmental accomplishments make accidents prevalent among toddlers?

Independence and desire to try things alone

Wanting to explore more away from parents

Walking well

Ability to climb

5. Effective discipline of a toddler includes

        A. consistent enforcement of well-defined boundaries or limits.
        B. punishment for poor behavior.
        C. allowing the child to learn the majority of the time by trial and error.
        D. consistently rewarding only good behavior.

Toddlers need to have consistent boundaries enforced for discipline to be effective. Behavior should not be enforced with only rewards or only punishments. Trial and error lacks consistent boundaries and may allow the toddler to experience unhealthy consequences.

6. A 20-month-old child is being discharged from the hospital. Which of the following potential health risks should be addressed with the parents? (Select all that apply.)

        _____ Cholesterol screening for cardiovascular disease
        _X_ Poisoning
        _____ Peer pressure
        _X_ Burns
        _X_ Falls

Poisoning, burns, and falls are all potential risks for this age group as the toddler becomes more curious and independent. Cholesterol screenings may begin as early as adolescence. Peer pressure usually begins during the school-age years, becoming more of a risk during adolescence.

7. A mother of a 2-year-old child states that her child has temper tantrums. The child says "No" every time the mother tries to help her. The nurse explains that developmentally, the toddler is

    A. trying to increase her independence.

    B. developing a sense of trust.

    C. manifesting an anger management problem.

    D. attempting to finish a project she set out to do.

The drive for independence is expressed by the toddler opposing the desires of those in authority and attempting to do everything for herself. Developing trust is a developmental task for infants, and finishing a project is a developmental task of the school-age child. This behavior is normal for a 2-year-old child and is not indicative of an anger management problem.

Unit 1 Foundations for Practice
Section: Nursing Throughout the Lifespan

Chapter 17: Preschooler (3 to 5 years)
Contributor: Sally Swenson, MA, RN

 NCLEX® Connections:

Learning Objective: Review and apply knowledge within **"Preschooler (3 to 5 years)"** in readiness for performance of the following nursing activities as outlined by the NCLEX® test plans:

Δ Assess/compare the preschooler's physical, cognitive, and psychosocial development to expected growth and development for age.

Δ Identify and report variances from expected growth and development.

Δ Plan and/or provide care to assist the preschooler to achieve expected growth and development outcomes.

Δ Plan and/or provide care appropriate to the preschooler's developmental level, inclusive of age-appropriate recreational/diversional activities.

Δ Teach children/family expected normal growth and development and age-appropriate health maintenance recommendations for the preschooler.

Δ Teach/reinforce accident prevention and health promotion activities for the preschooler.

 Key Points

Δ **Stages of Development** – The preschool years (3 to 5 years)

Theorist	Type of Development	Stage
Erikson	Psychosocial	Initiative vs guilt
Freud	Psychosocial	Phallic
Piaget	Cognitive	Preoperational

Expected Growth and Development:

Δ **Physical Development**

- **Weight**: The preschooler should gain about 2.25 kg (5 lb) per year.

- **Height**: The preschooler should grow 6.2 to 7.5 cm (2.5 to 3 in) per year.

- **Developmental** skills typically acquired by the preschooler include:

  ◊ Alternating feet on stairs.

  ◊ Going up and down steps easily.

  ◊ Hopping.

  ◊ Walking heel-to-toe.

  ◊ Dressing without help.

  ◊ Drawing copies of shapes on paper.

  ◊ Drawing a more detailed stick figure.

  ◊ Playing on playground equipment.

Δ **Cognitive Development**

- Preschoolers develop two phases of **preoperational thinking**, which include:

  ◊ **Preconceptual** thought (2 to 4 years) – Preschoolers make judgments based on visual appearances. **Misconceptions** in thinking during this stage include:

    ° Artificialism – Everything is made by humans.

    ° Animism – Inanimate objects are alive.

    ° Imminent justice – A universal code exists that determines law and order.

  ◊ **Intuitive** thought (begins around age 4) – Preschooler can classify information and become aware of cause and effect relationships.

- **Language** – The preschooler's vocabulary continues to increase. The preschooler can now speak in sentences, is able to identify colors, and enjoys talking.

- **Time** – The preschooler begins to understand the concepts of the past, present, and future. By the end of the preschool years, the child may comprehend days of the week.

Δ **Psychosocial Development**

- A preschooler may take on many new experiences despite not having all of the physical abilities necessary to be successful at everything. Guilt may occur when children are unable to accomplish a task and believe they have misbehaved. Guiding preschoolers to attempt activities within their capabilities while setting limits is appropriate.

Δ **Moral Development**

- Preschoolers continue in the good/bad orientation of the toddler years but begin to understand behaviors in terms of what is socially acceptable.

Δ **Self-concept Development**

- The preschooler feels good about self with regard to mastering skills such as dressing and feeding that allow independence. During stress, insecurity, or illness, a preschooler may regress to previous immature behaviors or develop habits such as nail biting or nose picking.

Δ **Body-image Changes**

- Mistaken perceptions of reality coupled with misconceptions in thinking lead to active fantasies and fears. The greatest fear is that of bodily harm.

- Sex-role identification is also occurring.

Δ **Age-appropriate Activities**

- Parallel play shifts to associative play during the preschool years. Play is not highly organized, but cooperation does exist between children. Appropriate activities include:

  ◊ Playing ball.

  ◊ Putting puzzles together.

  ◊ Riding tricycles.

  ◊ Pretend and dress-up activities.

  ◊ Role play.

  ◊ Painting.

  ◊ Sewing cards and beads.

  ◊ Reading books.

Δ **Nutrition**

- A preschooler consumes about half the amount of an adult (1,800 kcal).

- Preschoolers may continue to be picky eaters up to age 5.

- Parents need to ensure that their child is receiving a balance of nutrients.

Δ **Health Promotion and Prevention**

- **Child abuse** is a potential risk and may be **manifested as**

  ◊ **Physical neglect**: poor hygiene, failure to demonstrate adequate growth and development, injuries related to insufficient safe guards.

  ◊ **Emotional abuse and neglect**: failure to demonstrate adequate growth and development, poor social interactions, and fear of strangers.

◊ **Physical abuse**: bruising, welts, lacerations, burns, fractures, bite marks, fear of a parent(s) or lack of reactions, abdominal distension, vomiting, or missing hair.

◊ **Sexual abuse**: bruising; bleeding; abrasions around external genitalia, rectum, or mouth; STDs; urinary tract infections.

- **Upper respiratory tract infections and otitis media**: Acetaminophen (Tylenol) and cool mist vaporizers may be useful. Antibiotics or decongestants may be prescribed by a primary care provider. In general, becomes less prevalent as the child grows.

- **Sleep disturbances** frequently occur during early childhood, and problems range from difficulties going to bed to night terrors. Advise parents to:

    ◊ Assess whether or not the bedtime is too early or if the child is still taking a nap. The average preschooler requires around 12 hr of sleep a day. Some preschoolers still require a daytime nap.

    ◊ Keep a consistent bedtime routine.

    ◊ Try using a night light.

    ◊ Reassure the child who has been frightened, but avoid having the child sleep with the parents.

- **Vision screening** is routinely done in the preschool population as part of the prekindergarten physical exam. Myopia and amblyopia can be detected and treated before poor visual acuity impairs the learning environment.

- 2007 Centers for Disease Control and Prevention (CDC) **immunization recommendations** for healthy preschool children **3 to 5 years** include:

    ◊ 4 to 6 years – diphtheria and tetanus toxoids and pertussis (DTaP); inactivated poliovirus (IPV); measles, mumps, and rubella (MMR); and varicella.

    ◊ Yearly trivalent inactivated influenza vaccine (TIV) for preschoolers 36 to 59 months.

- **Injury prevention**

    ◊ **Drowning** – Do not leave the child unattended in the bathtub. Closely supervise the child at the pool or any other body of water.

    ◊ **Poisoning** – Avoid exposure to lead paint, elevate toxins and plants, and place safety locks on cabinets with cleaners and other chemicals. Keep poison control number near the phone. Keep medications in childproof containers.

    ◊ **Motor vehicles** – Use an approved car seat in the back seat (away from air bags). Preschool children should be in car seats appropriate for weight and height. The child should be restrained in a car seat or booster chair until seat belts fit correctly. Laws may vary from state to state and requirements may be up to 36.3 kg (80 lb) and height of 5 feet 9 inches.

Primary Reference:

Potter, P. A., & Perry, A. G. (2005). *Fundamentals of nursing* (6th ed.). St. Louis, MO: Mosby.

Additional Resources:

American Academy of Pediatrics. (2007, February). *Car safety seats: A guide for families 2007*. Retrieved March 15, 2007, from http://www.aap.org/family/carseatguide.htm

Centers for Disease Control and Prevention. (2007). *Recommended childhood and adolescent immunization schedule*. Retrieved January 17, 2007, from *http://www.cdc.gov/*

NANDA International (2004). *NANDA nursing diagnoses: Definitions and classification 2005-2006*. Philadelphia: NANDA.

Chapter 17: Preschooler (3 to 5 years)

Application Exercises

Scenario: A 4-year-old child is put to bed at 8:30 p.m. each evening and wakes up at about 7:30 a.m. Her parents report that she often lays in her bed talking to herself or gets up two to three times before finally getting to sleep 40 min later. The child attends preschool, where each afternoon the children take 2-hr naps.

1. What additional assessment information about the child's sleep patterns might be helpful?

2. What are some possible explanations for the child's behavior?

3. What teaching should the parents receive regarding their child's sleep problem?

Scenario: A 4-year-old child presents to the clinic with his father for a prekindergarten physical. The child is quiet and appears fearful. The father tells the nurse that his son has heard from other children at his preschool about the "shots" he has to get before going to kindergarten.

4. Developmentally, what other factors may be contributing to the child's fear?

5. The child's father states he is concerned that his child may not be ready for kindergarten. What developmental tasks should the child currently be doing to indicate that his growth and development is appropriate for his age? (Select all that apply.)

_____ He shows a good understanding of time.

_____ He is able to perform the heel-to-toe walk.

_____ He is able to hop.

_____ He demonstrates good coordination.

_____ He can draw copies of shapes on paper.

_____ He speaks in sentences.

6. A mother states that her 3-year-old daughter is not playing with the other children in their neighborhood play group. Instead, she sits near the other children but plays something else by herself. The nurse explains that it is normal for a 3-year-old to engage in

        A. associative play.

        B. cooperative play.

        C. imaginative play.

        D. parallel play.

7. Which of the following developmental tasks should be achieved during the preschool years?

        A. Sitting up alone

        B. Dressing independently

        C. Following several directions at once

        D. Comprehending satire

Chapter 17: Preschooler (3 to 5 years)

Application Exercises Answer Key

Scenario: A 4-year-old child is put to bed at 8:30 p.m. each evening and wakes up at about 7:30 a.m. Her parents report that she often lays in her bed talking to herself or gets up two to three times before finally getting to sleep 40 min later. The child attends preschool, where each afternoon the children take 2-hr naps.

1. What additional assessment information about the child's sleep patterns might be helpful?

   "Does your child awaken during the night?"

   "Does your child express being fearful of the dark? Or does she have a night light?"

   "What activity is your child engaged in just prior to bed?"

   "Have you put your child to bed at a later time with the same results? Or when your child has not had an afternoon nap, does she still have difficulty falling asleep?"

2. What are some possible explanations for the child's behavior?

   The child does not require as much sleep now as she did when she was a toddler.

   She may be outgrowing the need for an afternoon nap.

3. What teaching should the parents receive regarding their child's sleep problem?

   If the nap is necessary at preschool, then maybe her bedtime should be moved back. Also, make sure that the child is not engaging in stimulating activities just before bed. Place her in a room with low lighting and perform quiet activities prior to bedtime.

Scenario: A 4-year-old child presents to the clinic with his father for a prekindergarten physical. The child is quiet and appears fearful. The father tells the nurse that his son has heard from other children at his preschool about the "shots" he has to get before going to kindergarten.

4. Developmentally, what other factors may be contributing to the child's fear?

During the preschool years, the greatest fear children have is that of bodily harm.

Primary care providers may represent a source of that harm.

5. The child's father states he is concerned that his child may not be ready for kindergarten. What developmental tasks should the child currently be doing to indicate that his growth and development is appropriate for his age? (Select all that apply.)

_____ He shows a good understanding of time.

_X_ He is able to perform the heel-to-toe walk.

_X_ He is able to hop.

_____ He demonstrates good coordination.

_X_ He can draw copies of shapes on paper.

_X_ He speaks in sentences.

Walking heel-to-toe, hopping, drawing copies of shapes, and speaking in sentences are appropriate developmental tasks. Understanding of time and good coordination are usually achieved during the school-age years.

6. A mother states that her 3-year-old daughter is not playing with the other children in their neighborhood play group. Instead, she sits near the other children but plays something else by herself. The nurse explains that it is normal for a 3-year-old to engage in

        A. associative play.

        B. cooperative play.

        C. imaginative play.

        D. parallel play.

Preschool children engage in parallel play when they play around each other but are engaged in different activities. Older preschoolers may engage in associative play where they engage in the same activities, but there is no organization or rules. School-age children engage in cooperative play where roles are assigned to various children and play is done together. Imaginative play is not a recognized developmental level of play.

7. Which of the following developmental tasks should be achieved during the preschool years?

    A. Sitting up alone

    B. Dressing independently

    C. Following several directions at once

    D. Comprehending satire

A preschooler should be able to dress himself with occasional help in tying shoes or fastening complex buckles or closures. Sitting up alone is a developmental task of infancy. Following several directions at once and comprehending satire are developmental tasks of school-age children.

Unit 1   Foundations for Practice
Section: Nursing Throughout the Lifespan

Chapter 18:   School-Age Child (5 to 12 years)
Contributor: Sally Swenson, MA, RN

NCLEX® Connections:

Learning Objective: Review and apply knowledge within "**School-Age Child (5 to 12 years)**" in readiness for performance of the following nursing activities as outlined by the NCLEX® test plans:

Δ   Teach/reinforce accident prevention and health promotion activities for the school-age child.

Δ   Assess/compare the school-age child's physical, cognitive, and psychosocial development to expected growth and development for age.

Δ   Identify and report variances from expected growth and development.

Δ   Plan and/or provide care to assist the school-age child to achieve expected growth and development outcomes.

Δ   Teach children/family expected normal growth and development and age-appropriate health maintenance recommendations for the school-age child.

Δ   Teach/reinforce accident prevention and health promotion activities for the school-age child.

Key Points

Δ   **Stages of Development** – The school-age child (5 to 12 years)

Theorist	Type of Development	Stage
Erikson	Psychosocial	Industry vs inferiority
Freud	Psychosocial	Latency
Piaget	Cognitive	Concrete operations

Expected Growth and Development:

Δ **Physical Development**

- **Weight**: The school-age child will gain 2 to 4 kg (4.4 to 8.8 lb) per year.

- **Height**: The school-age child will grow by about 5 cm (2 in) per year.

- There is typically a weight gain between 10 to 12 years of age prior to the changes in height that come after this age.

- Changes related to puberty begin to appear in females, which include:

   ◊   Budding of breasts.

   ◊   Appearance of pubic hair.

   ◊   Menarche.

- Changes related to puberty begin to appear in males, which include:

   ◊   Enlargement of testicles with changes in scrotum, such as increased looseness.

   ◊   Appearance of pubic hair.

- Permanent teeth erupt.

- Coordination improves.

- Visual acuity improves to 20/20.

Δ **Cognitive Development**

- **Concrete** thought:

   ◊   Weight and volume seen as unchanging

   ◊   Is able to understand simple analogies

   ◊   Is able to understand time (days, seasons, etc.)

   ◊   Can define many words and understand rules of grammar

   ◊   Classifies more complex information

   ◊   Is able to understand various emotions people experience

Δ **Psychosocial development**

- A sense of industry is achieved through achievements in learning.

- Children at this age prefer the company of same-sex companions.

- Most relationships come from school associations.

- Children at this age may rival the same-sex parent.

- Fears of ridicule by peers and teachers over school related issues are common. Some children manifest nervous behaviors to deal with the stress such as nail biting.

Δ   **Moral Development**

- Early on, the school-age child may not understand the reasoning behind many rules and may try to find ways around them. Instrumental exchange is in place – "I'll help you if you help me." The child is out to make the best deal, and she does not really consider elements of loyalty, gratitude, or justice as she makes her decisions.

- In the later part of the school years, the child moves into a law-and-order orientation with more emphasis placed on justice being administered fairly.

Δ   **Self-concept Development**

- School-age children strive to develop a healthy self-respect through finding out in what areas they excel.

- School-age children need parents to encourage them regarding educational or extracurricular successes.

Δ   **Body-image Changes**

- This is the age at which solidification of body image occurs.

- Curiosity about sexuality should be addressed with education regarding sexual development and the reproduction process.

- School-age children are more modest and place more emphasis on privacy issues than preschoolers.

Δ   **Age-appropriate Activities**

- Competitive and cooperative play is predominant.

- 6 to 9 year olds:

    ◊   Play simple board and number games.

    ◊   Hopscotch.

    ◊   Jump rope.

    ◊   Collect rocks, stamps, cards, or coins.

    ◊   Ride bicycles.

    ◊   Build simple models.

    ◊   Join organized sports – skill building.

- 9 to 12 year olds:

    ◊   Make crafts.

    ◊   Build models.

    ◊   Collect/engage in hobbies.

    ◊   Solve jigsaw puzzles.

◊ Play board and card games.

◊ Join organized competitive sports.

Δ **Nutrition**

• By the end of the school-age years, the child is eating an adult proportion of food. He needs quality nutritious snacks.

Δ **Health Promotion and Prevention**

• Child abuse is a potential risk and may be manifested as:

◊ Physical neglect – poor hygiene, failure to demonstrate adequate growth and development, and injuries related to insufficient safe guards

◊ Emotional abuse and neglect – failure to demonstrate adequate growth and development, poor social interactions, and fear of strangers

◊ Physical abuse – bruising, welts, lacerations, burns, fractures, bite marks, fear of a parent(s) or lack of reactions, abdominal distension, vomiting, and/or missing hair

◊ Sexual abuse – bruising; bleeding; abrasions around external genitalia, rectum, or mouth; STDs; and urinary tract infections

• **Scoliosis** – School-age children should be screened for scoliosis by examining for a lateral curvature of the spine before and during growth spurts. Screening may take place at schools or at a health provider's office.

• **Obesity** is an increasing concern of this age group that predisposes them to low self-esteem, diabetes, heart disease, and high blood pressure. Advise parents to:

◊ Not use food as a reward.

◊ Emphasize physical activity.

◊ Make sure a balanced diet is consumed.

◊ Avoid frequent meals eaten in fast-food restaurants.

• **Cancers** such as leukemia are the second leading cause of death in children.

• **Respiratory infections** are still common at this age.

• **Asthma** accounts for many school absences. Parents, primary care providers, and school employees need to work together to manage the disease.

• 2007 Centers for Disease Control and Prevention (CDC) **immunization recommendations** for healthy school-age children **5 to 12** years of age include:

◊ If not given between the ages of 4 to 5, then by age 6: diphtheria and tetanus toxoids and pertussis (DTaP); inactivated poliovirus (IPV); measles, mumps, and rubella (MMR); and varicella.

◊ 11 to 12 years – Tetanus and diphtheria toxoids and pertussis vaccine (Tdap); measles, mumps, and rubella vaccine (MMR); human papillomavirus vaccine (HPV) in 3 doses; and meningococcal vaccine (MCV4).

- **Substance abuse** – Teach children to say "no" when offered drugs or alcohol.

- **Dental health** should be encouraged.

  ◊ Brushing

  ◊ Flossing

  ◊ Regular check-ups

  ◊ Appropriate snacks

- **Injury prevention**

  ◊ Fracture prevention – helmets and/or pads should be used when rollerblading, skateboarding, bicycling, riding scooters, and snowboarding.

  ◊ Avoid trampolines.

  ◊ Teach children to swim.

  ◊ Teach fire safety.

  ◊ Keep firearms locked up.

  ◊ Motor vehicles – The child should be restrained in a car seat or booster chair until adult seat belts fit correctly. Laws may vary from state to state and requirements may be up to 36.3 kg (80 lb) and a height of 5 feet 9 inches. Children less than 13 years of age are safest in the back seat.

Primary Reference:

Potter, P. A., & Perry, A. G. (2005). *Fundamentals of nursing* (6th ed.). St. Louis, MO: Mosby.

Additional Resources:

American Academy of Pediatrics. (2007, February). *Car safety seats: A guide for families 2007*. Retrieved March 15, 2007, from http://www.aap.org/family/carseatguide.htm

Centers for Disease Control and Prevention. (2007). *Recommended childhood and adolescent immunization schedule*. Retrieved January 17, 2007, from *www.cdc.gov/*

Hockenberry, M. (2005). *Wong's essentials of pediatric nursing*. (7th ed.). St. Louis, MO: Mosby.

NANDA International (2004). *NANDA nursing diagnoses: Definitions and classification 2005-2006*. Philadelphia: NANDA.

Chapter 18: School-Age Child (5 to 12 years)

Application Exercises

Scenario: A 10-year-old boy has been gaining weight without a proportional gain in height. His parents are concerned and talk to the school nurse.

1. What questions should be asked of the child's parents?

2. Should the school nurse consider the child's weight gain normal?

3. What information should the nurse share with the child's parents?

4. An 11-year-old girl is having her left wrist placed in a cast in the emergency department after falling at the skateboard park. What safety information should be discussed with the child prior to discharge?

5. A school nurse is preparing to talk to the 9- to 10-year-old girls about the physical changes that are, or soon will be, occurring with their bodies. List the sequence of changes the girls will experience with the onset of puberty.

6. An 8-year-old boy with a fractured femur is hospitalized in a two-bed room. With which of the following roommates should the boy share a room?

    A. A 14-year-old boy with colitis

    B. A 9-year-old boy with an appendectomy

    C. A 10-year-old girl with cancer

    D. A 6-year-old girl with asthma

7. Which of the following behaviors by a school-age child demonstrates appropriate psychosocial development?

    A. Seeking out a parent when feeling hungry

    B. Attempting to pour a glass of milk from a full gallon without assistance

    C. Bringing home a good grade on a math test and showing parents

    D. Endeavoring to spend more time with friends than with family

Chapter 18: School-Age Child (5 to 12 years)

Application Exercises Answer Key

Scenario: A 10-year-old boy has been gaining weight without a proportional gain in height. His parents are concerned and talk to the school nurse.

1. What questions should be asked of the child's parents?

   "Describe what a typical day is like for your child?"

   "What does your child typically eat at meals?"

   "Does your child snack in between meals, and what type of snacks does he consume?"

2. Should the school nurse consider the child's weight gain normal?

   Yes. If the child eats nutritious foods, does not consume many empty calories, and is active, this may be the normal weight gain experienced by 10- to 12-year old children.

3. What information should the nurse share with the child's parents?

   The weight gain can be hormonal and precede a growth spurt (height) surrounding puberty. Additionally, the child's metabolic rate will increase during the adolescent years, and he will require additional nutrients, so limiting intake at this time may not be warranted.

4. An 11-year-old girl is having her left wrist placed in a cast in the emergency department after falling at the skateboard park. What safety information should be discussed with the child prior to discharge?

   Wearing protective gear such as a helmet and elbow and knee pads when skateboarding will help prevent future injuries.

5. A school nurse is preparing to talk to the 9- to 10-year-old girls about the physical changes that are, or soon will be, occurring with their bodies. List the sequence of changes the girls will experience with the onset of puberty.

Budding of breasts

Pubic hair appears

Menarche

6. An 8-year-old boy with a fractured femur is hospitalized in a two-bed room. With which of the following roommates should the boy share a room?

    A. A 14-year-old boy with colitis

    B. A 9-year-old boy with an appendectomy

    C. A 10-year-old girl with cancer

    D. A 6-year-old girl with asthma

An 8-year-old boy would feel the most comfortable with a roommate of the same gender and close to the same age.

7. Which of the following behaviors by a school-age child demonstrates appropriate psychosocial development?

    A. Seeking out a parent when feeling hungry

    B. Attempting to pour a glass of milk from a full gallon without assistance

    C. Bringing home a good grade on a math test and showing parents

    D. Endeavoring to spend more time with friends than with family

School-age children are proud of their academic accomplishments. It is typical for a toddler or preschooler to seek out a parent when feeling hungry. School-age children would help themselves to the food. A preschooler who is developing hand-eye coordination and does not have realistic perceptions of his abilities is likely to attempt to pour a glass of milk from a full gallon. Adolescents often prefer to spend more time with friends than with family.

Unit 1   **Foundations for Practice**
Section: Nursing Throughout the Lifespan

Chapter 19:   Adolescent (12 to 20 years)
Contributor: Sally Swenson, MA, RN

 NCLEX® Connections:

Learning Objective: Review and apply knowledge within "**Adolescent (12 to 20 years)**" in readiness for performance of the following nursing activities as outlined by the NCLEX® test plans:

Δ   Assess/compare the adolescent's physical, cognitive, and psychosocial development to expected growth and development for age.

Δ   Identify and report variances from expected growth and development.

Δ   Plan and/or provide care to assist the adolescent to achieve expected growth and development outcomes.

Δ   Plan and/or provide care appropriate to the adolescent's developmental level, inclusive of age-appropriate recreational/diversional activities.

Δ   Teach children/family expected normal growth and development and age-appropriate health maintenance recommendations for the adolescent.

Δ   Teach/reinforce accident prevention and health promotion activities for the adolescent.

 Key Points

Δ   **Stages of Development** – The adolescent (12 to 20 years)

Theorist	Type of Development	Stage
Erikson	Psychosocial	Identity vs role confusion
Freud	Psychosocial	Genital
Piaget	Cognitive	Formal operations

Expected Growth and Development:

Δ   **Physical Development**

- Acne may appear during adolescence.

- Females reach 95% of their adult height by age 13. Hips widen throughout these years.

- Males reach 95% of their adult height by age 15. Shoulders widen throughout these years.

- In males, sexual maturation occurs in the following order:

    ◊   Increase in the size of the testes.

    ◊   Appearance of pubic hair.

    ◊   Rapid growth of genitalia.

    ◊   Growth of axillary hair.

    ◊   Appearance of downy hair on upper lip.

    ◊   Change in voice.

- Sleep habits change with puberty due to increased metabolism and rapid growth during the adolescent years. Changes are characterized by staying up late, sleeping in later in the morning, and perhaps sleeping longer than during the school-age years.

Δ   **Cognitive Development**

- The adolescent is capable of thinking at an adult level.

- Abstract thought is possible, and adolescents can deal with principles.

- The adolescent can evaluate the quality of his/her own thinking.

- Attention span becomes longer.

- **Language**: Adolescents develop jargon within the peer group. They are able to communicate one way with the peer group and another way with adults or teachers.

Δ   **Psychosocial Development**

- The adolescent develops a sense of **personal identity** that is influenced by expectations of the family.

- **Group** identity – The adolescent may become part of a peer-group that greatly influences his/her behavior.

- **Vocationally** – Work habits begin to solidify.

- **Sexually** – There is increased interest in the opposite sex.

- **Health perceptions** – Adolescents may view themselves as invincible to bad outcomes of risky behaviors.

Δ **Moral Development**

- Conventional law and order – Rules are not seen as absolutes. Each situation needs to be looked at, and perhaps the rules will need to be adjusted. Not all adolescents attain this level of moral development during these years.

Δ **Self-concept Development**

- A healthy self-concept is developed by having healthy relationships with peers, family, and teachers. Identifying a skill or talent helps maintain a healthy self-concept. Participation in sports, hobbies, or the community can have a positive outcome.

Δ **Body-image Changes**

- Adolescents seem particularly concerned with the lean bodies portrayed by the media. Changes that occur during puberty result in a great deal of comparisons among adolescents in the surrounding peer group. Parents also give their input as to hair styles, dress, and activity. Adolescents may require help if depression or eating disorders result due to poor body image.

Δ **Age-appropriate Activities**

- Nonviolent video games

- Nonviolent music

- Sports

- Caring for a pet

- Career-training programs

- Reading

- Social events (e.g., going to the movies, school dances)

Δ **Nutrition**

- Rapid growth and high metabolism require increases in quality nutrients. Nutrients that tend to be deficient during this stage of life are iron, calcium, and vitamins A and C.

- **Eating disorders** commonly develop during adolescence (more prevalent in girls than in boys) due to a fear of being overweight, fad diets, and/or as a mechanism of maintaining control over some aspect of life. Severe eating disorders include:

  ◊ **Anorexia nervosa** – extreme weight loss through severe dieting/ extreme exercising or binging and purging.

  ◊ **Bulimia nervosa** – severe binging and purging in between intense dieting.

  ◊ **Obesity** – diet high in fat without adequate physical activity.

Δ   **Health Promotion and Prevention**

- Child abuse is a potential risk and may be manifested as:

  ◊   Physical neglect – poor hygiene, failure to demonstrate adequate growth and development, and injuries related to insufficient safe guards

  ◊   Emotional abuse and neglect – failure to demonstrate adequate growth and development, poor social interactions, and fear of strangers

  ◊   Physical abuse – bruising, welts, lacerations, burns, fractures, bite marks, fear of a parent(s) or lack of reactions, abdominal distension, vomiting, and/or missing hair

  ◊   Sexual abuse – bruising; bleeding; abrasions around external genitalia, rectum, or mouth; STDs; and urinary tract infections

- Motor vehicle crashes **are the leading cause of death.**

- **Homicides are the second leading cause of death** and most prevalent among male adolescent acquaintances with a firearm. Violent media may influence this type of behavior.

- **Suicide is the third leading cause of death** among adolescents. Depressed and socially-isolated adolescents may demonstrate changes in behavior, which include:

  ◊   Poor school performance.

  ◊   Lack of interest.

  ◊   Tearfulness and not interacting with others.

  ◊   Disturbances in sleep or appetite.

  ◊   Expression of suicidal thoughts.

- **Substance abuse** – Adolescents are more likely to experiment with alcohol, tobacco, or illegal drugs to impress peers or because they believe it will help them feel better. Substance abuse is the leading contributor to motor vehicle fatalities. Drug Abuse Resistance Education (DARE) and other similar programs provide assistance in preventing experimentation.

- **Sexual experimentation** occurs in approximately 50% of adolescents. Abstinence is highly recommended. If sexual activity is occurring, the use of birth control is recommended.

- **Sexually transmitted diseases (STDs)** – Adolescents should undergo external genitalia examinations, Pap smears, and cervical and urethral cultures (specific to gender). Rectal and oral cultures may also need to be taken. The adolescent should be counseled about risk-taking behaviors and their exposure to STDs, as well as acquired immunodeficiency syndrome (AIDS), hepatitis, etc. The use of condoms will decrease the risk of STDs.

- **Pregnancy** – identification of pregnant adolescents should be done to ensure that nutrition and support is offered to promote the health of the adolescent and the infant. After the infant is delivered, education should be given to prevent future pregnancies.

- 2007 Centers for Disease Control and Prevention (CDC) **immunization recommendations** for the healthy adolescent **12 to 20** years include the following vaccines if not given at age 11 to 12: tetanus and diphtheria toxoids and pertussis (Tdap); human papillomavirus vaccine (HPV) series; hepatitis B (Hep B) series; inactivated poliovirus (IPV) series; measles, mumps, and rubella (MMR) series; varicella series; and meningococcal (MCV4).

- **Scoliosis** – Screening for scoliosis should continue during the adolescent years by examining for a lateral curvature of the spine before and during growth spurts. Screening may take place at schools or at a health provider's office.

- **Injury Prevention:**

  ◊ Encourage attendance at driver's education courses. Emphasize need for compliance with seat belt use.

  ◊ Teach the dangers of combining substance abuse with driving (Mothers Against Drunk Driving – MADD).

  ◊ Insist on helmet use with bicycles, motorcycles, skateboards, roller blades, and snowboards.

  ◊ Screen for substance use.

  ◊ Teach the adolescent not to swim alone.

  ◊ Teach proper use of sporting equipment prior to use.

Primary Reference:

Potter, P. A., & Perry, A. G. (2005). *Fundamentals of nursing* (6th ed.). St. Louis, MO: Mosby.

Additional Resources:

Centers for Disease Control and Prevention. (2007). *Recommended childhood and adolescent immunization schedule*. Retrieved January 17, 2007, from *www.cdc.gov/*

Hockenberry, M. (2005). *Wong's essentials of pediatric nursing*. (7th ed.). St. Louis, MO: Mosby.

NANDA International (2004). *NANDA nursing diagnoses: Definitions and classification 2005-2006*. Philadelphia: NANDA.

Chapter 19: Adolescent (12 to 20 years)

Application Exercises

1. Identify prevention strategies for the accidents that are common during the adolescent years.

Accidents	Prevention strategies
Motor vehicle crashes	
Drowning	
Sports injuries	
Substance abuse	
Head injuries	

2. What aspects of adolescent development increase the likelihood of accidents?

3. A mother of a 16-year-old adolescent reports that her son seems to require a lot of sleep. Is this a concern? Explain.

4. Place the following male puberty changes in the correct sequence.

_____ Appearance of pubic hair

_____ Change in voice

_____ Growth of axillary hair

_____ Increase in size of testes

_____ Appearance of downy hair on upper lip

_____ Rapid growth of genitalia

5. Which of the following interventions are appropriate for an adolescent male who is hospitalized with a broken femur? (Select all that apply.)

_____ Suggest that his parents room in with him.

_____ Provide a television and DVDs for him to watch.

_____ Restrict visitors.

_____ Encourage him to get enough rest.

_____ Allow him to perform his own morning care.

Chapter 19: Adolescent (12 to 20 years)

Application Exercises Answer Key

1. Identify prevention strategies for the accidents that are common during the adolescent years.

Accidents	Prevention strategies
Motor vehicle crashes	**Promote seatbelt use and driver's education courses.**
Drowning	**Teach adolescents not to swim alone.**
Sports injuries	**Teach proper use of athletic equipment and protective gear.**
Substance abuse	**Promote programs such as DARE and MADD.**
Head injuries	**Encourage helmet use with bicycles, skateboards, and snowboards.**

2. What aspects of adolescent development increase the likelihood of accidents?

Peer influences to abuse substances (e.g., nicotine, alcohol, marijuana)

An increase in risky behaviors because the adolescent views himself as invincible

Inexperienced drivers

3. A mother of a 16-year-old adolescent reports that her son seems to require a lot of sleep. Is this a concern? Explain.

Adolescents require more sleep due to increased metabolism and rapid growth. Sleep patterns may change with the adolescent staying up late and then sleeping later in the morning.

4. Place the following male puberty changes in the correct sequence.

    __2__   Appearance of pubic hair

    __6__   Change in voice

    __4__   Growth of axillary hair

    __1__   Increase in size of testes

    __5__   Appearance of downy hair on upper lip

    __3__   Rapid growth of genitalia

5. Which of the following interventions are appropriate for an adolescent male who is hospitalized with a broken femur? (Select all that apply.)

    _____   Suggest that his parents room in with him.

    __X__   **Provide a television and DVDs for him to watch.**

    _____   Restrict visitors.

    __X__   **Encourage him to get enough rest.**

    __X__   **Allow him to perform his own morning care.**

Movies and DVDs are appropriate diversional activities for an adolescent. It is important for him to get adequate rest, and allowing him to perform his own morning care will provide him with a sense of independence. Rooming in is most appropriate for the infant, toddler, preschooler, and school-age child. There is no reason to restrict visitors, and allowing his friends to visit can prevent feelings of isolation.

Unit 1   Foundations for Practice
Section: Nursing Throughout the Lifespan

Chapter 20:	Young Adult (20 to 40 years)

Contributor: Sally Swenson, MA, RN

 NCLEX® Connections:

Learning Objective: Review and apply knowledge within "**Young Adult (20 to 40 years)**" in readiness for performance of the following nursing activities as outlined by the NCLEX® test plans:

Δ   Assess/compare the young adult's physical, cognitive, and psychosocial development to expected growth and development for age.

Δ   Identify and report variances from expected growth and development.

Δ   Plan and/or provide care to assist the young adult to achieve expected growth and development outcomes.

Δ   Plan and/or provide care appropriate to the young adult's developmental level, inclusive of age-appropriate recreational/diversional activities.

Δ   Teach children/family expected normal growth and development and age-appropriate health maintenance recommendations for the young adult.

Δ   Teach/reinforce accident prevention and health promotion activities for the young adult.

 Key Points

Δ   **Stages of Development** – The young adult (ages 20 to 40)

Theorist	Type of Development	Stage
Erikson	Psychosocial	Intimacy vs isolation
Freud	Psychosocial	Genital
Piaget	Cognitive	Formal operations

Expected Growth and Development:

Δ   **Physical Development**

- Growth has concluded around age 20.

- Physical senses peak.

- Cardiac output and efficiency peak.

- Optimal muscle function occurs at ages 25 to 30.

- Metabolic rate decreases 2 to 4% every decade after age 20.

- Sex drive is high for men.

- Sex drive for women peaks during the later part of this stage.

- Optimal time for childbearing.

- Pregnancy-related changes occur, which include:

  ◊   Breast enlargement and tenderness.

  ◊   Amenorrhea.

  ◊   Morning sickness and fatigue.

  ◊   Pigmentation changes.

  ◊   Pruritus.

  ◊   Quickening.

  ◊   Abdominal distension.

  ◊   Urinary frequency.

  ◊   Changes in sex drive.

Δ   **Cognitive Development**

- The young adult years are an optimal time for education to occur – both formally and informally. In young adults:

  ◊   Critical thinking skills improve.

  ◊   Memory peaks in the 20s.

  ◊   There is a greater ability for creative thought.

Δ   **Psychosocial Development**

- Behaviors associated with the young adult include:

  ◊   Leaving home.

  ◊   Taking on more adult commitments and responsibilities.

  ◊   Going from being single to establishing a new family.

◊ Developing parenting skills.

◊ Making occupational choices that are characterized by:

° High goals/dreams.

° Exploration/experimentation.

- Young adults may encounter pregnancy-related changes.

◊ May question ability to parent

◊ May experience increased anxiety and/or depression, especially after the birth of the child

Δ **Moral Development**

- The young adult may personalize values and beliefs.

- Reasoning may be based on ethical fairness principles such as the principle of justice.

Δ **Self-concept Development**

- The formation of a healthy self-concept during the young adult years is influenced by:

◊ Avoidance of substance abuse.

◊ Late formation of a family.

◊ Frequent interactions with family and friends.

◊ Choosing to behave in an ethical manner.

Δ **Body-image Changes**

- Body-image changes are greatly influenced by what the young adult eats and how much exercise he gets.

- Pregnancy-related body image changes include:

◊ Mother may feel more feminine in the early stages.

◊ Mother may feel huge and unappealing in the last trimester.

◊ Mother may experience increased well-being with quickening.

Δ **Nutrition**

- Erratic schedules and busy lives can lead to eating an unbalanced diet.

- The following list indicates adequate calorie consumption for young adults.

◊ Active males – 2,800 kcal

◊ Sedentary females – 1,600 kcal

◊ Sedentary males and active females – 2,200 kcal

◊ Pregnant young adult women need to increase calorie consumption by 300 kcal for a total of 2,100 to 2,400 kcal

Δ   **Health Promotion and Prevention**

- Young adults tend to be free of illness. They may not seek health care on a regular basis or pay attention to signs and symptoms at an early stage. The leading cause of death in young adults is automobile crashes followed by homicide (including as a result of spousal abuse), suicide, cancer (testicular, cervical, ovarian), and heart disease.

- Other health risks for young adults include:

  ◊   Substance abuse.

  ◊   Periodontal disease due to poor oral hygiene.

  ◊   Unplanned pregnancies – high source of stress.

  ◊   Sexually transmitted diseases.

  ◊   Infertility.

  ◊   Work-related injuries or exposures.

- Pregnant women and their families should seek early prenatal care.

- With all of the life changes experienced during the young adult years, the client should be screened for stress and offered assistance as needed.

- Routine health care visits should include obtaining height, weight, and vital signs; screening for stress; education related to STDs, substance abuse, and contraception; and encouragement of good nutrition and regular physical activity.

- Young adults should follow age-related guidelines for screening.

  ◊   Females – starting at age 20 – at each routine health care visit:

   °   Blood pressure – minimum of every 2 years

   °   Body mass index

   °   Blood cholesterol – minimum of every 5 years

   °   Pap – yearly; after age 30 – every 1 to 3 years

   °   Clinical breast exam

  ◊   Males – starting at age 20 – at each routine healthcare visit:

   °   Blood pressure – minimum of every 2 years

   °   Body mass index

   °   Blood cholesterol – minimum of every 5 years

   °   Clinical testicular exam

- 2007 Centers for Disease Control and Prevention (CDC) **immunization recommendations** for healthy young adults **20 to 40** years include:

  ◊ Tetanus and diphtheria (Tdap) every 10 years, substituting with one dose of tetanus and diphtheria toxoids and pertussis (Tdap).

  ◊ One dose of measles, mumps, and rubella (MMR), or two doses if a college student, health care worker, or planning international travel.

  ◊ Two doses of varicella if no evidence of immunity.

  ◊ Females 26 years of age or younger not previously vaccinated should receive three doses of the human papillomavirus (HPV) vaccine.

- Injury prevention for the middle adult includes:

  ◊ Avoiding drugs that can lead to substance abuse.

  ◊ Avoiding taking drugs while driving a vehicle.

  ◊ Wearing a seat belt when operating a vehicle.

  ◊ Wearing helmets while bike riding.

  ◊ Installing smoking and carbon monoxide detectors in the home.

  ◊ Securing firearms in a safe location.

Primary Reference:

Potter, P. A., & Perry, A. G. (2005). *Fundamentals of nursing* (6th ed.). St. Louis, MO: Mosby.

Additional Resources:

Centers for Disease Control and Prevention. (2007). *Recommended adult immunization schedule.* Retrieved January 17, 2007, from *www.cdc.gov/*

NANDA International (2004). *NANDA nursing diagnoses: Definitions and classification 2005-2006.* Philadelphia: NANDA.

Chapter 20: Young Adult (20 to 40 years)

Application Exercises

1. List several developmental tasks that can assist a young adult to develop a positive self-concept.

2. What major life event may greatly alter the body image of a young adult female? Explain.

3. Which of the following statements made by a client indicates that he understands the health teaching related to health promotion and illness prevention?

    A. "I am young, so it does not matter what I eat and if I exercise."
    B. "It is important to schedule routine health care visits even if I am feeling well."
    C. "If I am having any discomfort, I will wait as long as possible before calling the doctor."
    D. If I am feeling stressed, I will just have a glass of wine to forget my troubles."

4. List several reasons that suggest the young adult years are a good time for childbearing.

5. Which of the following behaviors by a young adult demonstrates appropriate psychosocial development?

    A. Taking active involvement in providing guidance to the next generation
    B. Adjusting to major changes in roles and relationships due to losses
    C. Devoting a lot of time to establishing an occupation
    D. Finding oneself "sandwiched" in between and being responsible for two generations

Chapter 20: Young Adult (20 to 40 years)

Application Exercises Answer Key

1. List several developmental tasks that can assist a young adult to develop a positive self-concept.

   Satisfying career choice

   Late formation of a family

   Frequent interactions with family and friends

2. What major life event may greatly alter the body image of a young adult female? Explain.

   Pregnancy. This event causes significant physical changes in the female including:

   Breast enlargement and tenderness.

   Morning sickness and fatigue.

   Pigmentation changes.

   Pruritus.

   Abdominal distension.

3. Which of the following statements made by a client indicates that he understands the health teaching related to health promotion and illness prevention?

   A. "I am young, so it does not matter what I eat and if I exercise."

   B. "It is important to schedule routine health care visits even if I am feeling well."

   C. "If I am having any discomfort, I will wait as long as possible before calling the doctor."

   D. If I am feeling stressed, I will just have a glass of wine to forget my troubles."

   Young adulthood is a time of relative health, but routine screenings and health care visits are still important. Good nutrition and physical activity should be lifelong habits. It is important that the client not wait too long to seek medical care, as an illness/condition may be prevented or may be easier to manage by early detection. Using substances to manage stress can lead to substance abuse. Clients experiencing stress should seek professional assistance.

4. List several reasons that suggest the young adult years are a good time for childbearing.

Personal physical growth has concluded.

Physically, the body is at its peak.

Sex drive is high.

5. Which of the following behaviors by a young adult demonstrates appropriate psychosocial development?

    A. Taking active involvement in providing guidance to the next generation

    B. Adjusting to major changes in roles and relationships due to losses

    C. Devoting a lot of time to establishing an occupation

    D. Finding oneself "sandwiched" in between and being responsible for two generations

Exploring career options and then establishing oneself in a given occupation is a major developmental task for a young adult. Active involvement in the next generation and being responsible for two generations are developmental tasks for the middle adult. Adjusting to major role changes is a developmental task for an older adult.

Unit 1   Foundations for Practice
Section: Nursing Throughout the Lifespan

Chapter 21:   Middle Adult (40 to 60 years)
Contributor: Sally Swenson, MA, RN

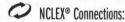 NCLEX® Connections:

Learning Objective: Review and apply knowledge within "**Middle Adult (40 to 60 years)**" in readiness for performance of the following nursing activities as outlined by the NCLEX ® test plans:

Δ Assess/compare the middle adult's physical, cognitive, and psychosocial development to expected growth and development for age.

Δ Identify and report variances from expected growth and development.

Δ Plan and/or provide care to assist the middle adult to achieve expected growth and development outcomes.

Δ Plan and/or provide care appropriate to the middle adult's developmental level, inclusive of age-appropriate recreational/diversional activities.

Δ Teach children/family expected normal growth and development and age-appropriate health maintenance recommendations for the middle adult.

Δ Teach/reinforce accident prevention and health promotion activities for the middle adult.

 Key Points

Δ   **Stages of Development** – The middle adult (ages 40 to 60)

Theorist	Type of Development	Stage
Erikson	Psychosocial	Generativity vs self-absorption
Freud	Psychosocial	Genital
Piaget	Cognitive	Formal operations

Δ The middle adult often has to balance his personal and professional life with providing assistance to:

• Aging parents.

• Adult children.

• Grandchildren.

Expected Growth and Development

Δ **Physical Development**

- Middle adults typically experience decreases in:
    - ◊ Skin turgor.
    - ◊ Melanin in hair (graying).
    - ◊ Hair.
    - ◊ Near vision.
    - ◊ Auditory acuity.
    - ◊ Sense of taste.
    - ◊ Skeletal muscle mass.
    - ◊ Range of motion.
    - ◊ Height.
    - ◊ Calcium/bone density.
    - ◊ Blood vessel elasticity.
    - ◊ Respiratory vital capacity.
    - ◊ Large intestine muscle tone.
    - ◊ Gastric secretions.
    - ◊ Estrogen/testosterone.
    - ◊ Glucose tolerance.

Δ **Cognitive Development**

- Reaction time/speed of performance slows slightly.
- Memory is intact.
- Crystallized intelligence remains (stored knowledge).
- Fluid intelligence (how one learns and processes new information) declines slightly.
- Creativity declines slightly.

Δ **Psychosocial Development**

- The middle adult may strive for generativity.
    - ◊ Uses life as an opportunity for creativity and productivity
    - ◊ Has concern for others
    - ◊ Parenting considered an important task
    - ◊ Strives to do well in one's own environment

- Other tasks include:
  ◊ Adjusting to changes in physical appearance and abilities.
  ◊ Maintaining/strengthening intimacy.

Δ **Moral Development**

- Religious maturity
  ◊ Spiritual beliefs and religion may take on added importance.
  ◊ The middle adult may become more secure in his/her convictions.
  ◊ The middle adult often has advanced moral development.

Δ **Self-concept Development**

- Women may experience issues related to menopause, empty nest, and sexuality. Men may have issues related to job performance and ability to provide. Middle adults may also experience:
  ◊ Depression.
  ◊ Irritability.
  ◊ Difficulty with sexual identity.
  ◊ Issues related to job performance and ability to provide (especially men).
  ◊ Marital changes with the death of a spouse or divorce.

Δ **Body-image Changes**

- Women – Symptoms of menopause may represent a:
  ◊ Loss of the reproductive role or femininity.
  ◊ New interest in intimacy.
- Men – Decreasing strength may be frustrating or frightening.
- Decreased sex drive may occur as a result of declining hormones, chronic diseases, or medications.
- Changes in physical appearance may raise concerns about desirability.

Δ **Nutrition**

- Most middle adults need to:
  ◊ Reduce calories.
  ◊ Reduce fats and protein.
  ◊ Increase calcium.
  ◊ Increase fiber.

Δ **Health Promotion and Prevention**

- The middle adult is especially at risk for alterations in health from:
  - ◊ Obesity and type 2 diabetes.
  - ◊ Cardiovascular disease.
  - ◊ Cancer.
  - ◊ Substance abuse (alcoholism).
  - ◊ Psychosocial stressors.

- Health screenings recommended for middle adults include:
  - ◊ Cardiovascular – blood pressure, cholesterol, lipid levels, and blood glucose levels.
  - ◊ Nutrition – height and weight.
  - ◊ Cancers:
    - ° Pap smears.
    - ° Mammograms.
    - ° Breast self-examination (BSE).

- Health screenings recommended for middle adults after age 50 include:
  - ◊ Stool for occult blood and/or sigmoidoscopy.
  - ◊ Prostate-specific antigen (PSA) and rectal exam.
  - ◊ Osteoporosis – bone density.

- 2007 Centers for Disease Control and Prevention (CDC) **immunization recommendations** for healthy middle adults **40 to 60** years include:
  - ◊ Tetanus and diphtheria (Td) every 10 years, substituting with one dose of tetanus and diphtheria toxoids and pertussis (Tdap).
  - ◊ One dose of measles, mumps, and rubella (MMR), or two doses if a college student, health care worker, or planning international travel.
  - ◊ Two doses of varicella if no evidence of immunity (up to age 50).
  - ◊ Starting at age 50, one dose annually of influenza vaccine.

- Mental health screenings for the middle adult can include:
  - ◊ Depression.
  - ◊ Stress.

- Nutrition counseling for the middle adult includes:
  - ◊ Increasing the consumption of whole grains.
  - ◊ Increasing the consumption of fresh fruits and vegetables.
  - ◊ Limiting fat and cholesterol.

◊ Increasing vitamin D and calcium supplementation (especially for women).

- Injury prevention for the middle adult includes:

  ◊ Avoiding drugs that can lead to substance abuse.

  ◊ Avoiding taking drugs while driving a vehicle.

  ◊ Wearing a seat belt when operating a vehicle.

  ◊ Wearing helmets while bike riding.

  ◊ Installing smoking and carbon monoxide detectors in the home.

  ◊ Securing firearms in a safe location.

Primary Reference:

Potter, P. A., & Perry, A. G. (2005). *Fundamentals of nursing* (6th ed.). St. Louis, MO: Mosby.

Additional Resources:

Centers for Disease Control and Prevention. (2007). *Recommended adult immunization schedule*. Retrieved January 17, 2007, from *www.cdc.gov/*

NANDA International (2004). *NANDA nursing diagnoses: Definitions and classification 2005-2006*. Philadelphia: NANDA.

Chapter 21: Middle Adult (40 to 60 years)

Application Exercises

1. What psychosocial developmental tasks may the middle adult strive to achieve?

2. What major life event may greatly alter the body image of a middle adult woman? Explain.

3. List cancer screenings that are recommended for the middle adult.

4. What cardiovascular screenings are recommended for the middle adult?

5. What nutritional recommendations should be taught to most middle adults? Explain.

6. When performing a psychosocial assessment, a nurse would expect a healthy middle adult to

    A. develop an acceptance of diminished strength and increased dependence on others.
    B. feel frustrated that time is too short for attempting to start another life.
    C. accept one's life as creative and productive.
    D. find someone to share one's life with.

7. Which of the following physical changes increases during the middle years?

    A. Muscle tone
    B. Hearing ability
    C. Blood pressure
    D. Cardiac efficiency

Chapter 21: Middle Adult (40 to 60 years)

Application Exercises Answer Key

1. What psychosocial developmental tasks may the middle adult strive to achieve?

   Using life as an opportunity for creativity and productivity

   Having concern for others

   Parenting

   Doing well in one's own environment

   Achieving civic and social responsibility for:

   - Δ **Children**
   - Δ **Parents**
   - Δ **Society**

   Achieving financial security

   Adjusting to changes in physical appearance and abilities

2. What major life event may greatly alter the body image of a middle adult woman? Explain.

   Menopause may represent a loss of the reproductive role or femininity. Women experiencing difficulties adjusting to menopause may experience the following symptoms: depression, irritability, and difficulty with sexual identity.

3. List cancer screenings that are recommended for the middle adult.

PAP smears

Mammograms

Breast self-examination (BSE)

After age 50:

    Δ   Stool for occult blood or sigmoidoscopy

    Δ   Prostate-specific antigen (PSA) and rectal exam

4. What cardiovascular screenings are recommended for the middle adult?

Blood pressure, cholesterol, lipids, and blood glucose levels

5. What nutritional recommendations should be taught to most middle adults? Explain.

Decrease caloric intake to decrease risk of diabetes and heart disease.

Increase the consumption of whole grains, fresh fruits, and vegetables. The increase in fiber will improve GI motility.

Limit fat and cholesterol intake to decrease cardiovascular disease and diabetes risks.

Vitamin D and calcium supplementation is recommended for women to decrease the risk of osteoporosis.

6. When performing a psychosocial assessment, a nurse would expect a healthy middle adult to

    A. develop an acceptance of diminished strength and increased dependence on others.

    B. feel frustrated that time is too short for attempting to start another life.

    C. accept one's life as creative and productive.

    D. find someone to share one's life with.

Healthy middle adults accept the life they have created for themselves and have a sense of social responsibility. Option A is true of older adults. Option B is true of adults who are having difficulties with the developmental tasks of middle age. Option D is true of young adults.

7. Which of the following physical changes increases during the middle years?

        A. Muscle tone

        B. Hearing ability

        C. Blood pressure

        D. Cardiac efficiency

Blood pressure typically increases during middle age. Muscle tone, hearing ability, and cardiac efficiency all decrease during middle age.

Unit 1
Section:

Foundations for Practice
Nursing Throughout the Lifespan

Chapter 22:	Older Adult (over 65 years)

Contributor: Sally Swenson, MA, RN

 NCLEX® Connections:

Learning Objective: Review and apply knowledge within "**Older Adult (over 65)**" in readiness for performance of the following nursing activities as outlined by the NCLEX® test plans:

Δ   Assess/compare the older adult's physical, cognitive, and psychosocial development to expected growth and development for age.

Δ   Identify and report variances from expected growth and development.

Δ   Plan and/or provide care to assist client to achieve expected growth and development outcomes.

Δ   Plan and/or provide care appropriate to the older adult's developmental level, inclusive of age-appropriate recreational/diversional activities.

Δ   Teach children/family expected normal growth and development and age-appropriate health maintenance recommendations for the older adult.

Δ   Teach/reinforce accident prevention and health promotion activities for the older adult.

 Key Points

Δ   **Stages of Development** – The older adult (over 60)

Theorist	Type of Development	Stage
Erikson	Psychosocial	Integrity vs despair
Freud	Psychosocial	Genital
Piaget	Cognitive	Formal operations

Expected Growth and Development:

Δ   **Physical Development**

- Physical changes related to the older adult include:

  ◊   A decrease in both skin turgor and subcutaneous fat, which leads to wrinkles and dry skin.

  ◊   Thinning hair.

  ◊   A decrease in chest wall movement, vital capacity, and an increase in cilia, which increases the risk for respiratory infections.

  ◊   Slower reaction time.

  ◊   A decrease in smell and taste sensations.

  ◊   A decline in near vision (presbyopia).

  ◊   The decreased ability for the eyes to adjust from light to dark can lead to night blindness while driving.

  ◊   An inability to hear high-pitched sounds (presbycusis).

  ◊   A decrease in muscle strength and tone.

  ◊   Decrease in digestive enzymes.

  ◊   Decrease in intestinal motility, which can lead to an increased risk of constipation.

  ◊   An increase in dental problems.

  ◊   Decalcification of bones.

  ◊   Degeneration of joints.

  ◊   Decrease in bladder capacity.

  ◊   Prostate hypertrophy in men.

  ◊   A decline in estrogen/testosterone production.

  ◊   A decline in thyroid hormone and insulin production.

  ◊   Atrophy of breast tissue in women.

Δ   **Cognitive Development**

- Many older adults maintain their cognitive function.

- Slowed neurotransmission, impaired vascular circulation, disease states, poor nutrition, and structural brain changes can result in the following cognitive disorders, which include:

  ◊   Delirium – acute, temporary, and usually the symptom of other physiologic problems (Delirium is often the first symptom of infection in the older adult.)

◊ Dementia – chronic, progressive, and possibly with an unknown cause (Alzheimer's disease)

◊ Depression – chronic, acute or gradual onset (present for at least 6 weeks)

Δ **Psychosocial Development**

- The developmental tasks of the older adult include:

  ◊ Adjustment to lifestyle changes related to retirement (e.g., decreased income, living situation, loss of work role).

  ◊ Adaptation to changes in family structure (may be role reversal in later years).

  ◊ Dealing with multiple losses (e.g., death of a spouse, friends, siblings).

  ◊ Finding ways not to become socially isolated and overcoming loneliness.

  ◊ Maintaining sexual health and the need to be touched.

  ◊ Facing death.

Δ **Self-concept Development**

- Older adults face difficulties in the area of self-concept, which include:

  ◊ Seeing oneself as an aging person.

  ◊ Finding ways to maintain a quality of life.

  ◊ Becoming more dependent on others for activities of daily living (ADLs).

Δ **Body-image Changes**

- Adjustments to decreases in physical strength and endurance may be difficult, especially for older adults who are cognitively active and engaged. Many older adults may feel frustrated that their bodies are limiting what they desire to do.

Δ **Nutrition**

- In addition to the gastrointestinal impairments that impact proper nutrition, other factors that influence nutrition in the older adult include:

  ◊ Difficulty getting to and from the supermarket to shop for food.

  ◊ Depression or dementia.

  ◊ Not wanting to eat alone.

  ◊ Medications that impact taste or appetite.

  ◊ Prescribed diets that usually do not taste good.

  ◊ Incontinence that may cause the person to limit fluid intake.

- Metabolic rates and activity decline as individuals age; therefore, total caloric intake should decrease to maintain a healthy weight.

- Nutritional recommendations for the older adult include:

  ◊ Increasing the intake of vitamins D, K, and calcium.

  ◊ Increasing fluid intake to minimize the risk of dehydration.

  ◊ Taking a low-dose multivitamin along with mineral supplementation.

  ◊ Limiting salt intake.

Δ **Health Risks**

- Cardiovascular diseases that can affect the older adult include:

  ◊ Coronary artery disease.

  ◊ Hypertension.

  ◊ Stroke.

- Factors affecting mobility of the older adult include:

  ◊ Arthritis.

  ◊ Osteoporosis.

  ◊ Falls.

- Mental health disorders that can affect the older adult include:

  ◊ Depression.

  ◊ Dementia.

  ◊ Suicide.

- Other disorders that can affect the older adult include:

  ◊ Diabetes.

  ◊ Cancers.

  ◊ Incontinence.

  ◊ Abuse and neglect.

  ◊ Cataracts.

  ◊ Alcoholism.

  ◊ Pain.

Δ **Health Promotion and Prevention**

- Health screenings recommended for the older adult include:

  ◊ Cardiovascular – blood pressure, cholesterol, lipid levels, and blood glucose levels.

◊ Nutrition – height and weight.

◊ Vision exams.

◊ Hearing exams.

◊ Cancers.

   ° Pap smears

   ° Mammograms

   ° Breast self-examination (BSE)

- Health screenings recommended for the older adult after age 60 include:

◊ Stool for occult blood or sigmoidoscopy.

◊ Prostate-specific antigen (PSA) and rectal exam.

◊ Osteoporosis (bone density).

- 2007 Centers for Disease Control and Prevention (CDC) **immunization recommendations** for healthy older adults **60** years of age and older include: tetanus and diphtheria (Td) every 10 years substituting with one dose of tetanus and diphtheria toxoids and pertussis (Tdap); one dose annually of influenza vaccine; and starting at age 65, one dose of the pneumococcal vaccine (PVC).

- Exercise – In addition to preserving respiratory and cardiovascular functioning, weight-bearing exercises are needed to increase bone density in the older adult.

- Nutritional supports for the older adult include:

◊ Vitamin D and calcium supplementation.

◊ Congregate meals.

◊ Meals on Wheels.

- Psychosocial interventions to improve self-concept and alleviate social isolation for the older adult include:

◊ Therapeutic communication.

◊ Touch.

◊ Reality orientation.

◊ Validation therapy.

◊ Reminiscence therapy.

◊ Attending to physical appearance.

◊ Assistive devices (e.g., hearing aids, canes, walkers).

- Accident prevention (fall prevention)

◊ Installing bath rails and grab bars

◊ Removing throw rugs

◊ Eliminating clutter from walkways/hallways

◊ Removing extension and phone cords from walkways/hallways

◊ Installing hand railings on all stairways

◊ Using ambulation-assistive devices (e.g., walkers, canes)

◊ Ensuring adequate lighting

Primary Reference:

Potter, P. A., & Perry, A. G. (2005). *Fundamentals of nursing* (6th ed.). St. Louis, MO: Mosby.

Additional Resources:

Centers for Disease Control and Prevention. (2007). *Recommended adult immunization schedule*. Retrieved January 17, 2007, from *www.cdc.gov/*

NANDA International (2004). *NANDA nursing diagnoses: Definitions and classification 2005-2006*. Philadelphia: NANDA.

Chapter 22: Older Adult (over 65 years)

Application Exercises

1. Which of the following are true regarding normal changes associated with aging? (Select all that apply.)

   _____ Increased urinary tract infections

   _____ Increased incidence of constipation

   _____ Decrease in muscle strength and tone

   _____ Decrease in digestive enzymes

   _____ Decrease in subcutaneous fat

   _____ Increase in bladder capacity

2. List several factors that place the older adult client at an increased risk for falls.

3. What measures can be implemented in the home to decrease the risk of falls for the older adult?

4. An older adult is admitted to the hospital. He has lost 4.5 kg (9.9 lb) since his last admission 6 months ago. What further assessment questions should the nurse ask of him to investigate the source of his weight loss?

5. Identify lifestyle recommendations for the older adult client in order to promote health and independence.

6. An older adult client who was treated for bronchitis 2 days ago is receiving home health care. The client's daughter tells the nurse providing the care that her father was fine yesterday, but was up several times during the night looking for his son who lives in another state, emptying desk drawers, and then accusing her of stealing. What is the most likely cause of this cognitive change?

7. Delirium, as opposed to dementia, is typically

   A. acute.

   B. chronic.

   C. progressive in nature.

   D. caused by unknown factors.

8. Presbyopia is a common visual age-related change that results in a decline in

        A. far vision.

        B. near vision.

        C. central vision.

        D. peripheral vision.

Chapter 22: Older Adult (over 65 years)

Application Exercises Answer Key

1. Which of the following are true regarding normal changes associated with aging? (Select all that apply.)

            Increased urinary tract infections

  X   **Increased incidence of constipation**

  X   **Decrease in muscle strength and tone**

  X   **Decrease in digestive enzymes**

  X   **Decrease in subcutaneous fat**

            Increase in bladder capacity

Normal aging leads to a decrease in muscle strength and tone, digestive enzymes, and subcutaneous fat. Constipation is often a problem due to decreased intestinal motility. There is a decrease in bladder capacity. Urinary tract infections are not an inevitable health problem, and measures should be taken to prevent them.

2. List several factors that place the older adult client at an increased risk for falls.

Impaired vision

Impaired mobility due to arthritis, muscle weakness, and pain

Slowed reaction time

Bowel or bladder incontinence

Side effects of medications (e.g., syncope, postural hypotension)

3. What measures can be implemented in the home to decrease the risk of falls for the older adult?

Remove throw rugs.

Make sure extension and phone cords are out of walkways/hallways.

Install bath railings or grab bars.

Install hand rails at stairways.

Eliminate clutter.

4. An older adult is admitted to the hospital. He has lost 4.5 kg (9.9 lb) since his last admission 6 months ago. What further assessment questions should the nurse ask of him to investigate the source of his weight loss?

"Do you eat alone or with someone?"

"How do you obtain your food?"

"Are you able to prepare your food?"

"Have you started any new diet or medication in the past 6 months?"

"What foods have you been eating within the past 24 hr?"

"Have you experienced any bowel changes, such as constipation or diarrhea?"

5. Identify lifestyle recommendations for the older adult client in order to promote health and independence.

Aerobic and weight-bearing exercises

Maintenance of appropriate body weight

Balanced diet with use of supplements as needed

Participation in socially satisfying activities

Regular physical examinations

6. An older adult client who was treated for bronchitis 2 days ago is receiving home health care. The client's daughter tells the nurse providing the care that her father was fine yesterday, but was up several times during the night looking for his son who lives in another state, emptying desk drawers, and then accusing her of stealing. What is the most likely cause of this cognitive change?

Because of the acute onset of cognitive changes, this is probably delirium. The client has a disease process (bronchitis) that could have progressed to pneumonia (infection) and/or decreasing oxygen saturation levels.

7. Delirium, as opposed to dementia, is typically

    A. acute.
    B. chronic.
    C. progressive in nature.
    D. caused by unknown factors.

Delirium is acute in nature, and once the cause is known and treated, the symptoms usually resolve. Dementia is chronic, progressive, and caused by unknown factors.

8. Presbyopia is a common visual age-related change that results in a decline in

    A. far vision.
    B. near vision.
    C. central vision.
    D. peripheral vision.

Presbyopia is a decline in near vision. Far vision is not related to presbyopia. Central vision impairment is true of macular degeneration, and impairment of peripheral vision is true of glaucoma.

Unit 2   **Health Assessment**

Section: Vital Signs

Chapter 23:	Temperature

Contributors: Jeanne Wissmann, PhD, RN, CNE
Sally Swenson, MA, RN

 NCLEX® Connections:

Learning Objective: Review and apply knowledge within "**Temperature**" in readiness for performance of the following nursing activities as outlined by the NCLEX® test plans:

Δ   Perform the appropriate assessment of the client's temperature within the nursing role, including:

- Preparing the client for the procedure.

- Client teaching (before and following the procedure).

- Using accurate equipment and technique based on the client's needs.

Δ   Assess/monitor the client's status by obtaining baseline data and comparing with subsequent findings.

Δ   Identify factors that influence the client's temperature.

Δ   Demonstrate appropriate actions necessary to manage a client with an abnormal temperature.

Δ   Document baseline and subsequent findings according to facility/agency protocol.

Δ   Assess/monitor and document the client's response to administration of pharmacological therapy.

 Key Points

Δ   **Physiological Responses**

- Temperature, measured in degrees, reflects the balance between heat produced and lost from the body.

- The neurological and cardiovascular systems work together to keep body temperature within a normal range.

- The rectum and tympanic membrane are core temperature measurement sites.

- The skin, mouth, and axillae are surface temperature measurement sites.

Δ **Normal Temperature Range** is:

- Orally 36 to 38° C (96.8 to 100.4° F). Average is 37° C (98.6° F).

- Rectal temperatures are usually 0.5° C (0.9° F) higher than oral temperatures.

- Axillary temperatures are usually 0.5° C (0.9° F) lower than oral temperatures.

- Normal temperature can vary among individuals. The client's usual temperature serves as a baseline for comparison.

Key Factors

Δ **Heat production** results from increases in basal metabolic rate, muscle activity, thyroxine output, and sympathetic stimulation, which increases heat production.

Δ **Heat loss** from the body occurs through:

- **Conduction** – transfer of heat from the body to another surface (when the body is immersed in cold water).

- **Convection** – dispersion of heat by air currents (wind blowing across exposed skin).

- **Evaporation** – dispersion of heat through water vapor (sweating and diaphoresis).

- **Radiation** – transfer of heat from one object to another object without contact between them (heat lost from the body to a cold room).

Δ **Newborns** have a large surface-to-mass ratio; therefore, **they lose heat rapidly to the environment**. Newborn temperature should be maintained between 35.5 to 37.5° C (95.9 to 99.5° F).

Δ **Older adult clients** have a loss of subcutaneous fat that results in **lower body** temperatures and feeling cold. Average body temperature is 36° C (96.8° F). Older adult clients are more likely to be adversely affected by extremes in environmental temperatures (e.g., heat stroke, hypothermia). It takes longer for body temperature to register on the thermometer due to changes in temperature regulation.

Δ **Hormone changes** may influence temperature. In general, temperature rises slightly with ovulation and menses. With menopause, intermittent body temperature may increase by up to 4° C (7.2° F).

Δ **Exercise, activity, and dehydration** can contribute to the development of hyperthermia.

Δ **Illness and injury** are often associated with elevations in temperature. Fever is the body's response to the infectious and/or inflammatory process that is occurring within.

Δ Recent food or fluid intake and smoking can interfere with accurate measurement of body temperature.

NANDA Nursing Diagnoses

- Δ Hyperthermia

- Δ Hypothermia

- Δ Ineffective thermoregulation

- Δ Risk for imbalanced body temperature

Nursing Interventions

- Δ Equipment

  - Electronic thermometers use a probe to measure body temperature. A disposable cover is placed on the probe prior to insertion. An audible signal occurs when temperature assessment is completed, and a digital reading of the temperature is provided. Oral, rectal, and axillary temperatures can be assessed using a similar device. Tympanic temperatures are obtained using a device specifically designed to assess temperature at the client's eardrum.

  - Disposable thermometers are designed for oral or axillary use. These thermometers are individually wrapped and discarded after one use. They offer a reduced risk of client cross-infection.

  - Glass, mercury-filled thermometers are rarely used due to the risk involved with mercury exposure. Shake the mercury level down to 95° F prior to use. If using a mercury-filled thermometer, follow facility/agency policy for proper disposable. Avoid contact with mercury, washing skin thoroughly if contact occurs.

- Δ Procedure

  - Wash hands and provide for privacy.

Oral Technique	Rectal Technique	Axillary Technique	Tympanic Technique
• Place the thermometer (with oral probe) under the client's tongue in posterior sublingual pocket lateral to center of lower jaw. • Leave in place until thermometer signal is heard. (Hold mercury thermometer in place for 3 min.)	• Provide privacy. • Place in Sims' position with upper leg flexed. Wearing gloves, spread buttock to expose anal opening. • Ask client to breathe slowly and relax, placing lubricated thermometer (with rectal probe) into the anus in direction of umbilicus 3.5 cm (1½ in) for adult. If resistance is encountered, remove immediately. Once inserted, hold the thermometer in place until thermometer signal is heard. (Hold mercury thermometer in place 3 min.)	• Place the thermometer (with oral probe) in the center of the client's clean, dry armpit. Lower arm over the probe. • Hold the arm down, keeping the thermometer in position until thermometer signal is heard. (Hold mercury thermometer in place 2 min.)	• Pull ear up and back (for adult) or down and back (for child). • Place the thermometer probe snugly into the client's outer ear canal and press the scan button. • Leave in place until the thermometer signal is heard. • Carefully remove the thermometer from the ear canal and read the temperature.
Safety measure: Do not use glass, mercury-filled thermometers for clients who might bite the thermometer (e.g., small children, confused clients).	Safety measure: Do not use for clients on bleeding precautions or who have rectal disorders.		

Oral Technique	Rectal Technique	Axillary Technique	Tympanic Technique
Age-specific: In general, this is the preferred method for individuals who are 4 years and older.	• Age-specific: A rectal measurement of temperature is more accurate than axillary. However, because of the possible risk of rectal perforation, the American Academy of Pediatrics recommends screening infants 3 months and younger by taking an axillary temperature initially. • Rectal temperature can be used to obtain a second measurement if the temperature is greater than 37.2° C (99° F).		• Age-specific: The American Academy of Pediatrics advises against the use of electronic ear thermometers for infants 3 months and younger due to inaccuracy of readings.
• Note: The oral site may not be appropriate for assessment of temperature in clients who breathe through their mouth or have experienced trauma to the face or mouth.	• Note: Stool in the rectum can cause inaccurate readings.		• Note: Excess earwax can impede the reading. If noted, use alternate ear or select another appropriate site for temperature assessment.

• Document findings and report abnormal findings to primary care provider.

Complications and Nursing Interventions

Δ **Fever** – Fever is usually not harmful unless it **exceeds 39° C (102.2° F).
 Hyperthermia** is an **abnormally elevated body temperature.**

- Obtain blood cultures if ordered.

- Assess/monitor white blood cell counts, sedimentation rates, and electrolytes
  as ordered.

- Administer antibiotics per order (after obtaining blood cultures).

- Provide fluids and rest.

- Provide antipyretics (e.g., aspirin, acetaminophen, ibuprofen). Aspirin use is
  not recommended for management of fever in children and adolescents who
  may have a viral illness (e.g., influenza, chickenpox) due to the risk of Reye
  syndrome associated with aspirin use in viral illnesses. Pediatric antipyretic
  dosages are calculated based on weight.

- A cooling blanket or tepid bath 29.4 to 32.2° C (85 to 90° F) may also be used.
  Offer blankets during chills and remove them when the client feels warm.

- Provide oral hygiene and dry clothing and linens.

Δ **Hypothermia** or a body temperature < 35 C (< 95° F) is an abnormally low body
 temperature.

- Provide a warm environmental temperature, heated humidified oxygen,
  warming blanket, friction to extremities, or warmed oral or intravenous
  fluids.

- Provide continuous cardiac monitoring.

- Have emergency resuscitation equipment on standby.

Primary Reference:

Potter, P. A., & Perry, A. G. (2005). *Fundamentals of nursing* (6th ed.). St. Louis, MO: Mosby.

Additional Resources:

For information about obtaining temperature for children, go to the American Academy
of Pediatrics Web site, *www.aafp.org/online/en/home.html*

NANDA International (2004). *NANDA nursing diagnoses: Definitions and classification
2005-2006*. Philadelphia: NANDA.

Chapter 23: Temperature

Application Exercises

Scenario: An 82-year-old man arrives at the emergency department with an oral body temperature of 38.3° C (101° F), pulse rate of 114/min, and respiratory rate of 22/min. He is restless and his skin is warm to the touch.

1. What implications does the aging process have on this client's temperature?

2. Identify possible causes for this client's elevated temperature.

3. Which of the following are appropriate nursing interventions for this client? (Select all that apply.)

_____ Obtain cultures (e.g., blood, sputum) prior to initiating antimicrobials as ordered.

_____ Restrict fluids.

_____ Allow for adequate rest.

_____ Provide oral care.

_____ Only change bed linens upon client request.

_____ Apply extra blanket if the client is chilling.

4. Based on the client assessment data provided, select the oral, axillary, or tympanic temperature-assessment site, and note the rationale for the selection. Some clients may have more than one option available to them.

Client Assessment	Site Selection	Rationale
A newborn		
A 6-month-old infant		
Healthy 60-year-old woman		
Confused 82-year-old man		
A client with hemorrhoids		
A client with a stuffy nose		
A client with a low platelet count secondary to chemotherapy		
A client immediately following mandibular surgery		

Chapter 23: Temperature

Application Exercises Answer Key

Scenario: An 82-year-old man arrives at the emergency department with an oral body temperature of 38.3° C (101° F), pulse rate of 114/min, and respiratory rate of 22/min. He is restless and his skin is warm to the touch.

1. What implications does the aging process have on this client's temperature?

> A baseline temperature in the older adult client is typically lower due to the loss of subcutaneous fat. An oral temperature of 38.3° C (101° F) would be an extremely high fever that the older adult client may not tolerate well.

2. Identify possible causes for this client's elevated temperature.

> A bacterial or viral infection, dehydration, or the inflammatory process can lead to an elevated body temperature.

3. Which of the following are appropriate nursing interventions for this client? (Select all that apply.)

   __X__ **Obtain cultures (e.g., blood, sputum) prior to initiating antimicrobials as ordered.**

   _____ Restrict fluids.

   __X__ **Allow for adequate rest.**

   __X__ **Provide oral care.**

   _____ Only change bed linens upon client request.

   __X__ **Apply extra blanket if the client is chilling.**

> **Cultures may be ordered to rule out the presence of infection and should be obtained prior to the initiation of antibiotic therapy. This prevents the antibiotic from interfering with the presence of the infection. Rest will help conserve energy and decrease metabolic rate. Oral care will provide comfort to the client with dry mucous membranes. Extra blankets will keep the client warm if he starts to chill. Fluids should be encouraged for the client with a fever. The client with a fever frequently sweats, so bed linens should be changed frequently and as needed.**

4. Based on the client assessment data provided, select the oral, axillary, or tympanic temperature-assessment site, and note the rationale for the selection. Some clients may have more than one option available to them.

Client Assessment	Site Selection	Rationale
A newborn	Axillary initially	Avoid risk of rectal perforation.
A 6-month-old infant	Tympanic	Child is older than 3 months.
A healthy 60-year-old woman	Oral	This is the preferred method for this age.
A confused 82-year-old man	Oral, tympanic or axillary	Oral is preferred if the client is able to close her mouth around the probe. A glass thermometer is contraindicated.
A client with hemorrhoids	Oral, tympanic, or axillary	Oral is the preferred method. Tympanic and axillary can also be used. The rectal method is contraindicated.
A client with a stuffy nose	Axillary or tympanic	This client is probably breathing through his mouth and will be unable to close his mouth around the probe.
A client with a low platelet count secondary to chemotherapy	Oral, tympanic, or axillary	Oral is the preferred method. Tympanic and axillary can also be used. The rectal method is contraindicated.
A client immediately following mandibular surgery	Axillary or tympanic	The oral route is contraindicated for a client with recent mouth trauma.

Unit 2   Health Assessment
Section: Vital Signs

Chapter 24:	Pulse
	Contributor: Sally Swenson, MA, RN

 NCLEX® Connections:

> **Learning Objective**: Review and apply knowledge within "**Pulse**" in readiness for performance of the following nursing activities as outlined by the NCLEX® test plans:
>
> Δ   Perform the appropriate assessment of the client's pulse/heart rate and rhythm within the nursing role, including:
>
> - Preparing the client for the procedure.
> - Client teaching (before and following the procedure).
> - Using accurate technique based on the client's needs.
>
> Δ   Assess/monitor the client's status by obtaining baseline data and comparing with subsequent findings.
>
> Δ   Identify factors that influence the client's pulse rate and rhythm.
>
> Δ   Demonstrate appropriate actions necessary to manage a client with an abnormal pulse/heart rate and rhythm.
>
> Δ   Document baseline and subsequent findings according to facility/agency protocol.
>
> Δ   Assess/monitor and document the client's response to administration of pharmacological therapy.

 Key Points

Δ   **Physiologic Responses**

- The cardiovascular system relies on the electrical and mechanical functioning of the heart. How much blood is pumped from the heart (the left ventricle) to the arterial circulation in 1 min is the cardiac output (CO).

- CO = heart rate (HR) x stroke volume (SV).

    ◊   HR = number of contractions of the heart/minute.

    ◊   SV = amount of blood that is pumped out of the heart with each contraction.

- The autonomic nervous system controls the heart rate. The parasympathetic nervous system lowers the heart rate, and the sympathetic nervous system raises the heart rate.

Δ **Pulse**, when discussed as a vital sign, is the measurement of heart rate and rhythm. The wave-like sensations or impulses felt in a peripheral arterial vessel or over the apex of the heart is assessed as a gauge of cardiovascular status.

- **Rate** – The number of times per minute the pulse is felt or heard.

- **Rhythm** – The regularity at which each impulse is felt. A premature or late heart beat can result in an irregular interval in which impulses are felt or heard and can indicate abnormal electrical activity of the heart. Normally, an impulse should be sensed at regular intervals.

- **Strength (amplitude)** – The strength of the impulse should be the same from beat to beat and can be graded on a scale of 0 to 4.

  ◊ This scale is as follows:

    ° 0 = absent, unable to palpate.

    ° 1+ = diminished, weaker than expected.

    ° 2+ = brisk, expected.

    ° 3+ = increased.

    ° 4+ = full volume, bounding.

- **Equality** – **Peripheral pulse** impulses should be symmetrical in quality and quantity from the right side of the body to the left. Assessments of strength and equality are for the purpose of evaluating the adequacy of the vascular system.

Δ **Normal pulse range** for the adult client is **60 to 100/min** at rest.

- **Tachycardia** = rate above the normal range or **> 100/min.**

- **Bradycardia** = rate below the normal range or **< 60/min.**

Key Factors

Δ **Dysrhythmia** – an irregular rhythm of the heart that frequently is noted as an irregular radial pulse.

Δ **A pulse deficit** occurs when the apical rate is greater than the radial rate. In the case of a dysrhythmia, the heart may contract ineffectively resulting in a beat being heard at the apical site, but a pulsation not being felt at the radial pulse point.

Δ **Age** – In infants, the pulse rate is 120 to 160/min. This rate gradually decreases as the child grows older. The average pulse for a 12 to 14 year old is 80 to 90/ min. The strength of the pulsation may weaken in the older adult client due to poor circulation or cardiac dysfunction, which makes the peripheral pulses more difficult to palpate.

Factors Leading to Tachycardia	Factors Leading to Bradycardia
Exercise	Long-term physical fitness
Fever	Hypothermia
Medications – epinephrine (Adrenaline), levothyroxine (Synthroid), beta$_2$-adrenergic agonists (albuterol [Proventil])	Medications – digoxin (Lanoxin), beta-blockers (propranolol [Inderal]), calcium channel blockers (Verapamil [Calan])
Changing position from lying down to sitting or standing	Changing position from standing or sitting to lying down
Acute pain	Chronic pain
Hyperthyroidism	Hypothyroidism
Anemia, hypoxemia	
Stress, anxiety, and fear	
Hypovolemia, shock and heart failure lead to ↓ CO with a compensatory ↑ HR	

NANDA Nursing Diagnoses

- Δ Acute pain

- Δ Deficient or excess fluid volume

- Δ Decreased cardiac output

- Δ Fatigue

- Δ Ineffective tissue perfusion

- Δ Risk for injury

Nursing Interventions

- Δ Equipment

  - A watch with a second hand or digital readout that allows for counting seconds

  - Stethoscope

- Δ Procedure

  - Wash hands and provide for privacy.

  - **Radial pulse** is located on the radial or thumb side of the forearm at the wrist.

    - ◊ Place index and middle finger of one hand gently but firmly over the pulse. Assess the pulsation for rate, rhythm, amplitude, and equality.

◊   If the peripheral pulsation is regular, then the rate is counted for 30 sec and multiplied by 2. If the pulsation is irregular, the rate should be counted for a full minute and compared to the apical pulse rate.

- **Apical pulse** is located at the fifth intercostal space at the left midclavicular line. Use this site for assessing the heart rate of an infant, rapid rates (> 100/min), irregular rhythms, or rates prior to the administration of cardiac medications.

  ◊   Place the stethoscope on the chest at the fifth intercostal space at the left midclavicular line. An apical pulse rate should always be counted for 1 min.

- Document findings and report abnormal findings to the primary care provider.

Complications and Nursing Interventions

Δ   Tachycardia

- Assess/monitor for other signs and symptoms (e.g., pain, anxiety, restlessness, fatigue, low blood pressure, oxygen saturation).

- Assess/monitor for potential medication side effects.

- Prevent injury.

- Notify primary care provider.

Δ   Bradycardia

- Assess/monitor for other signs and symptoms (e.g., hypotension, chest pain, diaphoresis, dyspnea, altered mental status).

- Assess/monitor for potential medication side effects.

- Prevent injury.

- Notify primary care provider.

Primary Reference:

Potter, P. A., & Perry, A. G. (2005). *Fundamentals of nursing* (6th ed.). St. Louis, MO: Mosby.

Additional Resources:

Bickley, L. S., & Szilagyi, P. G. (2003). *Bates' guide to physical examination and history taking* (8th ed.). Philadelphia: Lippincott Williams & Wilkins.

NANDA International (2004). *NANDA nursing diagnoses: Definitions and classification 2005-2006*. Philadelphia: NANDA.

Chapter 24: Pulse

Application Exercises

1. Determine which of the following factors increases or decreases the pulse rate. Check the appropriate box.

Factor	Increases	Decreases
Hyperthyroidism		
Calcium channel blockers		
Hypothermia		
Acute pain		
Blood loss		
Anxiety		
Walking on the treadmill		

2. Indicate the proper choice of pulse measurement site in each of the following situations. Choices may be used more than once.

_____ 2-month-old infant in for a routine checkup

_____ 76-year-old client showing tachycardia and an irregular rhythm on the cardiac monitor

_____ 56-year-old client with an order to receive a stat dose of digoxin (Lanoxin)

_____ 20-year-old client in the emergency department for stitches on her hand

_____ 16-year-old client who has been stable for 3 hr following an appendectomy

A. Apical

B. Radial

C. Simultaneous check of apical and radial

3. A client who is confused is brought into the emergency department by his son. The client's son tells the nurse he thinks his father may have been taking more of his digoxin (Lanoxin) than directed. Which of the following findings should the nurse assess for?

    A. Constipation

    B. Bradycardia

    C. Elevated blood pressure

    D. Agitation

4. A nurse is checking the vital signs of a 92-year-old client. The radial pulse has an irregular beat about every fifth or sixth beat. The rate is 92/min. The client is asymptomatic. The nurse's next step should be to

      A. report the findings to the primary care provider immediately.

      B. place the client on telemetry.

      C. obtain an electrocardiogram.

      D. check an apical pulse for 60 sec and note any pulse deficits.

Chapter 24: Pulse

Application Exercises Answer Key

1. Determine which of the following factors increases or decreases the pulse rate. Check the appropriate box.

Factor	Increases	Decreases
Hyperthyroidism	X	
Calcium channel blockers		X
Hypothermia		X
Acute pain	X	
Blood loss	X	
Anxiety	X	
Walking on the treadmill	X	

2. Indicate the proper choice of pulse measurement site in each of the following situations. Choices may be used more than once.

__A__ 2-month-old infant in for a routine checkup

__C__ 76-year-old client showing tachycardia and an irregular rhythm on the cardiac monitor

__A__ 56-year-old client with an order to receive a stat dose of digoxin (Lanoxin)

__B__ 20-year-old client in the emergency department for stitches on her hand

__B__ 16-year-old client who has been stable for 3 hr following an appendectomy

A. Apical

B. Radial

C. Simultaneous check of apical and radial

3. A client who is confused is brought into the emergency department by his son. The client's son tells the nurse he thinks his father may have been taking more of his digoxin (Lanoxin) than directed. Which of the following findings should the nurse assess for?

    A. Constipation

    B. Bradycardia

    C. Elevated blood pressure

    D. Agitation

A sign of digoxin (Lanoxin) toxicity is a slow heart rate or bradycardia.

4. A nurse is checking the vital signs of a 92-year-old client. The radial pulse has an irregular beat about every fifth or sixth beat. The rate is 92/min. The client is asymptomatic. The nurse's next step should be to

> A. report the findings to the primary care provider immediately.
>
> B. place the client on telemetry.
>
> C. obtain an electrocardiogram.
>
> **D. check an apical pulse for 60 sec and note any pulse deficits.**

This radial pulse does not require immediate medical treatment; therefore, the nurse should next assess the client's apical pulse to further assess the client's status. After the nurse assesses the client's apical pulse, the findings should be reported to the primary care provider. The primary care provider will decide if the client should be placed on telemetry and if an electrocardiogram should be obtained.

Unit 2   Health Assessment

Section: Vital Signs

Chapter 25:   Respirations and Pulse Oximetry

Contributor: Sally Swenson, MA, RN

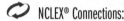 NCLEX® Connections:

Learning Objective: Review and apply knowledge within **"Respirations and Pulse Oximetry"** in readiness for performance of the following nursing activities as outlined by the NCLEX® test plans:

Δ   Perform the appropriate assessment of the client's respirations and pulse oximetry within the nursing role, including:

- Preparing the client for the procedure.

- Client teaching (before and following the procedure).

- Using accurate technique based on the client's needs.

Δ   Assess/monitor the client's status by obtaining baseline data and comparing with subsequent findings.

Δ   Identify factors that influence the client's respirations and pulse oximetry.

Δ   Document baseline and subsequent findings according to facility/agency protocol.

Δ   Assess/monitor and document the client's response to administration of pharmacological therapy.

 Key Points

Δ   **Physiological Responses**

- Chemoreceptors in the carotid arteries and aorta primarily monitor carbon dioxide (CO_2) levels of the blood. If carbon dioxide rises, the respiratory center of the brain is triggered to increase the respiratory rate. The increased respiratory rate rids the body of excess CO_2. For clients with chronic obstructive pulmonary disease (COPD), a low oxygen level becomes the primary respiratory drive.

Δ   The processes of respiration includes:

- **Ventilation** – the exchange of oxygen and carbon dioxide in the lungs. Measure ventilation with respiration rate, rhythm, and depth.

- **Diffusion** – the passage of oxygen and carbon dioxide between the alveoli and red blood cells. Measure diffusion with pulse oximetry.

- **Perfusion** – the flow of blood to and from the pulmonary capillaries. Measure perfusion with pulse oximetry.

Δ **Respiration** is the vital sign responsible for evaluating the effectiveness of the ventilatory process of oxygen and carbon dioxide exchange.

- **Rate** – the number of full inspirations and expirations in 1 min. Determine this by observing the number of times the client's chest rises and falls. **The normal range for adults is 12 to 20/min**.

- **Depth** – the amount of chest wall expansion that occurs with each breath. Abnormal depths are described as deep or shallow.

- **Rhythm** – the observation of breathing intervals. A regular rhythm with an occasional sigh is normal in adults.

Δ **Pulse Oximetry**

- This is a noninvasive measurement of the oxygen saturation of the blood.

- A pulse oximeter is a battery- or electric-operated device with a clip-on sensor probe that is clipped securely onto the client's finger, toe, nose, earlobe, or forehead.

- Pulse oximeter measures SaO_2 (arterial oxygen saturation) via a wave of infrared light that measures light absorption by oxygenated and deoxygenated hemoglobin in arterial blood. SaO_2 and SpO_2 are used interchangeably.

- Normal values are 95 to 100%. Acceptable levels may range from 91 to 100%. Some illness states may allow for an SaO_2 of 85 to 89%.

- Values may be slightly lower in the older adult client and those with dark skin.

- Additional reasons for low readings include hypothermia, poor peripheral blood flow, too much light (sun or infrared lamps), low hemoglobin levels, client movement, edema, and nail polish.

- Results less than 91% require nursing intervention to assist the client to regain normal SaO_2 levels. Results < 86% indicate an emergency. Life-threatening results may start at levels < 80%. The lower the SaO_2 level, the less accurate the value.

Key Factors

Δ **Age** – Respiratory rate decreases with age. Newborns have rates of 30 to 60/min. School-age children have a respiratory rate of 20 to 30/ min.

Δ **Gender** differences are noted when observing respirations. Men are diaphragmatic breathers, and abdominal movements are more noticeable. Women use more thoracic muscles, and chest movements are more pronounced when they breathe.

Δ **Pain** in the chest wall area may decrease the depth of respirations. At the onset of acute pain, the respiration rate will increase but will return to normal over time.

Δ **Anxiety** increases the rate and depth of respirations.

Δ **Smoking** causes the resting rate of respirations to increase.

Δ **Body position** – Upright positions allow the chest wall to expand more fully.

Δ **Medications** such as opioids, sedatives, bronchodilators, and general anesthetics will **decrease** the respiratory rate and depth. Respiratory depression can be a serious adverse effect. Amphetamines and cocaine may **increase** rate and depth.

Δ **Neurological injury** to the brain stem decreases respiratory rate and rhythm.

Δ **Illnesses** impacting the shape of the chest wall and changing the patency of passages, or those impairing muscle function, will consequently diminish normal respiratory effort. The use of accessory muscles with an increased rate will be seen.

Δ **Impaired oxygen carrying capacity of the blood** that occurs with anemia or at high altitudes results in increases in the respiratory rate and alterations in rhythm in order to compensate.

NANDA Nursing Diagnoses

Δ Impaired gas exchange

Δ Ineffective airway clearance

Δ Ineffective breathing pattern

Δ Ineffective tissue perfusion

Nursing Interventions

Δ Respiratory Rate

• Equipment

◊ A watch with a second hand or digital readout allows for counting seconds.

• Procedure

◊ Wash hands and provide for privacy.

◊ Place the client in semi-Fowler's position, being sure chest is visible.

◊ Have the client rest arm across abdomen, or place hand directly on the client's abdomen.

◊ Observe one full respiratory cycle, look at watch, and then begin counting rate.

◊ Regular rate can be counted for 30 sec and multiplied by 2. Count the rate for 1 min if irregular, > 20/min or < 12 /min.

◊ Document findings and report abnormal findings to the primary care provider.

Δ Pulse Oximetry

- Equipment

  ◊ Pulse oximeter is used.

- Procedure

  ◊ Wash hands and provide for privacy.

  ◊ Assess for appropriate probe site. Site must be dry and have adequate circulation.

  ◊ Be sure the client is in a comfortable position, supporting arm if finger is used as probe site.

  ◊ Apply sensor probe to site.

  ◊ Press power switch on oximeter.

  ◊ Note pulse reading and compare with the client's radial pulse. A discrepancy between the two pulse rates should be further assessed.

  ◊ Allow time for the readout to stabilize, and record this value as the oxygen saturation.

  ◊ Remove probe, turn off meter, and store equipment appropriately.

  ◊ If continuous monitoring is required, make sure alarms are set for a low and high limit. The alarms are turned on, and the sound level can be heard. Every 4 hr, assess skin under probe and move sensor to another location.

  ◊ Document findings and report abnormal findings to primary care provider.

Complications and Nursing Interventions

Δ Hypoxemia – SaO_2 < 90%

- Confirm that sensor probe is properly placed.

- Confirm that oxygen delivery system is functioning and that the client is receiving ordered oxygen levels.

- Place the client in semi-Fowler's or Fowler's position to maximize ventilation.

- Encourage deep breathing.

- Assess for signs of hypoxemia (e.g., tachypnea, tachycardia, restlessness).

- Assess/monitor vital signs. Report significant findings to the primary care provider.

- Remain with the client and provide emotional support to decrease anxiety.

Primary Reference:

Potter, P. A., & Perry, A. G. (2005). *Fundamentals of nursing* (6th ed.). St. Louis, MO: Mosby.

Additional Resources:

Bickley, L. S., & Szilagyi, P. G. (2003). *Bates' guide to physical examination and history taking* (8th ed.). Philadelphia: Lippincott Williams & Wilkins.

NANDA International (2004). *NANDA nursing diagnoses: Definitions and classification 2005-2006*. Philadelphia: NANDA.

Chapter 25: Respirations and Pulse Oximetry

Application Exercises

1. Determine whether each of the following factors increases or decreases the respiration rate. Check the appropriate box.

Factor	Increases	Decreases
Morphine		
Brisk walk on the treadmill		
Sickle cell disease		
Smoking		
Acute gallbladder attack		
Hiking in the mountains		
General anesthetic during surgery		

2. Which of the following nursing interventions are correct when assessing the client's respirations? (Select all that apply.)

_____ Always count the respiratory rate for 1 min.

_____ Place the client in semi-Fowler's position.

_____ Count the respiratory rate simultaneously with the pulse.

_____ Position the stethoscope on the anterior chest.

_____ Observe one full respiratory cycle before counting rate.

3. Place the following steps for obtaining an oxygen saturation level with a pulse oximeter in the correct order starting with 1 as the first step.

	Document findings and report abnormal findings to the primary care provider.
	Press power switch on oximeter.
	Wash hands and provide for privacy.
	Apply sensor probe to site.
	Note pulse reading and compare with the client's radial pulse.
	Remove probe, turn off meter, and store equipment appropriately.
	Assess for appropriate probe site.
	Allow time for the readout to stabilize and record this value as the oxygen saturation.

Chapter 25: Respirations and Pulse Oximetry

Application Exercises Answer Key

1. Determine whether each of the following factors increases or decreases the respiration rate. Check the appropriate box.

Factor	Increases	Decreases
Morphine		X
Brisk walk on the treadmill	X	
Sickle cell disease	X	
Smoking	X	
Acute gallbladder attack	X	
Hiking in the mountains	X	
General anesthetic during surgery		X

2. Which of the following nursing interventions are correct when assessing the client's respirations? (Select all that apply.)

_____ Always count the respiratory rate for 1 min.

__X__ **Place the client in semi-Fowler's position.**

_____ Count the respiratory rate simultaneously with the pulse.

_____ Position the stethoscope on the anterior chest.

__X__ **Observe one full respiratory cycle before counting rate.**

The best position for the client to be in when assessing the respiratory rate is semi-Fowler's with the chest being visible. Observing for one full respiratory cycle before starting to count assists in obtaining an accurate count. If the rate is regular, count for 30 sec and multiply by 2. Count the rate for 1 full min if irregular, > 20/min or < 12/min. It will be difficult to obtain an accurate reading of either the respiratory rate or the pulse if counted simultaneously. The respiratory rate is not auscultated with a stethoscope.

3. Place the following steps for obtaining an oxygen saturation level with a pulse oximeter in the correct order starting with 1 as the first step.

8	Document findings and report abnormal findings to the primary care provider.
4	Press power switch on oximeter.
1	Wash hands and provide for privacy.
3	Apply sensor probe to site.
5	Note pulse reading and compare with the client's radial pulse.
7	Remove probe, turn off meter, and store equipment appropriately.
2	Assess for appropriate probe site.
6	Allow time for the readout to stabilize and record this value as the oxygen saturation.

Unit 2   Health Assessment
Section: Vital Signs

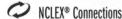

Chapter 26:	Blood Pressure
	Contributor: Sally Swenson, MA, RN

 NCLEX® Connections

> **Learning Objective**: Review and apply knowledge within "**Blood Pressure**" in readiness for performance of the following nursing activities as outlined by the NCLEX® test plans:
>
> Δ   Perform the appropriate assessment of the client's blood pressure within the nursing role, including:
>
> •   Preparing the client for the procedure.
>
> •   Client teaching (before and following the procedure).
>
> •   Using accurate technique based on the client's needs.
>
> Δ   Assess/monitor the client's status by obtaining baseline data and comparing with subsequent findings.
>
> Δ   Identify factors that influence the client's blood pressure.
>
> Δ   Demonstrate appropriate actions necessary to manage a client with an abnormal blood pressure.
>
> Δ   Document baseline and subsequent findings according to facility/agency protocol.
>
> Δ   Assess/monitor and document the client's response to administration of pharmacological therapy.

Key Points

Δ   **Blood pressure (BP)** reflects the force exerted by the blood in the arteries during heart contraction (systole) and relaxation (diastole).

•   **Systolic** BP (SBP) occurs during ventricular systole of the heart and represents the maximum amount of pressure exerted on the arteries.

•   **Diastolic** BP (DBP) occurs during ventricular diastole of the heart and represents the minimum amount of pressure exerted on the arteries.

Δ **Physiological responses**

- The principle determinants of BP are cardiac output (CO) and systemic vascular resistance (SVR).

- BP = CO x SVR.

CO is determined by: • HR. • Contractility. • Blood volume. • Venous return	• Systemic (peripheral) vascular resistance (SVR) is determined by the amount of constriction or dilation of the arteries.
• ↑ in any of these → ↑ CO → ↑ BP • ↓ in any of these → ↓ CO → ↓ BP	• ↑ in SVR → ↑ BP • ↓ in SVR → ↓ BP

Δ **Classifications of BP** according to the Seventh Report of the Joint National Committee on Prevention, Detection, Evaluation, and Treatment of High Blood Pressure (JNC 7):

BP Classification	Systolic BP (SBP) mm Hg	Diastolic BP (DPB) mm Hg
Normal	< 120	< 80
Prehypertension	120 to 139	80 to 89
Stage 1 hypertension	140 to 159	90 to 99
Stage 2 hypertension	≥ 160	≥ 100

Δ Classification is based on highest reading. A client with a blood pressure of 124/92 mm Hg has stage 1 hypertension because the DPB places the client in that category. A client with a blood pressure of 146/82 mm Hg also has stage 1 hypertension because the SPB places the client in that category.

Δ If the client has a SBP of ≥ 140 mm Hg and a DBP of ≥ 90 mm Hg when two or more BP measurements are averaged together, he should return for two or more visits for additional readings. A diagnosis of hypertension will be made if the readings are elevated on at least three separate occasions over several weeks.

Δ **Hypotension** is a BP that is below normal (**systolic< 90** mm Hg) and can be a result of fluid depletion, heart failure, or vasodilation.

Key Factors

Δ **Pulse pressure** is the difference between the systolic and the diastolic pressure readings.

Δ **Postural (orthostatic) hypotension** is a BP that falls when a client changes position from lying to sitting or standing, and it may result from various causes (e.g., peripheral vasodilation, medication side effects, or fluid depletion).

- Orthostatic changes are assessed by taking the client's BP and HR in the supine position. Next, have the client change to the sitting or standing position, wait 1 to 5 min, and reassess the BP and HR. The client is experiencing orthostatic hypotension if the SBP decreases more than 20 mm Hg and/or the DBP decreases more than 10 mm Hg with a 10 to 20% increase in the heart rate (HR).

Δ **Age**

- **Infants** have a low BP that gradually increases with age.

- **Older children and adolescents** will have varying BP based on body size. Larger children will have a higher BP.

- **Older adult clients** may have a slightly elevated systolic pressure due to decreased elasticity of blood vessels.

Δ **Circadian (diurnal) rhythms** affect BP with BP usually being lowest in the early morning hours and peaking during the later part of the afternoon or evening.

Δ **Stress** associated with fear, emotional strain, and acute pain can increase BP.

Δ **Ethnicity** – African Americans have a higher incidence of hypertension in general and at earlier ages.

Δ **Gender** – Adolescent to middle-age men have higher BPs than their female counterparts. Postmenopausal women have higher BPs than their male counterparts.

Δ **Medications** such as opiates, antihypertensives, and cardiac medications can lower BP. Some illicit drugs (cocaine), cold medications, oral contraceptives, and antidepressants can raise BP.

Δ **Exercise** can cause a decrease in BP for several hours afterwards.

NANDA Nursing Diagnoses

Δ Activity intolerance

Δ Decreased cardiac output

Δ Deficient fluid volume

Δ Excess fluid volume

Δ Ineffective tissue perfusion

Nursing Interventions

Δ **Equipment**

- **The ausculatory method** uses a

  ◊ **Sphygmomanometer** with a pressure manometer (aneroid or mercury) and appropriate size cuff. The width of the cuff should be 40% of the arm circumference at the point where the cuff will be wrapped. The bladder (inside the cuff) should surround 80% of the arm circumference of an adult and the whole arm for a child. Cuffs that are **too large** will give a **false low** reading, and cuffs that are **too small** will give a **false high** reading.

  ◊ **Stethoscope**

- **Automatic BP** devices may be used when available for monitoring clients that need to be evaluated frequently. A BP should be obtained first using the ausculatory method to make sure the automatic device readings are valid.

Δ **Procedure (Ausculatory Method)**

- Wash hands and provide for privacy.

- Initially take BP readings in both arms. If the difference is greater than 10 mm Hg, use the arm with the higher reading for subsequent measurements. In addition, this difference may indicate a vascular problem and should be reported to the primary care provider.

Client should	Primary care provider should
• Not smoke or drink any caffeine for 30 min prior to measurement. • Rest for 5 min before measurement.	• Use the ausculatory method with a properly calibrated and validated instrument. • Use an appropriate cuff size. • Not take a BP in an arm with a running IV or on the side where a mastectomy has occurred.
Be seated on a chair, with feet flat on floor, back and arm supported, and arm at heart level.	• Average two or more readings, separated by at least 2 min. (If first two readings differ by > 5 mm Hg, additional readings should be obtained and averaged.) • After initial readings, take BP and pulse in the standing position.

- Apply the BP cuff **2 cm above the antecubital space** with the brachial artery in line with the marking on the cuff.

- Estimate systolic pressure by palpating the radial pulse and inflating the cuff until the pulse disappears. Inflate the cuff another 30 mm Hg, and slowly release the pressure to note when the pulse is palpable again (the estimated systolic pressure).

- Deflate the cuff and wait 1 min.

- Position the stethoscope over the brachial artery.

- Quickly inflate the cuff to 30 mm Hg above the palpated systolic pressure.

- Release the pressure no faster than 2 to 3 mm Hg per second.

- The level at which the **first clear sounds** are heard is the systolic pressure.

- Continue to deflate the cuff until the sounds **muffle and disappear** and note the **diastolic pressure**.

- Record systolic over diastolic (e.g., 110/70 mm Hg).

Δ   **Unexpected BP Readings**

- It is frequently helpful to retake the BP near the end of an encounter with the client. Earlier pressures may be higher due to the stress of being in an office setting or hospital.

- Recheck BPs that have been taken by assistive personnel or when an automatic device is used.

- The cuff needs to be completely deflated between attempts. Wait at least 1 full min before reinflating the cuff. Air trapped in the bladder can cause a false high reading.

- Notify the primary care provider if BP is above or below the client's usual value.

Complications and Nursing Interventions

Δ   **Orthostatic (Postural) Hypotension**

- Assess/monitor the client's BP.

- Instruct the client to press the call light button and not to get out of bed without assistance.

- Have the client sit at the edge of the bed for at least 1 min before standing up for at least 1 min.

- Assist with ambulation.

- Home care instructions include:

  ◊   Instructing the client that lightheadedness and dizziness can occur.

  ◊   Advising the client to sit or lie down if these symptoms occur.

  ◊   Advising the client to **get up slowly** when lying or sitting and **to avoid sudden changes in position**.

Δ   **Hypertension**

- Assess/monitor the client for other signs and symptoms (e.g., tachycardia, bradycardia, pain, anxiety). Primary hypertension is usually asymptomatic.

- Assess for identifiable causes of hypertension (e.g., renal disease, thyroid disease, medication).

- Administer pharmacological therapy as ordered by the primary care provider.

- Assess for risk factors.

- Encourage lifestyle modifications, which include:

  ◊ Smoking cessation.

  ◊ Dietary modifications – DASH (Dietary Approaches to Stop Hypertension) diet.

    ° Restrict sodium.

    ° Consume adequate potassium, calcium and magnesium. These minerals play a role in lowering BP.

    ° Restrict cholesterol and saturated fats.

  ◊ Weight control.

  ◊ Modification of alcohol intake.

  ◊ Physical activity.

  ◊ Stress reduction.

- Encourage the client to follow-up with the primary care provider for medication monitoring.

Primary Reference:

Potter, P. A., & Perry, A. G. (2005). *Fundamentals of nursing* (6th ed.). St. Louis, MO: Mosby.

Additional Resources:

Department of Health and Human Services, National Institutes of Health, and National Heart, Lung, and Blood Institute (2003). Seventh report of the joint national committee on prevention, detection, evaluation, and treatment of high blood pressure (JNC 7). Retrieved September 26, 2006, from *www.nhlbi.nih.gov/guidelines/hypertension/*

NANDA International (2004). *NANDA nursing diagnoses: Definitions and |classification 2005-2006.* Philadelphia: NANDA.

Chapter 26: Blood Pressure

Application Exercises

1. Determine whether each of the following factors increases or decreases the BP. Check the appropriate box.

Factor	Increases	Decreases
Cocaine		
A brisk walk on the treadmill		
Antihypertensives		
Acute gallbladder attack		
Postoperative pain		

2. For each of the following readings, identify the classification of BP according to the JNC 7.

_____ 132/94 mm Hg   A. Normal

_____ 108/72 mm Hg   B. Prehypertension

_____ 148/86 mm Hg   C. Stage 1 hypertension

_____ 172/92 mm Hg   D. Stage 2 hypertension

_____ 126/82 mm Hg

3. Which of the following techniques are correct when assessing a client's BP? (Select all that apply.)

_____ Have the client drink a cup of coffee prior to the check.

_____ Make sure the client has been sitting quietly for at least 5 min.

_____ Average two or more readings, separated by at least 2 min.

_____ Keep the room cold to ensure vasoconstriction.

_____ Avoid taking BP readings in an arm with a running IV.

4. A 30-year-old client presents to the clinic for the first time for a routine check-up. His health history is insignificant for any acute or chronic health problems. The client's initial averaged BP on arrival is 138/92 mm Hg. Is this reading significant? Why or why not? What course of action should the nurse take in regards to this reading?

5. A nurse is checking the vital signs of a newly admitted client with a broken femur. The client's BP is 140/94 mm Hg. The client denies a prior history of hypertension. The nurse's next step should be to

        A. ask the client if she is having pain.

        B. report the elevated BP to the primary care provider.

        C. return in 30 min to recheck the BP.

        D. check orthostatic BP.

6. A client is discovered to be hypovolemic with a BP of 80/48 mm Hg. Pulse rate is 98/min and regular, respirations are 28/min, oxygen saturation is 94% with oxygen at 2 L, and temperature is 37.5° C (99.5° F) axillary. Fluid boluses are being given while blood is being prepared by the laboratory. To monitor the client's response to the fluid boluses, the nurse should

        A. obtain an electrocardiogram.

        B. monitor blood glucose levels.

        C. obtain frequent BP readings using an automatic BP device.

        D. monitor urine output every hour by inserting a Foley catheter.

Chapter 26: Blood Pressure

Application Exercises Answer Key

1. Determine whether each of the following factors increases or decreases the BP. Check the appropriate box.

Factor	Increases	Decreases
Cocaine	X	
A brisk walk on the treadmill		X
Antihypertensives		X
Acute gallbladder attack	X	
Postoperative pain	X	

2. For each of the following readings, identify the classification of BP according to the JNC 7.

  __C__   132/94 mm Hg   A. Normal

  __A__   108/72 mm Hg   B. Prehypertension

  __C__   148/86 mm Hg   C. Stage 1 hypertension

  __D__   172/92 mm Hg   D. Stage 2 hypertension

  __B__   126/82 mm Hg

3. Which of the following techniques are correct when assessing a client's BP? (Select all that apply.)

  _____ Have the client drink a cup of coffee prior to the check.

  __X__ **Make sure the client has been sitting quietly for at least 5 min.**

  __X__ **Average two or more readings, separated by at least 2 min.**

  _____ Keep the room cold to ensure vasoconstriction.

  __X__ **Avoid taking BP readings in an arm with a running IV.**

When assessing the client's BP, it is important for the client to be resting quietly for at least 5 min, as activity increase BP. Two readings should be taken initially and averaged together. If the first two readings differ by > 5 mm Hg, additional readings should be obtained and averaged. The nurse should avoid using an arm with a running IV as the BP cuff pressure can cause damage to the vein. The client should refrain from drinking caffeine for 30 min prior to having BP checked. A cold environment can cause vasoconstriction that can cause a false high diastolic reading.

4. A 30-year-old client presents to the clinic for the first time for a routine check-up. His health history is insignificant for any acute or chronic health problems. The client's initial averaged BP on arrival is 138/92 mm Hg. Is this reading significant? Why or why not? What course of action should the nurse take in regards to this reading?

The reading is elevated but may not be significant. The BP should be taken again later during the exam. The client may have been anxious initially, and the BP may be lower later in the visit. If the averaged reading remains elevated, it should be reported to the primary care provider. This client will probably be asked to return in a week for a follow up BP check.

5. A nurse is checking the vital signs of a newly admitted client with a broken femur. The client's BP is 140/94 mm Hg. The client denies a prior history of hypertension. The nurse's next step should be to

      A. ask the client if she is having pain.

      B. report the elevated BP to the primary care provider.

      C. return in 30 min to recheck the BP.

      D. check orthostatic BP.

This client has a broken femur, and his BP may be elevated due to pain. The nurse should ask if he is having pain and continue a full pain assessment. If after treating his pain the client's BP is still elevated, the nurse should report this finding to the primary care provider. This client needs further assessment at this time, and coming back in 30 min is not appropriate. There is no indication for orthostatic pressures, and it might be difficult to have the client sit or stand with a broken femur.

6. A client is discovered to be hypovolemic with a BP of 80/48 mm Hg. Pulse rate is 98/min and regular, respirations are 28/min, oxygen saturation is 94% with oxygen at 2 L, and temperature is 37.5° C (99.5° F) axillary. Fluid boluses are being given while blood is being prepared by the laboratory. To monitor the client's response to the fluid boluses, the nurse should

      A. obtain an electrocardiogram.

      B. monitor blood glucose levels.

      C. obtain frequent BP readings using an automatic BP device.

      D. monitor urine output every hour by inserting a Foley catheter.

The client is hypotensive and is being treated with fluid boluses. The nurse will be monitoring for an increase in BP. After obtaining an initial BP by the ausculatory method, this client's BP needs to be monitored frequently. The use of an automatic BP device will facilitate obtaining these readings. There is no indication for an electrocardiogram or to monitor blood glucose levels. Hourly output may be an important assessment, but the desired response is an elevated BP. Also, there is no indication for insertion of a Foley catheter.

Unit 2   Health Assessment

Section: System-Specific Assessment

Chapter 27:   Health History

Contributor: Sally Swenson, MA, RN

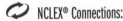 NCLEX® Connections:

> **Learning Objective**: Review and apply knowledge within "**Health History**" in readiness for performance of the following nursing activities as outlined by the NCLEX® test plans:
>
> Δ   Obtain health history information by collecting relevant health care data from the client and family.
>
> Δ   Use therapeutic communication to assess the client's current health status.
>
> Δ   Identify the client's response to past/current health problems and prescribed treatments.
>
> Δ   Recognize the client's risk for acute and chronic health complications.
>
> Δ   Identify the client's lifestyle practices and how they impact illness prevention and early detection.
>
> Δ   Document a comprehensive health history and review of systems using appropriate agency format.
>
> Δ   Maintain confidentiality of all client information.

 Key Points

Δ   Comprehensive health histories are part of the health assessment process.

Δ   The health history provides subjective data relevant to the client's health status and is best obtained from the client. Additional sources include the family, medical records, and other primary care providers.

Δ   Data collected should be descriptive, concise, complete, and relevant.

Δ   Assessment is the first step of the nursing process, beginning with the first encounter, continuing throughout the nurse-client relationship.

Δ   The health history is obtained during a client interview, which is part of the assessment step of the nursing process.

Δ   Health history information is usually obtained using agency format and protocols.

Key Procedural Points

Δ **Interviewing techniques** involve introducing the purpose of the interview to the client, information gathering, testing hypotheses by asking for more specific information, and then concluding the interview by summarizing the findings with the client.

- **Therapeutic communication techniques** assist the nurse in developing rapport with the client. The techniques encourage a trusting relationship, whereby the client feels comfortable telling her story.

  ◊ Therapeutic techniques include active listening, use of open-ended questions, clarifying, and summarizing.

  ◊ **Active listening** – shows the client that he has the nurse's undivided attention.

  ◊ **Open-ended questions** – used initially to encourage the client to tell her story in her own way. Questions should be asked using a language the client can understand.

  ◊ **Clarifying** – allows the nurse to question the client about specific details in greater depth or direct the client toward relevant parts of the history.

  ◊ **Summarizing** – allows the client to validate the story the nurse has gathered as accurate.

Δ Nontherapeutic techniques include giving advice, ignoring feelings, and offering false reassurance.

Components of the Health History

Demographic information	• Identifying data includes: ◊ Name, address, and phone number. ◊ Birth date and age. ◊ Gender. ◊ Race and ethnic origin. ◊ Marital status. ◊ Occupation. ◊ Family/significant others living at home.
Source of history	• This usually comes from the client, but family members or other medical records can provide useful information. • Note the reliability of the historian.
Chief concern	This is a brief statement in the client's own words of why he is seeking care.
History of present illness	• This history is a detailed, chronological description of the problem(s) that led to the chief complaint. The description should start at the farthest point in time and work toward the present. • Details about the symptom(s), such as location, quality, quantity, setting, timing, alleviating or aggravating factors, and associated phenomenon are important aspects to explore with the client.

Past health history and current health status	• Childhood illnesses – both communicable and chronic • Medical, surgical, obstetrical, gynecological, and psychiatric history including time frames, diagnoses, hospitalizations, and treatments • Current immunization status and the dates and results of any screening tests • Allergies – medication, environmental, food • Current medications – prescription, over-the-counter, vitamins, supplements, and time of last dose(s) taken.
Family history	• This history includes health information of immediate relatives such as grandparents, parents, siblings, children, and grandchildren. Current ages or age at death are recorded, as well as diseases or conditions that were or are present in family members.
Social history	• This is information regarding the relationships important to the client, concerns regarding his present living or work situations, financial status, and ability to perform activities of daily living (ADLs).
Health promotion behaviors	• Exercise/activity, diet, sun exposure, wearing of safety equipment, substance use, stress

Δ   **Review of systems** ascertains information about the functioning of all the client's body systems. Related or other health problems may be discovered at this time. This part of the history is usually very extensive and can be incorporated into the physical exam as each body system is examined.

System	Questions to Be Asked
Integumentary	• Do you have any skin diseases? • Do you have any itching, bruising, lumps, hair loss, nail changes, or sores? • Do you have any allergies? • How do you care for your hair, skin, and nails? • Do you use lotions, soaps, and/or sunscreen?
Head and neck	• Are you having any pain? • Are you able to move your head and shoulders with ease? • Are any of your lymph nodes swollen? • Have you noticed any unusual facial movements?
Eyes	• How is your vision? • Have you noticed any changes? • Do you ever have discharge from your eyes? • Do you wear glasses or contact lenses? • When was your last eye exam?

Ears, nose, mouth and throat	• How well do you hear? • Have you noticed any changes in your hearing? • Do you wear a hearing aid? • Do you ever experience tinnitus, discharge, vertigo, or pain? • Do you have a history of ear infections? • Are you having any pain, stuffiness, or discharge from your nose? • Do you ever experience nose bleeds? • Have you noticed any change in your sense of smell or taste? • How often do you go to the dentist? • Do you have dentures? • Do you have any problems with your gums? • Do you have any difficulty swallowing or problems with hoarseness or sore throat?
Breasts	• Do you perform self-breast exams? • Do you have any tenderness or lumps in your breast(s)? • Do you have any discharge from the nipples?
Respiratory	• Do you have any difficulties breathing? • Do you need to sit up to breath? • Are you ever short of breath? • Have you been around anyone who has a cold, flu, or cough? • Do you smoke?
Cardiovascular	• Do you have any problems with your heart? • Do you ever have pain in your chest? • Do you have high cholesterol or high blood pressure? • Do you have any swelling in your feet and ankles?
Gastrointestinal	• Do you have any problems with your stomach, such as nausea, vomiting, or pain? • Do you have any problems with your bowels, such as diarrhea or constipation? • When was your last bowel movement? • Have you had any recent weight changes? • Do you have any food intolerances? • What is your 24-hr food history?
Genitourinary	• Do you have any difficulties voiding, such as burning, incontinence, urgency, frequency, nocturia, or hesitancy? • Have you noticed any change in the color of your urine? • Have you noticed any changes in your menstrual cycle, such as cramps, discharge, or itching? • Have you experienced painful intercourse? • Have you experienced any sexual dysfunction? • Have you had any pain in the scrotum or testes?
Musculoskeletal	• Have you noticed any pain in your joints or muscles? • Have you experienced any weakness or twitching? • Have you had any recent falls? • Are you able to care for yourself?

Neurological	• Do you have any problems with dizziness or headaches? • Do you ever have seizures? • Do you ever have any weakness, tremors, numbness, or tingling anywhere?
Mental health	• Is there anything stressful going on at work or at home? • Do you feel as though you are having any problems with depression? • Have you experienced any recent losses? • Are you having any problems concentrating?
Endocrine	• Have you noticed any change in voiding patterns? • Have you noticed any change in your energy level? • Have you noticed any change in your ability to handle stress? • Have you experienced any change in weight or appetite? • Have you had any visual disturbances? • Have you experienced any palpitations?
Allergic/ immunologic	• Do you have any allergies to medications, foods, or environmental substances? • Did you receive a flu or pneumonia shot? • Have you ever received a blood transfusion? If so, did you suffer any reaction?

Documentation

Δ   Inform the client that note taking will take place during the interview.

Δ   To facilitate note taking during the interview, summarize information for future clarification. Do not rely on total memory recall.

Δ   Document descriptive, concise, complete, and relevant data.

Δ   Reassure client that confidentiality will be maintained.

Δ   Use guidelines for good charting.

Primary Reference:

Potter, P. A., & Perry, A. G. (2005). *Fundamentals of nursing* (6th ed.). St. Louis, MO: Mosby.

Additional Resources:

Bickley, L. S., & Szilagyi, P. G. (2003). *Bates' guide to physical examination and history taking* (8th ed.). Philadelphia: Lippincott Williams & Wilkins.

Jarvis, C., (2004). *Physical examination & health assessment.* (4th ed.). St. Louis, MO: Saunders.

NANDA International (2004). *NANDA nursing diagnoses: Definitions and classification 2005-2006.* Philadelphia: NANDA.

Chapter 27: Health History

Application Exercises

1. Which of the following is an effective technique to use when interviewing a client?

    A. Start the interview with "nonthreatening" topics.

    B. Use only nondirective questions.

    C. Have the client fill out a printed nursing history form.

    D. Ask questions word for word from the history form.

2. A client presents with severe headache pain. Identify what questions the nurse should ask to obtain information regarding a symptom analysis.

Location	
Quality	
Quantity	
Timing	
Setting	
Alleviating or aggravating factors	
Associated phenomenon	

3. The history of the present illness is

    A. information about family members with the same health problem.

    B. extensive information about a body system.

    C. the primary care provider's report of the client.

    D. a chronological description of the client's chief concern.

4. A client expresses concern to the nurse over the confidentiality of the information she is providing during her health history. The nurse should respond by telling the client

    A. exactly with whom the information will be shared.

    B. that it is required for her to give any information that is requested.

    C. a confidential piece of information about herself.

    D. not to worry about anything.

5. A client has come in for a routine health assessment without having a specific health concern. Identify open-ended questions that the nurse could ask to encourage the client to talk further about his health.

6. Which of the following is the most important reason for a nurse to obtain a health history from a client who has just been admitted to the medical unit?

    A. The client's health history must be documented for insurance reimbursement.

    B. The health history assists the primary care provider to categorize clients with similar health problems.

    C. The health history gives the nurse an opportunity to provide health promotion teaching.

    D. The client's health history facilitates development of a mutually agreed-upon plan of care.

Chapter 27: Health History

Application Exercises Answer Key

1. Which of the following is an effective technique to use when interviewing a client?

   A. Start the interview with "nonthreatening" topics.
   B. Use only nondirective questions.
   C. Have the client fill out a printed nursing history form.
   D. Ask questions word for word from the history form.

   Starting the interview with nonthreatening topics will facilitate establishing rapport and trust between the client and nurse. Using nondirective questions may make the client feel comfortable, but may allow the client to avoid discussing important details. Having the client fill out a history form and asking questions word for word may discourage the establishment of a therapeutic relationship with the client.

2. A client presents with severe headache pain. Identify what questions the nurse should ask to obtain information regarding a symptom analysis.

Location	**Where is your headache? Point to where it hurts.**
Quality	**What does the pain feel like? Is it dull, stabbing, throbbing, and/or achy?**
Quantity	**On a scale of 0 to 10, with 0 being no pain and 10 being the worst pain you have ever experienced, how would you rate the pain?**
Timing	**When did the pain start? How long have you had it? Is it constant or intermittent?**
Setting	**Where are you when you experience the pain? Does it happen at work? At home?**
Alleviating or aggravating factors	**What makes the pain better or worse? Have you taken any medications for the pain?**
Associated phenomenon	**Do you have any nausea? Are you dizzy?**

3. The history of the present illness is

> A. information about family members with the same health problem.
>
> B. extensive information about a body system.
>
> C. the primary care provider's report of the client.
>
> **D. a chronological description of the client's chief concern.**

The history of the present illness is a chronological description of the client's chief concern starting from the farthest point in time moving to the present. Family member information is part of the family history. Information about body systems is part of the review of systems. The primary care provider's report is more inclusive than the history of the present illness.

4. A client expresses concern to the nurse over the confidentiality of the information she is providing during her health history. The nurse should respond by telling the client

> **A. exactly with whom the information will be shared.**
>
> B. that it is required for her to give any information that is requested.
>
> C. a confidential piece of information about herself.
>
> D. not to worry about anything.

The client has a right to confidentiality and the right to know with whom her information will be shared. The client has the right to refuse to reveal information if she chooses. The nurse telling the client confidential information about herself is not professional. Telling the client not to worry discounts the client's concerns.

5. A client has come in for a routine health assessment without having a specific health concern. Identify open-ended questions that the nurse could ask to encourage the client to talk further about his health.

Was there a specific reason you wanted a physical exam done at this time?

What made you decide to come in for your physical exam?

What concerns do you have about your health?

6. Which of the following is the most important reason for a nurse to obtain a health history from a client who has just been admitted to the medical unit?

    A. The client's health history must be documented for insurance reimbursement.

    B. The health history assists the primary care provider to categorize clients with similar health problems.

    C. The health history gives the nurse an opportunity to provide health promotion teaching.

    D. The client's health history facilitates development of a mutually agreed-upon plan of care.

The nurse obtains a health history to identify current health problems and uses the information to set mutually agreed-upon goals and plan care. Documentation for insurance reimbursement may be required but is not the most important reason for obtaining the client's health history. The primary care provider will use personal health information only for the care of that individual. Health teaching may take place while the nurse is obtaining the health history, but the nurse first needs to know what health promotion teaching the client needs. This is identified during the health history.

Unit 2   Health Assessment
Section: System-Specific Assessment

Chapter 28:   General Survey
                Contributor: Sally Swenson, MA, RN

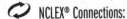 **NCLEX® Connections:**

Learning Objective: Review and apply knowledge within **"General Survey"** in readiness for performance of the following nursing activities as outlined by the NCLEX® test plans:

Δ   Perform the appropriate assessment of the client's general health status, measurements, and vital signs.

Δ   Assess/monitor the client's physical appearance, body structure, mobility, and behavior.

Δ   Assess/monitor measurements and vital signs by obtaining baseline data and comparing with subsequent findings.

Δ   Use therapeutic communication to assess the client's current health status.

Δ   Identify emergent health concerns and intervene as appropriate.

Δ   Document baseline and subsequent findings according to hospital protocol.

 Key Points

Δ   **Therapeutic techniques for health assessment** are meant to foster communication and create an environment conducive for an optimal health assessment experience for the client.

•   The nurse introduces himself/herself and the various parts of the assessment to the client.

•   For very ill or older adult clients, perform assessments in several shorter segments to avoid overtiring them.

•   When possible, start by asking for the health history, performing the general survey, and taking vital signs to build a rapport with the client prior to doing more sensitive parts of the exam.

•   Avoid the use of medical jargon, and use therapeutic communication techniques to encourage the client to talk freely about his health.

- When observing verbal or nonverbal expressions of discomfort, try to position the client comfortably before proceeding with the rest of the assessment.

- Provide privacy while performing the exam, using a gown or draping the client with a sheet to visualize only one section of the body at a time.

- Inform or warn the client as to the various techniques to be used prior to performing those parts of the exam.

- Ensure for adequate lighting and room temperature.

- Reduce environmental noises (TV, radio, visitors talking) to enhance communication and eliminate distractions.

- Share findings with the client, taking cues to determine how much information the client desires.

Δ **General survey** is a written summary of the nurse's impression of the client's overall state of health. The nurse gathers this information from the first encounter with the client and continues to make observations throughout the assessment process. The nurse will assess:

- **Physical appearance**.

  ◊ Age

  ◊ Gender and race

  ◊ Level of consciousness

  ◊ Color of skin

  ◊ Facial features

  ◊ Signs of distress (e.g., pallor, labored breathing, guarding)

- **Body structure**.

  ◊ Body build, stature, height, and weight

  ◊ Nutritional status

  ◊ Symmetry of body parts

  ◊ Posture and usual position

  ◊ Gross abnormalities (e.g., skin lesions, amputations)

- **Mobility**.

  ◊ Gait

  ◊ Range of motion

  ◊ Motor activity

- **Behavior** to include:
  - ◊ Facial expression and mannerisms.
  - ◊ Mood and affect.
  - ◊ Speech.
  - ◊ Dress, hygiene, grooming, and odors (body and breath).
- **Vital signs**.
  - ◊ Temperature
  - ◊ Pulse
  - ◊ Respiration
  - ◊ Blood pressure

Sample Documentation

Client – 16-year-old male, alert and oriented x 3. No distress noted. Personal hygiene and grooming slightly unkept but appropriate to age. Weight appropriate to height, good posture and steady gait. Does not maintain good eye contact. Volunteers no information but answers questions appropriately when asked.

Primary Reference:

Potter, P. A., & Perry, A. G. (2005). *Fundamentals of nursing* (6th ed.). St. Louis, MO: Mosby.

Additional Resources:

Bickley, L. S., & Szilagyi, P. G. (2003). *Bates' guide to physical examination and history taking* (8th ed.). Philadelphia: Lippincott Williams & Wilkins.

Jarvis, C. (2004). *Physical examination & health assessment* (4th ed.). St. Louis, MO: Saunders.

NANDA International (2004). *NANDA nursing diagnoses: Definitions and classification 2005-2006*. Philadelphia: NANDA.

Chapter 28: General Survey

Application Exercises

1. Which of the following therapeutic techniques is/are used to provide a comfortable environment for performing a health assessment? (Select all that apply.)

_____ Provide privacy.

_____ Examine sensitive areas first.

_____ Reduce environmental noises.

_____ Explain various techniques before they are performed.

_____ Use medical jargon to save time.

2. Place the number of the general survey component next to the area to be assessed. Each component can be used twice.

_____ Level of consciousness

_____ Gait

_____ Symmetry of body parts

_____ Facial features

_____ Speech

_____ Motor activity

_____ Dress and grooming

_____ Posture

1. Physical appearance

2. Body structure

3. Mobility

4. Behavior

Chapter 28: General Survey

Application Exercises Answer Key

1. Which of the following therapeutic techniques is/are used to provide a comfortable environment for performing a health assessment? (Select all that apply.)

  X   **Provide privacy.**

        Examine sensitive areas first.

  X   **Reduce environmental noises.**

  X   **Explain various techniques before they are performed.**

        Use medical jargon to save time.

Providing for privacy, reducing environmental noises, and explaining techniques to be used will facilitate establishing a trusting relationship and performing a health assessment. Sensitive areas should be examined after the client has developed some trust and feels more comfortable. Medical jargon may confuse the client and lead to misunderstanding of the intended message.

2. Place the number of the general survey component next to the area to be assessed. Each component can be used twice.

1 Level of consciousness		1. Physical appearance
3 Gait		
2 Symmetry of body parts		2. Body structure
1 Facial features		
4 Speech		3. Mobility
3 Motor activity		
4 Dress and grooming		4. Behavior
2 Posture		

Unit 2   Health Assessment
Section: System-Specific Assessment

Chapter 29:   Physical Assessment Techniques
                 Contributor: Sally Swenson, MA, RN

 NCLEX® Connections:

> **Learning Objective**: Review and apply knowledge within "**Physical Assessment Techniques**" in readiness for performance of the following nursing activities as outlined by the NCLEX® test plans:
>
> Δ   Perform physical assessments using the techniques of inspection, palpation, percussion, and auscultation.
>
> Δ   Recognize normal and abnormal findings when performing a physical assessment on a client.
>
> Δ   Identify the appropriate equipment needed to perform a physical assessment.

 Key Points

Δ   Guidelines to facilitate performing a physical assessment include:

   •   Using good lighting.

   •   Providing a quiet and comfortable environmental temperature.

   •   Looking and observing before touching.

   •   Keeping nails short and hands and stethoscope warm.

   •   Completely exposing the body part to be inspected while draping the client appropriately.

   •   Abstaining from feeling or listening through clothing (Clothing can obscure or create sounds.).

   •   Preparing all necessary equipment and having it readily available.

   •   Using standard precautions when in contact with body fluids, wound drainage, and open lesions.

   •   Writing down any values that may be forgotten by the end of the exam.

Δ   Assessment techniques are done in the **order of inspection, palpation, percussion, and auscultation** when all four techniques are needed. The **exception is the abdomen,** which is examined using **inspection, auscultation, percussion, and palpation**. Percussion and palpation are delayed to avoid changing normally occurring bowel sounds.

Key Procedural Points

Δ   Inspection

- **Inspection**, which is the first step in an assessment, begins the minute the nurse first interacts with the client and continues throughout the rest of the examination.

- A penlight, an otoscope, ophthalmoscopes, or another lighted instrument may enhance the process.

- Inspection involves using the sense of vision, smell, and hearing to observe and detect any normal or abnormal findings in the client.

Δ   **Palpation** is the touching of the client to determine the size, consistency, texture, temperature, location, and tenderness of an organ or body part.

- Light palpation, < 1 cm, is required for most body surfaces. Deeper palpation is used to assess abdominal organs or masses.

- Various parts of the hands are used to detect the different sensations.

  ◊   The **dorsal surface** is the most sensitive to temperature.

  ◊   The **ulnar surface and base of fingers** are sensitive to vibration.

  ◊   **Finger tips** are sensitive to pulsation, position, texture, size, and consistency.

  ◊   The **fingers and thumb** are used to grab an organ or mass.

- Starting with light palpation, be systematic, calm, and gentle. Proceed to deep palpation if indicated.

Δ   **Percussion** involves the tapping of body parts with fingers, fists, or small instruments to evaluate the size, location, tenderness, and presence or absence of fluid or air in body organs.

- **Techniques for percussion include:**

  ◊   **Direct percussion,** which involves the examiner producing sounds by striking the client's body to illicit sounds.

  ◊   Indirect **percussion,** which uses the examiner's hand placed flatly on the client's body as the striking surface for sound production.

  ◊   **Fist percussion,** which is used to assess for tenderness over the kidneys, liver, and gallbladder.

- The sounds produced are evaluated for amplitude or intensity (loud or soft), pitch or frequency (high or low), duration (time the sound lasts), and quality (what it sounds like).

Δ **Auscultation** is the technique used to listen to sounds produced by the body. Some sounds may be loud enough to be heard unaided, but most sounds require a stethoscope, and on occasion, a Doppler technique to assess accurately (e.g., heart sounds, air moving through the respiratory tract, blood moving through blood vessels). The examiner must learn to isolate the various sounds produced by the body to make accurate assessments.

- The sounds produced are evaluated for amplitude or intensity (loud or soft), pitch or frequency (high or low), duration (time the sound lasts), and quality (what it sounds like).

- The diaphragm of the stethoscope is used to listen to high-pitched sounds (e.g., normal heart sounds, bowel sounds, breath sounds).

  ◊ The diaphragm should be placed firmly on the body part being examined.

- The bell of the stethoscope is used to listen to low-pitched sounds (e.g., abnormal heart sounds, bruits).

  ◊ The bell should be placed lightly on the body part being examined.

Equipment

Δ Equipment needed for a screening exam includes:

- Scale with height measurement.
- Thermometer.
- Stethoscope with diaphragm and bell.
- Sphygmomanometer.
- Reading chart.
- Otoscope/ophthalmoscope and nasal speculum.
- Penlight (can use ophthalmoscope).
- Cotton balls.
- Sharp/dull object.
- Tuning fork.
- Glass of water.
- Items to test smell and taste.
- Clean gloves.
- Tongue depressor.

- Reflex hammer.

- Marking pen.

- Measuring tape and clear, flexible ruler with measurements in centimeters.

Primary Reference:

Potter, P. A., & Perry, A. G. (2005). *Fundamentals of nursing* (6th ed.). St. Louis, MO: Mosby.

Additional Resources:

Bickley, L. S., & Szilagyi, P. G. (2003). *Bates' guide to physical examination and history taking* (8th ed.). Philadelphia: Lippincott Williams & Wilkins.

Jarvis, C. (2004). *Physical examination & health assessment.* (4th ed.). St. Louis, MO: Saunders.

NANDA International (2004). *NANDA nursing diagnoses: Definitions and classification 2005-2006.* Philadelphia: NANDA.

Chapter 29: Physical Assessment Techniques

Application Exercises

1. Identify the location where the following percussion sounds are normally produced in the body.

Percussion Sound	Expected Location to be Heard
Tympany	
Resonance	
Dull	
Flat	

2. Put an X in the box for the appropriate assessment technique(s) used to assess each of the following. (Select all that apply.)

Assessment	Inspection	Palpation	Percussion	Auscultation
Pupil size				
Ankle edema				
Skin temperature				
Bowel sounds				
Loose teeth				
Liver size				
External ear				
Kidney tenderness				

3. The nurse should use which part of the hand to assess for vibration?

        A. Ulnar surface

        B. Finger pads

        C. Dorsal surface

        D. Palmar surface

4. Which of the following is true regarding inspection?

    A. Very little information is provided.

    B. Adequate time should be allowed.

    C. It must be done quickly to avoid making the client uncomfortable.

    D. It can be eliminated if the client is too modest.

5. The correct order for performing assessment techniques for the abdomen is

    A. inspection, palpation, percussion, and auscultation.

    B. inspection, auscultation, percussion, and palpation.

    C. auscultation, inspection, percussion, and palpation.

    D. auscultation, palpation, percussion, and inspection.

Chapter 29: Physical Assessment Techniques

Application Exercises Answer Key

1. Identify the location where the following percussion sounds are normally produced in the body.

Percussion Sound	Expected Location to be Heard
Tympany	**Gastric bubble**
Resonance	**Lungs**
Dull	**Liver**
Flat	**Muscles**

2. Put an X in the box for the appropriate assessment technique(s) used to assess each of the following. (Select all that apply.)

Assessment	Inspection	Palpation	Percussion	Auscultation
Pupil size	X			
Ankle edema	X	X		
Skin temperature		X		
Bowel sounds				X
Loose teeth	X	X		
Liver size		X	X	
External ear	X	X		
Kidney tenderness			X	

3. The nurse should use which part of the hand to assess for vibration?

A. Ulnar surface

B. Finger pads

C. Dorsal surface

D. Palmar surface

The ulnar surface of the hand is the most sensitive to vibration.

4. Which of the following is true regarding inspection?

    A. Very little information is provided.

    B. Adequate time should be allowed.

    C. It must be done quickly to avoid making the client uncomfortable.

    D. It can be eliminated if the client is too modest.

Inspection reveals a great deal of information, and the nurse should devote adequate time during the physical examination for inspection. It is a necessary component of the physical exam.

5. The correct order for performing assessment techniques for the abdomen is

    A. inspection, palpation, percussion, and auscultation.

    B. inspection, auscultation, percussion, and palpation.

    C. auscultation, inspection, percussion, and palpation.

    D. auscultation, palpation, percussion, and inspection.

The abdomen is examined using inspection, auscultation, percussion, and palpation. Percussion and palpation are delayed to avoid changing normally occurring bowel sounds.

Unit 2   Health Assessment
Section: System-Specific Assessment

Chapter 30:	Skin, Hair, and Nails
	Contributor: Sally Swenson, MA, RN

 NCLEX® Connections:

Learning Objective: Review and apply knowledge within "**Skin, Hair, and Nails**" in readiness for performance of the following nursing activities as outlined by the NCLEX® test plans:

Δ   Use effective communication to collect history assessment data related to the client's skin, hair, and nails.

Δ   Perform the appropriate assessment of the client's skin, hair, and nails within the nursing role, including:

- Preparing the client for the procedure.

- Client teaching (before and following the procedure).

- Using accurate equipment and technique based on the client's needs.

Δ   Assess/monitor the client's status by obtaining baseline data and comparing with subsequent findings.

Δ   Identify factors that influence the client's skin, hair, and nails.

Δ   Document baseline and subsequent findings according to hospital protocol.

Δ   Maintain confidentiality of all client information.

 Key Points

Δ   In the case of infants, skin assessment can be done all at once. In adults, it is generally easier to complete the skin assessment in segments as other parts of the body are being evaluated. Examine the upper extremities when the client is sitting or recumbent. Remove stockings/socks, and drape the client to expose the entire lower extremity at once.

Δ   Comparisons should be made from **side to side** to evaluate for any variations.

Δ   **Lesions** should be examined **individually**, using appropriate terminology when documenting.

Δ   **Braden scale** or a similar assessment tool can be used to predict the risk for pressure ulcer formation.

Key Procedural Points

Δ   **Inspection and palpation** are typically performed simultaneously.

Δ   Equipment needed for a thorough skin assessment includes:

◊   Adequate lighting.

◊   Gloves, which are used for the palpation of open or draining lesions.

◊   A flexible ruler or tape measure to measure the size and depth of lesions in centimeters.

Health History – Review of systems

Δ   Questions the nurse should ask include:

- Have you noticed any changes in your skin color? If so, is the change generalized or localized?

- Do you have a rash? Where is it located? Does it itch? How long has it been present? What have you used to treat the rash?

- Is your skin excessively dry or oily? Does this change with the seasons? Do you use anything to treat it?

- Have you developed any new moles or lesions? Have any of the moles or lesions changed in any way (e.g., color, borders, and/or size)?

- How often are you out in the sun? Do you use sunscreen?

- Do you have any swelling? If in your legs, is it present in both legs? Does the swelling cause pain? What do you do to relieve the swelling? Does it occur at any particular time of day?

Inspection and Palpation

Δ   **Assess color** of the client's hair, nails, and skin for uniformity. Hair color may vary due to dyes or from aging changes. The nails should appear pink. Normal skin color varies from ivory to ruddy to deep brown. Common color variations in the skin can occur as follows:

Color Change	Description	Indication
Pallor	Loss of color	Anemia or lack of blood flow
Cyanosis	Bluish	Hypoxia or impaired venous return
Jaundice	Yellow-orange of skin, sclera, and mucous membranes	Liver dysfunction, red blood-cell destruction
Erythema	Redness	Inflammation

Δ Palpate **temperature** of the skin with the dorsal part of the hand; check for symmetry. The client's skin should feel warm. Changes may reflect circulation impairment or environmental temperature.

Δ **Texture** of the client's skin should be smooth, soft, and even when palpated. The nails should be firm and smooth. Hair texture should be smooth and coarse or fine.

Δ Assess **skin turgor** by lifting and releasing a fold of skin on the forearm or sternum to evaluate that it returns quickly into place. Tenting is a delay in the skin returning to its normal place. Poor turgor may indicate dehydration or be a sign of aging.

Δ **Moisture** in the axillae can be a normal finding. Otherwise, the skin should be dry. Diaphoresis, oiliness, or excessive dryness should be noted.

Δ **Edema** is the presence of fluid in the tissues causing swollen, tight, and shiny skin surfaces. The swelling should be assessed for discoloration, location, and tenderness. In the extremities, the circumference of the swollen body area should be measured and compared to the other side.

• Common clinical practice includes grading the level of pitting edema present. Use agency grading scale. This grading is somewhat subjective as findings may vary from examiner to examiner. Findings are most reliable when performed as serial exams by the same examiner.

• Evaluate pitting by compressing the skin for at least 5 sec over a bony prominence (e.g., behind medial malleolus, dorsum of foot, or over shin) and then assess.

Four-point Scale	Degree	Response
1+	2 mm – trace	Rapid
2+	4 mm – mild	10 to 15 sec
3+	6 mm – moderate	1 to 2 min
4+	8 mm – severe	2 to 5 min

Δ **Examine lesions** for size, color, shape, consistency, elevation, location, distribution, configuration, tenderness, and presence of fluid or drainage. Any change noted should be reported to the primary care provider. Lesions commonly occur in healthy individuals.

• **Primary lesions** arise from healthy skin tissue. Common examples include:

Lesions	Descriptions	Examples
Macule	Nonpalpable, skin color change, < 1 cm	Freckle
Papule	Palpable, circumscribed , < 0.5 cm	Elevated nevi
Nodule/tumor	Palpable, circumscribed, 0.5 cm or >	Wart
Vesicle	Serous fluid-filled, < 1 cm	Blister
Pustule	Pus filled	Acne
Wheal	Palpable, irregular borders, edematous	Mosquito bite

- **Secondary lesions** result from a change in a primary lesion. Common examples include:

Lesions	Descriptions	Examples
Erosion	Lost epidermis, moist surface, no bleeding	Ruptured vesicle
Crust	Dried blood, serum, or pus	Scab
Scale	Flakes of skin that exfoliate	Dandruff or psoriasis
Fissure	Linear crack	Tinea pedis
Ulcer	Loss of epidermis and dermis with possible bleeding and scarring	Venous stasis ulcer

Δ   Common examples of skin lesions in various age groups include:

Children	Adults	Older Adults
• Diaper dermatitis • Intertrigo • Impetigo • Atopic dermatitis (eczema)	• Primary contact dermatitis • Tinea pedis (ringworm of the foot) • Psoriasis • Labial herpes simplex (cold sores)	• Lentigines (liver spots) • Seborrheic keratosis • Acrochordons (skin tags) • Sebaceous hyperplasia

- **Vascular lesions** are created with aging changes or when damage occurs to the blood vessels in or near the skin. Common examples include:

Lesions	Descriptions
Spider angioma	Red center with radiating legs that are red, up to 2 cm, and can be raised
Cherry angioma	Red, 1 to 3 cm, round, and can be raised
Spider vein	Bluish, spider-shaped or may be linear, with up to several inches in size
Petechia/purpura	Deep reddish purple, flat, petechia = 1 to 3 mm, purpura > 3 mm
Ecchymosis	Purple fading to green or yellow over time, variable in size, and flat
Hematoma	Raised ecchymosis

Δ   Note **cleanliness** of the client's hair, skin, and nails, as well as any odors. The nail base should be firm to palpation. Note the curvature of the nail plate in relationship to the tissue just before the cuticle. The angles should be ≤ 160 **Clubbing** is an abnormal curvature of the nail with an angle ≥ 160°. This can result from conditions with chronic low oxygen saturation (e.g., emphysema, chronic bronchitis).

Δ   Document **infestations** of the hair or skin.

Δ   Note **hair distribution** patterns. If hair loss is present, it should be symmetrical as with male pattern baldness.

Δ   **Capillary refill** assesses circulation to the periphery. Blanching the nail bed with firm pressure and then quick release should result in a brisk return of pink color.

NANDA Nursing Diagnoses

Δ   Impaired skin integrity

Δ   Risk for infection

Δ   Pain

Δ   Disturbed body image

Δ   Deficient knowledge

Sample Documentation

Skin is pink, warm, and dry. Turgor is brisk and skin is elastic. Rough, thickened skin over heels, elbows, and knees, otherwise, skin is smooth. A 0.5 cm brown papule on right forearm and a 2.5 cm long scar on left knee that is well-healed. Scalp is dry with slight dandruff noted. Hair is brown, clean, smooth, straight, and evenly distributed on the head. Axillary and pubic hair is evenly distributed with no infestations noted. Nails are short and firm with no clubbing noted. Capillary refill is < 3 sec. No edema is noted.

Primary Reference:

Potter, P. A., & Perry, A. G. (2005). *Fundamentals of nursing* (6th ed.). St. Louis, MO: Mosby.

Additional Resources:

Bickley, L. S., & Szilagyi, P. G. (2003). *Bates' guide to physical examination and history taking* (8th ed.). Philadelphia: Lippincott Williams & Wilkins.

Jarvis, C. (2004). *Physical examination & health assessment.* (4th ed.). St. Louis, MO: Saunders.

NANDA International (2004). *NANDA nursing diagnoses: Definitions and classification 2005-2006.* Philadelphia: NANDA.

          Fundamentals for Nursing

Chapter 30: Skin, Hair, and Nails

Application Exercises

1. Match the type of lesion commonly seen on a skin assessment with its correct assessment terminology.

_____	Freckle	A. Wheal
_____	Wart	B. Macule
_____	Blister	C. Nodule
_____	Acne	D. Pustule
_____	Psoriasis	E. Scale
_____	Mosquito bite	F. Vesicle

2. A client presents to the clinic wanting a lesion on his neck evaluated. List the assessments that should be documented about the lesion.

3. Which of the following assessments should be considered an abnormal finding during a skin assessment?

   A. No clubbing noted

   B. Brisk capillary refill

   C. 3+ pitting edema in feet bilaterally

   D. Numerous light brown macules, < 3 mm in size, located on nose and cheeks

4. A client's skin temperature is best assessed by using which part of the hand?

   A. Fingertips

   B. Dorsal surface

   C. Palmar surface

   D. Base of the hand

5. Match the term in the left column with its definition from the right column. Each letter can only be used once.

_____	Jaundice	A. Paleness, absence of color
_____	Erythema	B. Yellowish appearance of the skin
_____	Cyanosis	C. Redness of the skin
_____	Pallor	D. Grayish blue tone

6. Which of the following questions should the nurse ask the client to assess health promotion patterns related to the skin?

    A. "How does your skin feel?"

    B. "Have you noticed skin changes in other areas?"

    C. "How does the affected area look to you?"

    D. "How would you describe your usual skin exposure to the sun?"

7. Which of the following lesion characteristics indicates the need for further assessment?

    A. Round shape with distinct borders

    B. Bleeds easily

    C. Light brown in color

    D. Nonpalpable

8. Assessment of an older adult client reveals significant tenting of the skin over his forearm. Which of the following best explains this finding?

    A. Loss of adipose tissue and elasticity

    B. Parchment-like skin

    C. Significant flaking and dryness

    D. Skin tags

Chapter 30: Skin, Hair, and Nails

Application Exercises Answer Key

1. Match the type of lesion commonly seen on a skin assessment with its correct assessment terminology.

   <u>**B**</u>   Freckle   A. Wheal

   <u>**C**</u>   Wart   B. Macule

   <u>**F**</u>   Blister   C. Nodule

   <u>**D**</u>   Acne   D. Pustule

   <u>**E**</u>   Psoriasis   E. Scale

   <u>**A**</u>   Mosquito bite   F. Vesicle

2. A client presents to the clinic wanting a lesion on his neck evaluated. List the assessments that should be documented about the lesion.

   Location

   Size

   Shape

   Color

   Consistency

   Presence of fluid or drainage

   Elevation

   Tenderness

3. Which of the following assessments should be considered an abnormal finding during a skin assessment?

   A. No clubbing noted

   B. Brisk capillary refill

   C. 3+ pitting edema in feet bilaterally

   D. Numerous light brown macules, < 3 mm in size, located on nose and cheeks

   An abnormal finding is 3+ bilateral pitting edema. Normal findings include no clubbing, brisk capillary refill, and light brown macules noted on the nose and cheeks.

4. A client's skin temperature is best assessed by using which part of the hand?

    A. Fingertips

    B. Dorsal surface

    C. Palmar surface

    D. Base of the hand

The dorsal surface of the hand is the most sensitive to temperature changes.

5. Match the term in the left column with its definition from the right column. Each letter can only be used once.

B	Jaundice	A. Paleness, absence of color
C	Erythema	B. Yellowish appearance of the skin
D	Cyanosis	C. Redness of the skin
A	Pallor	D. Grayish blue tone

6. Which of the following questions should the nurse ask the client to assess health promotion patterns related to the skin?

    A. "How does your skin feel?"

    B. "Have you noticed skin changes in other areas?"

    C. "How does the affected area look to you?"

    D. "How would you describe your usual skin exposure to the sun?"

Excessive sun exposure can lead to skin caner. Teaching/reinforcing the use of sunscreen is recommended to decrease the amount of exposure.

7. Which of the following lesion characteristics indicates the need for further assessment?

    A. Round shape with distinct borders

    B. Bleeds easily

    C. Light brown in color

    D. Nonpalpable

A lesion that bleeds easily needs further assessment, as it is not normal for lesions to bleed. Normal findings of lesions include roundness in shape with distinct borders. A nonpalpable lesion that is light brown in color is also a normal finding.

8. Assessment of an older adult client reveals significant tenting of the skin over his forearm. Which of the following best explains this finding?

A. Loss of adipose tissue and elasticity

B. Parchment-like skin

C. Significant flaking and dryness

D. Skin tags

Tenting is a result of loss of adipose tissue and elasticity of the skin. Thin, parchment-like skin, dryness, and skin tags do not cause tenting.

Unit 2   **Health Assessment**

Section: System-Specific Assessment

Chapter 31:   **Head and Neck**
         Contributor: Sally Swenson, MA, RN

 NCLEX® Connections:

> **Learning Objective**: Review and apply knowledge within "**Head and Neck**" in readiness for performance of the following nursing activities as outlined by the NCLEX® test plans:
>
> Δ   Use effective communication to collect history assessment data related to the client's head and neck.
>
> Δ   Perform the appropriate assessment of the client's head and neck within the nursing role, including:
>
> > •   Preparing the client for the procedure.
> >
> > •   Client teaching (before and following the procedure).
> >
> > •   Using accurate technique based on the client's needs.
>
> Δ   Assess/monitor the client's status by obtaining baseline data and comparing with subsequent findings.
>
> Δ   Document baseline and subsequent findings according to hospital protocol.
>
> Δ   Maintain confidentiality of all client information.

 Key Points

Δ   **Head** – The skull and face are the primary targets of the head exam. The skin and hair of the head should be also be examined *(Refer to chapter 30, Skin, Hair and Nails.)*. Inspection and palpation of the head are usually done together.

Δ   **Neck** – The shoulders, range of motion, lymph nodes, thyroid gland, and trachea position are part of the neck exam. The carotid arteries and jugular veins of the neck can be examined at this time.

Key Procedural Points

Δ   Use the techniques of inspection, palpation, and auscultation to examine the client's head and neck.

Δ   Use a stethoscope.

Δ   Test the following cranial nerves during the head and neck exam:

Assessment	Cranial Nerves (CN)
Assess face for strength and sensation.	CN V (trigeminal)
Assess face for movement.	CN VII (facial)
Assess shoulders for strength.	CN XI (spinal accessory)

Health History – Review of Systems

Δ   Questions the nurse should ask include:

• Do you experience headaches? If so, how often, and where are they located?

• Do you experience any pain in your neck?

• Are you able to move your head and shoulders with ease?

• Have you noticed any unusual facial movements?

• Are any of your lymph nodes swollen?

Inspection and Palpation

Δ   **Head**

• **Skull**

◊   Size (Normal is normocephalic.)

◊   Depressions

◊   Deformities

◊   Masses

◊   Tenderness

◊   Overall contour and symmetry

• **Face**

◊   Symmetry of facial features

◊   Symmetry of expressions

◊   Involuntary movements (abnormal)

◊   Proportionate features (no thickening as in acromegaly)

◊ **CN V**

    ° Motor – Test the **strength** of the muscle contraction by asking the client to clench teeth while palpating the masseter and temporal muscles and then the temporomandibular joint.

    ° Sensory – Test **light touch** by having the client close her eyes, gently touching her face with a cotton swab, and asking her to tell you when the touch is felt.

◊ **CN VII**

    ° Motor – Test facial movement by having the client smile, frown, puff out cheeks, raise eyebrows, close eyes tightly, and show teeth.

Δ **Neck**

• **Muscles**

◊ Shoulders should be equal in height and with normal muscle mass.

◊ Range of motion (ROM) – The client should be able to move his head smoothly and without distress in the following directions:

    ° Chin to chest (flexion).

    ° Ear to shoulder bilaterally (lateral flexion).

    ° Chin up (hyperextension).

◊ **CN XI** – Place hands on the client's shoulders and ask the client to shrug the shoulders against resistance.

Δ **Lymph nodes** – Chains of lymph nodes extend from the lower half of the head down into the neck and should be palpated for enlargement. Lymph nodes to be palpated include:

Occipital lymph node	Base of the skull
Preauricular lymph node	In front of the ear
Postauricular lymph node	Over the mastoid
Submandibular lymph node	Along the base of the mandible
Tonsillar (retropharyngeal) lymph node	Angle of the mandible
Submental lymph node	Midline under the chin
Anterior cervical lymph nodes	Along the sternocleidomastoid muscle
Posterior cervical lymph nodes	Posterior to sternocleidomastoid muscle

• Lymph nodes should be nonpalpable and nontender.

• Use the pads of the index and middle fingers and move the skin over the underlying tissue in a circular motion. Compare from side to side.

- If an enlargement is found, the node should be further evaluated for

  ◊ Location.

  ◊ Tenderness.

  ◊ Size.

  ◊ Shape.

  ◊ Consistency.

  ◊ Mobility.

  ◊ Discreteness.

Δ The **thyroid gland** is bilobed. The nurse should examine the gland by:

- First, inspecting the lower half of the client's neck to see if an enlargement of the gland is visible.

- Having the client take a sip of water and watching the thyroid tissue move up.

- Approaching the client from behind and having the client tip her head forward and to the right. Use the left hand to displace the trachea slightly to the right while placing your right fingers between the sternomastoid muscle and the trachea.

- Instructing the client to take a sip of water and feeling for the movement of the thyroid gland as it moves up with the trachea and larynx.

- Repeating this procedure for the other side, palpating it for:

  ◊ Size.

  ◊ Masses.

  ◊ Smoothness.

Δ **Trachea** – Inspect and palpate the trachea for any deviation. The trachea should be midline.

Auscultation

Δ If the thyroid is enlarged, the nurse should auscultate the gland using a stethoscope. The presence of a bruit indicates an abnormal increase in blood flow to the area.

NANDA Nursing Diagnoses

Δ Acute pain

Δ Body-image disturbance

Sample Documentation

Skull is normocephalic, symmetrical, and nontender. Client has symmetrical facial features and movements. Trachea is midline. Thyroid lobes are palpable but not enlarged; no nodules noted. Neck is supple with no palpable lymph nodes. Client has full range of motion of the neck. CN V, VII, and XI are intact.

Primary Reference:

Potter, P. A., & Perry, A. G. (2005). *Fundamentals of nursing* (6th ed.). St. Louis, MO: Mosby.

Additional Resources:

Bickley, L. S., & Szilagyi, P. G. (2003). *Bates' guide to physical examination and history taking* (8th ed.). Philadelphia: Lippincott Williams & Wilkins.

Jarvis, C. (2004). *Physical examination & health assessment.* (4th ed.). St. Louis, MO: Saunders.

NANDA International (2004). *NANDA nursing diagnoses: Definitions and classification 2005-2006.* Philadelphia: NANDA.

Chapter 31: Head and Neck

Application Exercises

1. Match the examination technique needed to perform each assessment. (Each technique can be used more than once.)

_____ Thyroid	A. Inspection only
_____ Facial symmetry	B. Palpation only
_____ Lymph nodes	C. Inspection and palpation
_____ Trachea position	
_____ Movement of chin to chest	
_____ Left occipital skull deformity	

2. Match each lymph node of the head and neck with its location for palpation.

_____ Occipital lymph node	A. Along the base of the mandible
_____ Preauricular lymph node	B. Midline under the chin
_____ Postauricular lymph node	C. Base of the skull
_____ Submandibular lymph node	D. Along the sternocleidomastoid muscle
_____ Tonsillar (retropharyngeal) lymph node	E. Posterior to sternocleidomastoid muscle
_____ Submental lymph node	F. Over the mastoid
_____ Anterior cervical lymph nodes	G. Angle of the mandible
_____ Posterior cervical lymph nodes	H. In front of the ear

3. Which of the following should be assessed when examining the face? (Select all that apply.)

_____ Lymph nodes

_____ Perception of light touch of the face

_____ Symmetry of facial features

_____ ROM of the neck

_____ Presence of involuntary movements

4. Asking a client to tip her head to one side and slightly forward, palpating either side of the trachea at the lower half of the neck, and then asking the client to swallow is the correct technique for examining

        A. lymph nodes.

        B. ROM of the neck.

        C. symmetry of the skull.

        D. the thyroid gland.

5. A nurse asks a client to smile, frown, and puff out his cheeks. If the client is unable to follow these commands, it is most likely that there has been damage to the

        A. facial nerve.

        B. trigeminal nerve.

        C. hypoglossal nerve.

        D. glossopharyngeal nerve.

Chapter 31: Head and Neck

Application Exercises Answer Key

1. Match the examination technique needed to perform each assessment. (Each technique can be used more than once.)

C	Thyroid	A. Inspection only
A	Facial symmetry	B. Palpation only
B	Lymph nodes	C. Inspection and palpation
C	Trachea position	
A	Movement of chin to chest	
C	Left occipital skull deformity	

2. Match each lymph node of the head and neck with its location for palpation.

C	Occipital lymph node	A. Along the base of the mandible
H	Preauricular lymph node	B. Midline under the chin
F	Postauricular lymph node	C. Base of the skull
A	Submandibular lymph node	D. Along the sternocleidomastoid muscle
G	Tonsillar (retropharyngeal) lymph node	E. Posterior to sternocleidomastoid muscle
B	Submental lymph node	F. Over the mastoid
D	Anterior cervical lymph nodes	G. Angle of the mandible
E	Posterior cervical lymph nodes	H. In front of the ear

3. Which of the following should be assessed when examining the face? (Select all that apply.)

_____	Lymph nodes
X	**Perception of light touch of the face**
X	**Symmetry of facial features**
_____	ROM of the neck
X	**Presence of involuntary movements**

Assessment of the perception of light touch to the face indicates that the sensory portion of the trigeminal nerve (CN V) is intact. Symmetry of facial movements and presence of involuntary movements of the face are also assessed. Lymph nodes and ROM of the neck are assessed while examining the neck.

4. Asking a client to tip her head to one side and slightly forward, palpating either side of the trachea at the lower half of the neck, and then asking the client to swallow is the correct technique for examining

> A. lymph nodes.
>
> B. ROM of the neck.
>
> C. symmetry of the skull.
>
> **D. the thyroid gland.**

This is the correct technique for examining the thyroid gland.

5. A nurse asks a client to smile, frown, and puff out his cheeks. If the client is unable to follow these commands, it is most likely that there has been damage to the

> **A. facial nerve.**
>
> B. trigeminal nerve.
>
> C. hypoglossal nerve.
>
> D. glossopharyngeal nerve.

The facial nerve controls movements of the face. The trigeminal nerve controls muscle strength of the jaw and light touch sensation. The hypoglossal nerve controls movement of the soft palate. The glossopharyngeal nerve controls movement of the tongue.

Unit 2   Health Assessment

Section: System-Specific Assessment

Chapter 32:   Eyes
Contributor: Sally Swenson, MA, RN

 NCLEX® Connections:

Learning Objective: Review and apply knowledge within "**Eyes**" in readiness for performance of the following nursing activities as outlined by the NCLEX® test plans:

Δ   Use effective communication to collect history assessment data related to the client's eyes.

Δ   Perform the appropriate assessment of the client's eyes within the nursing role, including:

•   Preparing the client for the procedure.

•   Client teaching (before and following the procedure).

•   Using accurate technique based on the client's needs.

Δ   Assess/monitor the client's status by obtaining baseline data and comparing with subsequent findings.

Δ   Document baseline and subsequent findings according to hospital protocol.

Δ   Maintain confidentiality of all client information.

 Key Points

Δ   The sense of vision is controlled by the eyes.

Δ   The examination of the eyes includes external anatomy, internal anatomy, visual pathways, fields, and reflexes.

Δ   Abnormal findings include loss of visual fields, asymmetric corneal light reflex, periorbital edema, conjunctivitis, and corneal abrasion.

Key Procedural Points

Δ   The primary technique for examination of the eyes is inspection. A limited amount of palpation is done wearing gloves.

Δ   Perform the eye exam in the following sequence, using the appropriate equipment.

Test	Equipment
Visual acuity	Snellen and Rosenbaum charts, eye cover, and Ishihara test
Extraocular movements (EOMs)	Penlight or ophthalmoscope light and eye cover
Visual fields	Eye cover
External structures	Penlight or ophthalmoscope light and gloves
Internal structures	Ophthalmoscope

Δ   Test cranial nerves during the eye exam.

Assessment	Cranial Nerves (CN)
Visual acuity	CN II (optic)
Extraocular movements	CN III (oculomotor), CN IV (trochlear), CN VI (abducens)
Visual fields	CN II (optic)
Corneal light reflex Pupillary reaction to light	CN II (optic), CN III (oculomotor)

Health History – Review of Systems

Δ   Questions the nurse should ask include:

- How is your vision? Have you noticed any changes?

- Do you ever experience double vision? Do you ever see spots or halos?

- Do you ever experience discharge from your eyes?

- Do you wear glasses or contact lenses?

- When was your last eye exam?

Inspection

Δ   **Visual Acuity** – CN II

- Use the **Snellen chart** with the client standing 20 ft from the chart.

- Evaluate both eyes and then each eye separately with and without correction.

- For each eye, the opposite eye is covered.

- The client is asked to read the smallest line of print visible.

- The line for which two or fewer letters are missed is recorded as the visual acuity (20/20 is normal).

- The first number indicates **the number of feet from the chart** that the client is standing, and the second number is the **distance at which a normal-sighted person can read the line.**

Δ Screen for **myopia** (impaired far vision) using the Snellen chart.

Δ Screen for **presbyopia** (impaired near vision or farsightedness) using the Rosenbaum eye chart held **14 in** from the client's face. Readings correlate with the Snellen chart.

Δ Assess for **color vision** using the Ishihara test. The client should be able to identify the various shaded shapes.

Δ **Extraocular movements** (EOMs) – Assess EOMs to determine the coordination of the eye muscles using three different tests (CN III, CN IV, CN VI).

- Test the **corneal light reflex** by directing a light onto the client's eyes and looking to see if the reflection is seen symmetrically on the corneas.

- Screen for **strabismus** with the cover/uncover test. While covering one eye, the client is asked to look in another direction. The cover is removed and both eyes should be gazing in the same direction.

- **The six cardinal positions of gaze** require the client to follow the examiner's finger with his eyes without moving his head. The examiner moves his finger in a wide "H" pattern about 20 to 25 cm from the client's eyes. Eye movements should be smooth and symmetrical with no jerky or tremor-like movements (**nystagmus**).

Δ Evaluate **visual fields** (CN II) by facing the client at a distance of 60 cm. The client covers one eye while the nurse covers the direct opposite eye (e.g., client's right eye and nurse's left eye are covered). The client is asked to look at the nurse and report when she can see the fingers on the examiner's outstretched arm coming in from four directions (up, down, temporally, and nasally). The expected finding is that the client should see the examiner's fingers at the same time as the examiner.

Δ **External Structures**

- **Eyebrows** should be symmetrical and evenly distributed from the inner to the outer canthus.

- **Eyelids** should close completely and open to allow the lower border and most of the upper portion of the iris to be seen. No **ptosis** (covering of the pupil by the upper eyelid) should be noted.

- **Eyelashes** should curve outward and be evenly distributed with no inflammation around any of the hair follicles.

- **Conjunctiva**
  - ◊ **Palpebral** is pink.
  - ◊ **Bulbar** is transparent.
- **Sclera** should be white.
- **Corneas** are clear.
- **Lenses** are clear. Cloudiness occurs with **cataracts.**
- **PERRLA** (CN II, CN III)
  - ◊ **P – Pupils**
  - ◊ **E – Equal** in size and between 3 to 5 mm
  - ◊ **R – Round** in shape
  - ◊ **R – React to light** both directly and consensually when a light is directed into one pupil and then the other
  - ◊ **A – Accommodation** of the pupils when they dilate to look at an object far away and then converge and constrict to focus on a near object

Δ **Irises** should be round and illuminate fully when a light is shined across from the side. A partially illuminated iris may be indicative of **glaucoma**. The color of the irises should also be noted.

Δ **Internal Exam Technique and Expected Findings**

- Darken the surrounding room.

- Turn on the ophthalmoscope, and use the lens selector disc to find the large white disc.

- The diopter is set at 0. The examiner can change the setting to bring structures into focus during the exam.

- The examiner should use his right eye to examine the client's right eye and vice versa.

- The client should be instructed to stare at a point somewhere behind the examiner.

- The examiner starts slightly lateral and 25 to 30 cm from the client finding and following the **red reflex**, to within a distance of 2 to 3 cm of the client's eye.

- Expected findings include:

  ◊ **Optic disc** is light pink or more yellow than the surrounding retina.

  ◊ **Retina** should be without lesions, and color will be dark pink in those with a dark complexion and light pink in fair-skinned clients.

  ◊ **Arteries and veins** are found in a 2 to 3 ratio and without nicking.

  ◊ **Macula** may not be readily visible without pupil dilation but may be briefly glimpsed when the client looks directly at the light.

Palpation

Δ The **lacrimal apparatus** is palpated to assess for tenderness and to see if any discharge can be expressed from the lacrimal duct. No tenderness and no discharge should be noted. Clear fluid (tears) is an expected finding.

NANDA Nursing Diagnoses

Δ Altered sensory perception (visual)

Δ Risk for injury

Sample Documentation

Visual acuity is 20/30 in the left eye, 20/20 in the right eye, and 20/20 in both eyes without correction. EOM's are symmetrical with no strabismus or nystagmus noted. Peripheral fields are full bilaterally. Eyebrows are evenly distributed. Eyelids close completely with no ptosis. No discharge noted. Bulbar conjunctiva are clear, palpebral conjunctiva are pink, sclera are white, and irises are blue bilaterally. Corneas and lenses are clear. PERRLA is intact bilaterally. Red reflex is present bilaterally. Retinas are yellowish orange with no nicking or hemorrhaging of vessels.

Primary Reference:

Potter, P. A., & Perry, A. G. (2005). *Fundamentals of nursing* (6th ed.). St. Louis, MO: Mosby.

Additional Resources:

Bickley, L. S. (2003). *Bates' guide to physical examination and history taking.* New York: Lippincott Williams & Wilkins.

Jarvis, C. (2004). *Physical examination & health assessment.* (4th ed.). St. Louis, MO: Saunders.

NANDA International (2004). *NANDA nursing diagnoses: Definitions and classification 2005-2006.* Philadelphia: NANDA.

Chapter 32: Eyes

Application Exercises

1. Match the examination technique or tool needed to screen for the following conditions.

_____ Color blindness	A. Illumination of the iris
_____ Myopia	B. Cover/uncover test
_____ Nystagmus	C. Six cardinal positions of gaze
_____ Presbyopia	D. Snellen chart
_____ Strabismus	E. Rosenbaum chart
_____ Glaucoma	F. Ishihara test

2. Which of the following are expected eye findings. (Select all that apply.)

_____ No discharge is noted when palpating the lacrimal apparatus.

_____ Ptosis is noted bilaterally.

_____ PERRLA are intact bilaterally.

_____ Sclera are pink.

_____ Nystagmus is noted on upward gaze bilaterally.

_____ Irises are brown bilaterally.

_____ Nicking of vessels is noted bilaterally.

_____ Corneas are clear bilaterally.

_____ Visual acuity in right, left, and both eyes together is 20/20 with correction.

3. A client asks what her Snellen eye test results mean. Her acuity for both eyes together is 20/30. Which of the following is the nurse's best response?

A. "You see at 20 ft what the normal-sighted person sees at 30 ft."

B. "You see at 30 ft what the normal-sighted person sees at 20 ft."

C. "You see at 10 ft what the normal-sighted person sees at 50 ft."

D. "You see at 50 ft what the normal-sighted person sees at 20 ft."

4. A client with nystagmus will demonstrate

A. one eye gazing in a different direction during the cover/uncover test.

B. jerky eye movements during the six cardinal positions of gaze test.

C. droopy eyelids that partially or completely cover the pupil.

D. nicking of the retinal blood vessels during the internal eye exam.

5. What part of the eye exam should occur first?

        A. Extraocular movements

        B. Internal structures

        C. Visual acuity

        D. Visual fields

6. An ophthalmoscope is necessary to examine which of the following eye structures? (Select all that apply.)

     _____ Cornea

     _____ Retina

     _____ Sclera

     _____ Iris

     _____ Optic disc

     _____ Arteries

Chapter 32: Eyes

Application Exercises Answer Key

1. Match the examination technique or tool needed to screen for the following conditions.

   F   Color blindness   A. Illumination of the iris

   D   Myopia   B. Cover/uncover test

   C   Nystagmus   C. Six cardinal fields of gaze

   E   Presbyopia   D. Snellen chart

   B   Strabismus   E. Rosenbaum chart

   A   Glaucoma   F. Ishihara test

2. Which of the following are expected eye findings. (Select all that apply.)

   X   **No discharge is noted when palpating the lacrimal apparatus.**

   _____   Ptosis is noted bilaterally.

   X   **PERRLA are intact bilaterally.**

   _____   Sclera are pink.

   _____   Nystagmus is noted on upward gaze bilaterally.

   X   **Irises are brown bilaterally.**

   _____   Nicking of vessels is noted bilaterally.

   X   **Corneas are clear bilaterally.**

   X   **Visual acuity in right, left, and both eyes together is 20/20 with correction.**

The eyes should not have any discharge. The pupils should be equal, round, and they should react to light and accommodation bilaterally. Brown is a normal color for irises. Corneas should be clear, and 20/20 vision is normal. Ptosis, which is covering of the eye with the eyelids, is not a normal finding. The sclera should be white. Nystagmus should not be present, and there should not be any nicking of blood vessels.

3. A client asks what her Snellen eye test results mean. Her acuity for both eyes together is 20/30. Which of the following is the nurse's best response?

A. "You see at 20 ft what the normal-sighted person sees at 30 ft."

B. "You see at 30 ft what the normal-sighted person sees at 20 ft."

C. "You see at 10 ft what the normal-sighted person sees at 50 ft."

D. "You see at 50 ft what the normal-sighted person sees at 20 ft."

The first number indicates the number of feet from the Snellen eye chart that the client is standing, and the second number is the distance at which a normal-sighted person can read the line of the Snellen eye chart.

4. A client with nystagmus will demonstrate

A. one eye gazing in a different direction during the cover/uncover test.

B. jerky eye movements during the six cardinal fields of gaze test.

C. droopy eyelids that partially or completely cover the pupil.

D. nicking of the retinal blood vessels during the internal eye exam.

Nystagmus is demonstrated with jerky eye movements during the six cardinal fields of gaze test. Strabismus is demonstrated by one eye gazing in a different direction than the other eye. Ptosis is demonstrated by droopy eyelids that partially or completely cover the pupil. Nicking of the retinal blood vessels indicates damage to the blood vessels of the eye.

5. What part of the eye exam should occur first?

A. Extraocular movements

B. Internal structures

C. Visual acuity

D. Visual fields

Visual acuity should be assessed first during an eye exam. Assessing extraocular movements, internal structures, and visual fields may interfere with the ability of the client to read and demonstrate accurate visual acuity.

6. An ophthalmoscope is necessary to examine which of the following eye structures? (Select all that apply.)

_____ Cornea

__X__ **Retina**

_____ Sclera

_____ Iris

__X__ **Optic disc**

__X__ **Arteries**

The retina, optic disc, and arteries are internal structures of the eye and must be examined with an ophthalmoscope. The cornea, sclera, and iris are all external structures of the eye and can be examined with the nurse's eye.

Unit 2   Health Assessment

Section: System-Specific Assessment

Chapter 33:   Ears, Nose, Mouth, and Throat
                 Contributor: Sally Swenson, MA, RN

 NCLEX® Connections:

Learning Objective: Review and apply knowledge within "**Ears, Nose, Mouth, and Throat**" in readiness for performance of the following nursing activities as outlined by the NCLEX® test plans:

Δ   Use effective communication to collect history assessment data related to the client's ears, nose, mouth, and throat.

Δ   Perform the appropriate assessment of the client's ears, nose, mouth, and throat within the nursing role, including:

   • Preparing the client for the procedure.

   • Client teaching (before and following the procedure).

   • Using accurate technique based on the client's needs.

Δ   Assess/monitor the client's status by obtaining baseline data and comparing with subsequent findings.

Δ   Document baseline and subsequent findings according to facility/agency protocol.

Δ   Maintain confidentiality of all client information.

Key Points

Δ   The sense of hearing and equilibrium is controlled by the ears.

Δ   The examination of the ears includes assessment of the external, middle, and internal ear and evaluation of hearing.

Δ   Abnormal findings include otitis externa, osteoma, polyp, retracted drum, decreased hearing acuity, and lateralization.

Key Procedural Points

Δ   Use the techniques inspection and palpation to examine the ears, nose (sinuses), mouth, and throat.

Δ   Equipment

- Otoscope

- Wristwatch with a second hand

- Tuning fork

- Nasal speculum

- Tongue blade

- Penlight

- Gauze square

- Cotton-tipped applicators

Δ   Test the following cranial nerves during the ears, nose, mouth, and throat exam.

Assessment	Cranial Nerves (CN)
Assess ears for hearing.	CN VIII (acoustic)
Assess nose for smell.	CN I (olfactory)
Assess mouth for taste.	CN VII (facial) and CN IX (glossopharyngeal)
Assess tongue for movement and strength.	CN XII (hypoglossal)
Assess mouth for movement of soft palate and gag reflex. Assess swallowing and speech.	CN IX (glossopharyngeal) and CN X (vagus)

Health History – Review of Systems

Δ   Questions the nurse should ask include:

- How well do you hear?

- Have you noticed any changes in your hearing? Do you wear a hearing aid?

- Do you ever experience tinnitus, discharge, vertigo, or pain? Do you have a history of ear infections?

- Do you ever have pain, stuffiness, or discharge from your nose?

- Do you ever experience nose bleeds?

- Have you noticed any change in your sense of smell or taste?

- How often do you go to the dentist? Do you have dentures? Do you have any problems with your gums?

- Do you have any difficulty swallowing or problems with hoarseness or sore throat?

Inspection and Palpation

Δ   **Ears**

- **External ear**

  ◊   **Alignment** – The top of the auricles should meet an imaginary horizontal line that extends from the outer canthus of the eye.

  ◊   **Lesions and tenderness** in the ears are unexpected findings.

  ◊   The **ear canal** should be free of foreign bodies or discharge.

  ◊   **Cerumen** is an expected finding.

- **Internal ear**

  ◊   Straighten the ear canal by pulling the auricle up and back in adults and older children, and down and back in younger children. Using the otoscope, insert the speculum 1 to 1.5 cm following, but not touching, the ear canal to visualize:

  - **Tympanic membranes** that are pearly gray and intact.

  - **Light reflex** that is visible and in a well-defined cone shape.

  - **Umbo and manubrium landmarks** that are readily visible.

  - **Ear canal** that is pink with fine hairs.

- **Auditory screening tests**

Test	Technique	Expected Finding
Whisper test (CNV III)	• One ear is occluded and the other ear is tested to see if the client can hear whispered sounds without seeing the examiner's mouth move. • Repeat with the other ear.	The client can hear the examiner whisper softly 30 to 60 cm away.
Rinne test	• Place a vibrating tuning fork firmly against the mastoid bone and note the time. • Have the client state when he can no longer hear the sound, note the time, and then move the tuning fork in front of the ear canal. When the client can no longer hear the tuning fork, note the time.	Air conduction (AC) > bone conduction (BC); 2 to 1 ratio.
Weber test	Place a vibrating tuning fork on top of the client's head. Ask the client if the sound is heard best in the right ear, left ear, or both ears equally.	Sound is heard equally in both ears (negative Weber test).

Δ **Nose**

- **Position** – should be midline and symmetrical

- **Patency** should be present for each nostril without excessive flaring.

- Examine **internal structures** using a nasal speculum barely inserted into each nostril as the client tips his head back. Inspect should indicate that the:

  ◊ Septum is midline and intact.

  ◊ Mucosa is deep pink and moist with no discharge or lesions.

- Assess **smell** (CN I) by asking the client to occlude one nare at a time and identifying a familiar smell with eyes closed.

Δ **Mouth and Throat**

- **Lips** are darker pigmented skin than the face, symmetrical, smooth, soft with no lesions, and nontender.

- **Gums** are coral pink and tight against the teeth with no bleeding on gloves when palpated.

- **Mucous membranes** are without lesions, moist, and pink.

- **Tongue** – Use a gauze pad to hold the tip and move the tongue from side to side. The dorsum surface is pink, with the presence of papillae, and symmetrical. The underside of the tongue should be smooth with a symmetrical vascular pattern. Assess taste (CN VII, CN IX) by identification of different foods placed on tongue with eyes closed. Ask the client to move his tongue up, down, and side to side. Test strength (CN XII) by applying resistance against each cheek while the client sticks his tongue into each cheek.

- Assess **teeth** for malocclusions by asking the client to clench his teeth. Missing or loose teeth, as well as any discoloration, should be noted. Teeth should be shiny, white, and smooth.

- **Hard palate** is pink, intact, symmetrical, firm, and concave.

- **Soft palate** is lighter pink than the hard palate, intact, symmetrical, and moves with vocalization (CN IX, CN X).

- **Uvula** is pink, midline, intact, and should move with vocalization.

- **Tonsils** that are visible should be the same color as the surrounding mucosa and graded on a scale of 1 to 4.

  ◊ +1 barely visible

  ◊ +2 halfway to the uvula

  ◊ +3 touching the uvula

  ◊ +4 touching each other or midline

- Elicit **gag reflex** by using a tongue blade to stimulate the back of the throat (CN IX, CN X). Warn the client prior to performing this assessment.

- Note **speech** during the course of the examination. Note whether or not the client's speech is clear and articulate.

Palpation – Sinuses

Δ **Technique**

- Palpate frontal sinuses by pressing upward with thumbs from just below the eyebrows on either side of the bridge of the nose.

- Palpate maxillary sinuses by pressing upward at the skin crevices that run from the sides of the nose to the corner of the mouth.

Δ **Expected finding**: Nontender

NANDA Nursing Diagnoses

Δ Altered sensory perception (auditory)

Δ Impaired oral mucous membranes

Δ Impaired swallowing

Sample Documentation

No lesions or tenderness noted on external ears. Top of ears align with outer canthus of eyes. Tympanic membranes pearly gray and translucent with well-defined cone of light. Light yellow cerumen present in ear canals bilaterally. Auditory acuity intact to whispered voice bilaterally. Negative Weber test and AC > BC bilaterally. Nose is midline and symmetrical. Nares are patent. Nasal mucosa is pink, septum intact and midline; no discharge noted. No sinus tenderness. Lips are darker pink and intact; symmetrical. Oral mucosa is pink, no dental caries noted; no missing teeth. Tongue is pink and midline. Papilla present on dorsum, and symmetrical vascular pattern noted on the underside of the tongue. Gums are tight against the teeth with no bleeding noted. Hard and soft palates are intact with no lesions. Uvula is midline. Gag reflex is present. Tonsils are +1 bilaterally. Taste and smell sensations are intact. Speech is clear. CN I, VII, VIII, IX, X, XII intact.

Primary Reference:

Potter, P. A., & Perry, A. G. (2005). *Fundamentals of nursing* (6ᵗʰ ed.). St. Louis, MO: Mosby.

Additional Resources:

Bickley, L. S., & Szilagyi, P. G. (2003). *Bates' guide to physical examination and history taking* (8ᵗʰ ed.). Philadelphia: Lippincott Williams & Wilkins.

Jarvis, C. (2004). *Physical examination & health assessment.* (4ᵗʰ ed.). St. Louis, MO: Saunders.

NANDA International (2004). *NANDA nursing diagnoses: Definitions and classification 2005-2006*. Philadelphia: NANDA.

Chapter 33: Ears, Nose, Mouth, and Throat

Application Exercises

1. When a nurse performs an internal ear exam, what are the expected findings?

2. Match the appropriate technique for each of the following assessments.

_____ Vibrating tuning fork is placed on the
mastoid process and then placed near
the ear when the sound is no longer heard.

A. Whisper test

B. Weber test

_____ Vibrating tuning fork is placed midline
on top of the head, and the client is asked
where the sound is heard best.

C. Gag reflex

_____ The back of the throat is stimulated with a
tongue depressor.

D. Rinne test

_____ The client occludes one ear while the nurse
whispers in the other ear from 30 cm away.

3. Note whether each of the following notations are expected or unexpected findings during an assessment of the ears, nose, mouth, and throat.

Notation	Expected	Unexpected
Pale, boggy nasal mucosa		
White plaques on tongue bilaterally		
Ear canals patent with slight amount of amber cerumen present in the right ear		
Reddened, bulging tympanic membranes		
Gag reflex present and speech clear		
Air conduction less than bone conduction in both ears bilaterally		
Auricles nontender and without lesions		
Auditory acuity intact to the spoken voice but not to a whisper in the right ear		

4. When inspecting the internal ear of an adult with the otoscope, the nurse should pull the ear
_____ to straighten the ear canal.

5. The expected finding for a negative Weber test is

        A. sound heard equally in both ears.

        B. sound lateralizes to one ear or the other.

        C. air conduction is greater than bone conduction.

        D. bone conduction is greater than air conduction.

Chapter 33: Ears, Nose, Mouth, and Throat

Application Exercises Answer Key

1. When a nurse performs an internal ear exam, what are the expected findings?

   Tympanic membranes are pearly gray and intact.

   Light reflex is visible in a well-defined cone shape.

   Umbo and manubrium landmarks are readily visible.

   Ear canal is pink with fine hairs.

2. Match the appropriate technique for each of the following assessments.

   D Vibrating tuning fork is placed on the
         mastoid process and then placed near
         the ear when the sound is no longer heard.

   B Vibrating tuning fork is placed midline
         on top of the head, and the client is asked
         where the sound is heard best.

   C The back of the throat is stimulated with a
         tongue depressor.

   A The client occludes one ear while the nurse
         whispers in the other ear from 30 cm away.

   A. Whisper test

   B. Weber test

   C. Gag reflex

   D. Rinne test

3. Note whether each of the following notations are expected or unexpected findings during an assessment of the ears, nose, mouth, and throat.

Notation	Expected	Unexpected
Pale, boggy nasal mucosa		X
White plaques on tongue bilaterally		X
Ear canals patent with slight amount of amber cerumen present in the right ear	X	
Reddened, bulging tympanic membranes		X
Gag reflex present and speech clear	X	
Air conduction less than bone conduction in both ears bilaterally		X
Auricles nontender and without lesions	X	
Auditory acuity intact to the spoken voice but not to a whisper in the right ear		X

Normal findings include patent ear canals with a slight amount of cerumen noted, negative Weber test, present gag reflex, clear speech, and nontender auricles without lesions. The nasal mucosa should be pink and moist. There should not be any lesions on the tongue. The tympanic membrane should be pearly gray and intact, and air conduction should be greater than bone conduction bilaterally.

4. When inspecting the internal ear of an adult with the otoscope, the nurse should pull the ear _____ to straighten the ear canal.

Up and back: The ear is pulled up and back to straighten the ear canal of an adult and older child, and it is pulled down and back for a child.

5. The expected finding for a negative Weber test is

A. sound heard equally in both ears.

B. sound lateralizes to one ear or the other.

C. air conduction is greater than bone conduction.

D. bone conduction is greater then air conduction.

The Weber test is examining for lateralization. If the sound is heard equally in both ears, it is considered a negative test.

Unit 2   Health Assessment
Section: System-Specific Assessment

Chapter 34:   Breasts
                Contributor: Sally Swenson, MA, RN

 NCLEX® Connections:

> **Learning Objective**: Review and apply knowledge within **"Breasts"** in readiness for performance of the following nursing activities as outlined by the NCLEX® test plans:
>
> Δ   Use effective communication to collect history assessment data related to the client's breasts.
>
> Δ   Perform the appropriate assessment of the client's breasts within the nursing role, including:
>
> - Preparing the client for the procedure.
> - Client teaching (before and following the procedure).
> - Using accurate technique based on the client's needs.
>
> Δ   Assess/monitor the client's status by obtaining baseline data and comparing with subsequent findings.
>
> Δ   Document baseline and subsequent findings according to facility/agency protocol.
>
> Δ   Maintain confidentiality of all client information.

 Key Points

Δ   Clients who have had a mastectomy, **breast augmentation, and/or reconstruction** should have the incisional lines palpated. Lymphedema may be noted in clients who have impaired lymphatic drainage on the affected side.

Δ   **Self-breast exam (SBE)** should be addressed with the client during the exam. Ask the client whether or not she performs a monthly SBE, and if not, instruct the client on the necessity of it and/or how to perform the exam. At home, inspection can be done in front of the mirror, and palpation can be done in the shower.

Δ   Breast exams should be performed on both female and male clients.

	Expected Findings	Normal Abnormal Findings
Female	• Breasts should be firm, elastic, and without lesions or nodules. • Breast tissue may feel granular or lumpy bilaterally in some women. • **Age-related changes** – With menopause, the breast tissue atrophies and is replaced with adipose tissue, making it feel softer and more pendulous. The atrophied ducts may feel like thin strands.	• **Fibrocystic breast disease** is characterized by tender cysts that are often more prominent during menstruation.
Male	• No edema, masses, or tenderness should be present. • Areolas are round and darker pigmented.	• Unilateral or bilateral (but asymmetrical) **gynecomastia** in adolescent boys or bilateral **gynecomastia** in older adult males may be present.

Key Procedural Points

Δ Use the techniques of **inspection and palpation** to examine the breasts.

- Equipment
    - ◊ Gloves
    - ◊ Lotion
    - ◊ Drape
    - ◊ Small pillow or folded towel

Δ **Documentation of nodules** should include:

- Location (quadrant or clock method).
- Size (actual centimeters).
- Shape.
- Consistency (soft, firm, or hard).
- Discreteness (well-defined borders of mass).
- Tenderness.
- Erythema.
- Dimpling or retraction over the mass.
- Lymphadenopathy.
- Mobility.

Health History – Review of Systems

Δ   Questions the nurse should ask include:

- Do you perform self-breast exams? How often?

- Have you noticed any tenderness or lumps? Does this change with your menstrual cycle?

- Have you experienced any discharge from the nipples?

Inspection

Female	Male
• **Four positions** (done sitting or standing) ◊ Arms at the side ◊ Arms above head ◊ Hands on hips pressing firmly ◊ Leaning forward (arms out in front or can remain on hips)	In sitting or lying position (with arms at the side only)

Δ   **Inspect For**

- Size and symmetry (One breast is often slightly larger than the other.).

- Shape (e.g., convex, conical, pendulous).

- Symmetrical venous patterns and consistency of skin color.

- Absence of lesions, edema, or erythema.

- Round shape of areola.

- Darker-pigmented areola and nipple.

- Direction of nipples (Nipples are usually everted; recent inversion is abnormal.).

Palpation

Δ   **Axillary and clavicular lymph nodes** are best palpated in the sitting position. Lymph nodes should not be palpable or tender. The following lymph nodes should be assessed:

- **Supraclavicular.**

- **Infraclavicular.**

- **Pectoral.**

- **Central or deep** (may be normal to palpate if < 1 cm and nontender).

- **Lateral.**

- **Subscapular.**

- **Epitrochlear.**

Δ **Breast exam** – Wear gloves if skin is not intact. Feel for lumps using the finger pads of four fingers (Use lotion as a lubricant if needed). The best position is for the client to be lying down with the arm up by her head and a small pillow or folded towel placed under the shoulder of the side being examined. This position spreads the breast tissue more evenly over the chest wall allowing for easier palpation.

- Palpate each breast from the sternum to posterior axillary line, and from the clavicle to the bra line (including the areola, nipple, and tail of Spence) using one of three techniques:

    ◊ Circular pattern.

    ◊ Wedge pattern.

    ◊ Vertical strip pattern.

Δ **Nipples** should be carefully compressed between the thumb and index finger to check for discharge. Discharge is not expected in nonlactating women. Note color, consistency, and odor of any discharge.

Δ **Pendulous breasts** require that a **bimanual technique** be used to support the lower portion of the breast while the tissue is palpated against the supporting hand.

NANDA Nursing Diagnoses

Δ Disturbed body image

Δ Acute pain

Sample Documentation

Breasts are conical, symmetrical in size, and without masses or lesions. Nipples and areola are darker pigmented and symmetrical. Everted nipples are without discharge. No palpable axillary or clavicular lymph nodes.

Primary Reference:

Potter, P. A., & Perry, A. G. (2005). *Fundamentals of nursing* (6th ed.). St. Louis, MO: Mosby.

Additional Resources:

Bickley, L. S., & Szilagyi, P. G. (2003). *Bates' guide to physical examination and history taking* (8th ed.). Philadelphia: Lippincott Williams & Wilkins.

Jarvis, C. (2004). *Physical examination & health assessment.* (4th ed.). St. Louis, MO: Saunders.

NANDA International (2004). *NANDA nursing diagnoses: Definitions and classification 2005-2006.* Philadelphia: NANDA.

Chapter 34: Breasts

Application Exercises

1. Identify the four positions the female client should be in when the nurse is examining her breasts.

2. What information should be documented when describing a breast mass?

3. True or False: It is not necessary to perform a breast exam on a male client.

4. Which of the following are expected changes of the breast tissue after menopause? (Select all that apply.)

    _____ Clear discharge from nipples

    _____ More pendulous

    _____ Breast tissue replaced by adipose tissue

    _____ Firmer

    _____ Nodular

5. During palpation of the breast, the client is instructed to extend an arm over her head, and a small pillow or folded towel is placed under her shoulder to

    A. spread the tissue more evenly over the chest wall for easier palpation.

    B. avoid the client from guarding during the exam.

    C. expose the tail of Spence for easier inspection.

    D. determine whether or not a breast mass is consistently irregular when palpating a nodule.

Chapter 34: Breasts

Application Exercises Answer Key

1. Identify the four positions the female client should be in when the nurse is examining her breasts.

   The client can be standing or sitting

   Δ   **with her arms at her sides.**

   Δ   **with her arms over her head.**

   Δ   **with her hands pressed against her hips.**

   Δ   **leaning forward.**

2. What information should be documented when describing a breast mass?

   Location, size, shape, consistency, discreteness, tenderness, erythema, dimpling or retraction over the lump, lymphadenopathy, and mobility

3. True or False: It is not necessary to perform a breast exam on a male client.

   False: Breast exams should be performed on male and female clients.

4. Which of the following are expected changes of the breast tissue after menopause? (Select all that apply.)

   _____   Clear discharge from nipples
   _**X**_   **More pendulous**
   _**X**_   **Breast tissue replaced by adipose tissue**
   _____   Firmer
   _____   Nodular

   The breasts become more pendulous, breast tissue is replaced by adipose tissue, and breasts may feel more nodular and softer. Discharge from the nipples is an abnormal finding.

5. During palpation of the breast, the client is instructed to extend an arm over her head, and a small pillow or folded towel is placed under her shoulder to

A. spread the tissue more evenly over the chest wall for easier palpation.

B. avoid the client from guarding during the exam.

C. expose the tail of Spence for easier inspection.

D. determine whether or not a breast mass is consistently irregular when palpating a nodule.

This position spreads the tissue more evenly over the chest wall for easier palpation.

Unit 2   Health Assessment
Section: System-Specific Assessment

Chapter 35:   Thorax and Lungs
Contributor: Sally Swenson, MA, RN

 NCLEX® Connections:

Learning Objective: Review and apply knowledge within "**Thorax and Lungs**" in readiness for performance of the following nursing activities as outlined by the NCLEX® test plans:

Δ   Use effective communication to collect history assessment data related to the client's thorax and lungs.

Δ   Perform the appropriate assessment of the client's thorax and lungs, within the nursing role, including:

- Preparing the client for the procedure.
- Client teaching (before and following the procedure).
- Using accurate technique based on the client's needs.

Δ   Assess/monitor the client's status by obtaining baseline data and comparing with subsequent findings.

Δ   Document baseline and subsequent findings according to facility/agency protocol.

Δ   Maintain confidentiality of all client information.

 Key Points

Δ   **Age-related Changes**

- Chest shape changes so that the anteroposterior (AP) diameter becomes similar to the transverse diameter (barrel chest).
- Chest excursion or expansion diminishes.

Key Procedural Points

Δ   Use the techniques of inspection, palpation, percussion, and auscultation to examine the anterior and posterior thorax and lungs.

Δ   Equipment

- Stethoscope

- Centimeter ruler

- A wristwatch with a second hand or digital readout that allows for counting seconds

Δ   **Anatomical reminder**: The **right** lung has **three** lobes, while the **left** lung has **two** lobes. Auscultating the right middle lobe is done using the axillary sites.

Δ   **Chest landmarks** are used to perform assessments correctly and describe findings. The following vertical landmarks are used:

- **Midsternal line** is through the center of the sternum.

- **Midclavicular line** is through the midpoint of the clavicle.

- **Anterior axillary line** is through the anterior axillary folds.

- **Midaxillary line** is through the apex of the axillae.

- **Posterior axillary line** is through the posterior axillary fold.

- **Right and left scapular lines** are through the inferior angle of the scapula.

- **Vertebral line** is along the center of the spine.

Δ   **Percussion and auscultatory sites** are in the intercostal spaces (ICS).

- **Posterior thorax** – the sites are between the scapula and the vertebrae on the upper portion of the back. Below the scapula, the sites are along the right and left scapular lines.

- **Anterior thorax** – the sites are along the midclavicular lines bilaterally, with several sites at the anterior/midaxillary lines bilaterally in the lower portions of the chest wall and on either side of the sternum following along the rib cage.

- Percussion and auscultation should occur so that **side-to-side** comparisons can be made.

- Maximize sounds heard by:

  ◊   Having the client take deep breaths with open mouth each time the stethoscope is moved.

  ◊   Placing the stethoscope directly on the client's skin to prevent muffling or distortion of sounds.

◊   Facilitating client breathing by medicating for pain, giving clear
directions, and assisting the client to a sitting position.

Δ   **Positioning** – The posterior thorax is best assessed with the client sitting or
standing. The anterior thorax can be assessed with the client sitting, lying, or
standing.

Health History – Review of Systems

Δ   Questions the nurse should ask include:

- Do you have any chronic lung conditions such as asthma or emphysema? Do
you take any medications for your respiratory condition?

- Have you ever had pneumonia? If so, when and how often?

- Do you get frequent upper respiratory infections?

- Do you ever experience shortness of breath or difficulty breathing with
activity?

- Do you have a cough? Is it productive of sputum? If so, what does it look
like?

- Do you currently or have you ever smoked? If you no longer smoke, when
did you quit? How long did you smoke? If you do currently smoke, when did
you start and how much do you smoke?

Inspection

Δ   **Shape** – The AP diameter should be half of the transverse diameter.

Δ   **Symmetry** – The chest should be symmetrical with no deformities of the ribs,
sternum, scapula, or vertebrae with equal movements during respiration.

Δ   **ICS** – should not see excessive retractions.

Δ   **Respiratory Effort**

- Rate and pattern – should be regular with 16 to 20/min

- Character of breathing (e.g., diaphragmatic, abdominal, thoracic)

- Use of accessory muscles

- Chest wall expansion

- Depth of respirations – unlabored, quiet breathing being the expected finding

Δ   **Cough** – if productive, note the color/consistency of sputum.

Δ   **Trachea** should be midline.

Palpation

Δ   **Surface characteristics** include tenderness, lesions, lumps, and deformities. Tenderness is an unexpected finding.

Δ   **Chest Excursion or Expansion** of Posterior Thorax

   •   With thumbs aligned parallel along the spine at the level of the tenth rib, and the hands flattened around the client's back, instruct the client to take a deep breath. Thumbs should move outward approximately 5 cm when the client takes a deep inspiration.

Δ   **Vocal (Tactile) Fremitus**

   •   Palpate the chest wall using the ulnar surface of both hands comparing side to side.

   •   Ask the client to say **"99"** each time the hands are moved.

   •   **Expected findings** – Vibration is symmetrical and more pronounced over larger airways.

Percussion

Δ   Compare sounds that are produced from side to side.

Δ   Normal percussion of the thorax should result in **resonance.**

Δ   **Abnormal Findings and Significance**

   •   **Dullness** – caused by fluid or solid tissue which may be indicative of pneumonia or a tumor

   •   **Hyperresonance** – caused by the presence of air which may be indicative of pneumothorax or emphysema

Auscultation

Δ   **Expected Sounds**

   •   Bronchial – loud, high-pitched, expiration heard longer than inspiration over trachea

   •   Bronchovesicular – medium pitch and intensity, equal inspiration and expiration, and heard over larger airways

   •   Vesicular – soft, low-pitched, inspiration heard; longer expiration heard over most of the lungs

Δ   **Adventitious Sounds**

   •   Crackles or rales – fine to coarse popping heard as air passes through fluid or re-expands collapsed small airways

- Wheezes – high-pitched whistling, musical sounds heard as air passes through narrowed airways
- Pleural friction rub – grating sound produced as the inflamed visceral and parietal pleura rub against each other during inspiration

NANDA Nursing Diagnoses

Δ   Ineffective airway clearance

Δ   Ineffective breathing pattern

Δ   Fatigue

Sample Documentation

Respiratory rate is 16/min and regular. Respirations are easy and unlabored. Thorax has a greater transverse than AP diameter. No chest wall deformities noted. Trachea is midline. Movement is symmetrical with 5 cm of expansion. Equal tactile fremitus noted. Resonant sounds percussed throughout. Vesicular sounds heard primarily over the bases bilaterally. No adventitious sounds noted.

Primary Reference:

Potter, P. A., & Perry, A. G. (2005). *Fundamentals of nursing* (6th ed.). St. Louis, MO: Mosby.

Additional Resources:

Bickley, L. S., & Szilagyi, P. G. (2003). *Bates' guide to physical examination and history taking* (8th ed.). Philadelphia: Lippincott Williams & Wilkins.

Jarvis, C. (2004). *Physical examination & health assessment.* (4th ed.). St. Louis, MO: Saunders.

NANDA International (2004). *NANDA nursing diagnoses: Definitions and classification 2005-2006.* Philadelphia: NANDA.

Chapter 35: Thorax and Lungs

Application Exercises

1. Match each of the following sounds with its correct description.

_____ Bronchial sounds

A. Fine, coarse popping sounds produced by sudden opening of collapsed alveoli

_____ Bronchovesicular

B. High-pitched whistling, musical sounds produced by narrowed airways

_____ Vesicular

C. Grating sound produced by inflamed moving pleura

_____ Crackles/rales

D. The expected percussion sound over the thorax

_____ Pleural friction rub

E. Inspiration > expiration, softer, and lower-pitched

_____ Wheezes

F. Percussion sound heard over air-filled lung tissue

_____ Resonance

G. Expiration = inspiration, medium pitch and intensity

_____ Hyperresonance

H. Expiration > inspiration, loud and high-pitched, and heard over trachea

2. Which of the following is assessed when performing palpation of the thorax and lungs? (Select all that apply.)

_____ Breath sounds

_____ Respiratory effort

_____ Tactile fremitus

_____ Surface characteristics

_____ Chest excursion

3. When auscultating breath sounds, the nurse should instruct the client to

   A. repeat "99" continuously.

   B. count the number of respirations for a full minute.

   C. take a deep breath through his mouth each time the stethoscope is moved.

   D. breathe rapidly for 30 sec.

4. When auscultating breath sounds, the nurse should

   A. listen to the top of the anterior chest and then the top of the posterior chest.

   B. compare side to side proceeding from top to bottom.

   C. listen only to the posterior chest.

   D. complete one side of the chest before proceeding to the other side.

Chapter 35: Thorax and Lungs

Application Exercises Answer Key

1. Match each of the following sounds with its correct description.

__H__	Bronchial sounds	A. Fine, coarse popping sounds produced by sudden opening of collapsed alveoli
__G__	Bronchovesicular	B. High-pitched whistling, musical sounds produced by narrowed airways
__E__	Vesicular	C. Grating sound produced by inflamed moving pleura
__A__	Crackles/rales	D. The expected percussion sound over the thorax
__C__	Pleural friction rub	E. Inspiration > expiration, softer, and lower-pitched
__B__	Wheezes	F. Percussion sound heard over air-filled lung tissue
__D__	Resonance	G. Expiration = inspiration, medium pitch and intensity
__F__	Hyperresonance	H. Expiration > inspiration, loud and high-pitched, and heard over trachea

2. Which of the following is assessed when performing palpation of the thorax and lungs? (Select all that apply.)

_____ Breath sounds

_____ Respiratory effort

__X__ **Tactile fremitus**

__X__ **Surface characteristics**

__X__ **Chest excursion**

Tactile fremitus, surface characteristics, and chest excursion are all assessed during palpation. Breath sounds are assessed by auscultation. Respiratory effort is assessed by inspection.

3. When auscultating breath sounds, the nurse should instruct the client to

    A. repeat "99" continuously.

    B. count the number of respirations for a full minute.

    C. take a deep breath through his mouth each time the stethoscope is moved.

    D. breathe rapidly for 30 sec.

This instruction will allow the nurse to listen to a full inspiration and expiration. Having the client say "99" is used to assess tactile fremitus. It is not necessary to listen to a full minute of respirations. Rapid breathing will not allow the nurse to adequately assess breath sounds.

4. When auscultating breath sounds, the nurse should

    A. listen to the top of the anterior chest and then the top of the posterior chest.

    B. compare side to side proceeding from top to bottom.

    C. listen only to the posterior chest.

    D. complete one side of the chest before proceeding to the other side.

Comparing side-to-side breath sounds is the correct technique to use. This allows the nurse to make comparisons between right and left lungs in a systematic way.

Unit 2   Health Assessment

Section: System-Specific Assessment

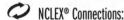

Chapter 36:	Circulatory System

Contributor: Sally Swenson, MA, RN

 NCLEX® Connections:

Learning Objective: Review and apply knowledge within "**Circulatory System**" in readiness for performance of the following nursing activities as outlined by the NCLEX® test plans:

Δ   Use effective communication to collect history assessment data related to the client's circulatory system.

Δ   Perform the appropriate assessment of the client's circulatory system, within the nursing role, including:

• Preparing the client for the procedure.

• Client teaching (before and following the procedure).

• Using accurate technique based on the client's needs.

Δ   Assess/monitor the client's status by obtaining baseline data and comparing with subsequent findings.

Δ   Document baseline and subsequent findings according to facility/agency protocol.

Δ   Maintain confidentiality of all client information.

Key Points

Δ   **Cardiac Cycle and Heart Sounds**

• Closure of the mitral and tricuspid valves signals the beginning of ventricular systole (contraction) and produces the S_1 sound (lub). This is heard best with the diaphragm of the stethoscope.

• Closure of the aortic and pulmonic valves signals the beginning of ventricular diastole (relaxation) and produces the S_2 sound (dub). This is heard best with the diaphragm of the stethoscope.

• An S_3 sound is produced by rapid ventricular filling and can be a normal finding in children and young adults. This is heard best with the bell of the stethoscope.

- An S_4 sound is produced by a strong atrial contraction and can be a normal finding in older and athletic adults and children. This is heard best with the bell of the stethoscope.

- **Murmurs** are heard when blood volume is increased in the heart, or the flow of blood is impeded or altered from normal. A murmur is heard in the heart as a blowing or swishing sound. This is heard best with the bell of the stethoscope.

  ◊ **Systolic murmurs** are heard just after S_1.

  ◊ **Diastolic murmurs** are heard just after S_2.

- **Thrills** are a palpable vibration that may be present with murmurs or cardiac malformation.

- **Bruits** are produced by obstructed peripheral blood flow and are heard as a blowing or swishing sound with the **bell** of the stethoscope.

Δ **Age-Related Changes**

- **Systolic murmurs** – Mitral regurgitation is a common physiologic change that will produce a systolic murmur in the older adult client.

- **Systolic hypertension (widened pulse pressure)** – This is a common finding with atherosclerosis in the older adult client.

- **Point of maximal impulse (PMI)** becomes more difficult to palpate because the anteroposterior diameter of the chest widens.

Key Procedural Points

Δ **Equipment**

- Stethoscope

- Blood pressure cuff

- A wristwatch with a second hand or digital readout that allows for counting seconds

- Ruler and straight edge

Δ **Auscultatory Sites for the Heart**

- **Aortic** – just right of the sternum at the second intercostal space (ICS)

- **Pulmonic** – just left of the sternum at the second ICS

- **Erb's point** – just left of the sternum at the third ICS

- **Tricuspid** – just left of the sternum at the fourth ICS

- **Apical/mitral** – left midclavicular line at the fifth ICS

Health History – Review of Systems

Δ   Questions the nurse should ask include:

- Do you have any problems with your heart? Do you take any medications?

- Do you have high blood pressure or high cholesterol?

- Do your feet and ankles ever swell?

- Do you experience chest pain? When? How long does it last? How often does it occur? Describe the pain.

- What are you doing before the pain begins?

- Are there any other symptoms associated with the pain (nausea, shortness of breath, sweating, dizziness)?

- What have you tried to relieve the pain?

- Describe your energy level. Are you frequently tired? Do you have unusual fatigue?

- Do you experience fainting spells? If so, how often? When was the last time it occurred?

Inspection and Palpation

Δ   **Vital signs** – Pulse and blood pressure are indicators of cardiovascular status. *(Refer to chapter 24: Pulse, and chapter 26: Blood Pressure.)*

Δ   **Heart**

- **Apical pulse or PMI**

  ◊   May be visible just lateral to the left midclavicular line at the fifth ICS. In female clients, the breast tissue will need to be displaced.

  ◊   Palpate where it was visualized. If not visualized, try to palpate the location and the size.

  ◊   Expected finding – The apical pulse should be just lateral to the left midclavicular line at the fifth ICS and no larger than 2.5 cm in diameter.

- **Heaves (or lifts)** are abnormal, visible elevations of the chest wall that are seen with heart failure, and are often located along the left sternal border or at the PMI.

- **Thrills** – use the ulnar surface of the hand to feel for vibrations similar to that of a purring kitten. This is not an expected finding.

Δ **Peripheral Vascular System**

- Inspect jugular **veins** with the client in bed with the head of the bed at a 30 to 45° angle to assess for right-sided heart failure.

  ◊ **Appearance** – no neck vein distension should be noted.

  ◊ **Jugular venous pressure (JVP)** – should be measured at less than 2.5 cm above the sternal angle using the following technique:

    ° Place one ruler vertically at the sternal angle.

    ° Locate the pulsation in the external jugular vein and place the straight edge of another ruler parallel to the floor at the level of the pulsation.

    ° Line up the two rulers as a T square keeping the horizontal ruler at the level of pulsation.

    ° The level where the horizontal ruler intersects the vertical ruler is where the JVP is measured.

Δ **Peripheral Arteries**

- Palpate peripheral pulses for strength (amplitude) and equality (symmetry).

  ◊ **Strength (amplitude)** – The strength of the impulse should be the same from beat to beat and can be graded on a scale of 0 to 4.

  ◊ A common scale to use is

    ° 0 = absent, unable to palpate.

    ° 1+ = diminished, weaker than expected.

    ° 2+ = brisk, expected.

    ° 3+ = increased.

    ° 4+ = full volume, bounding.

  ◊ **Equality** – **Peripheral pulse** impulses should be symmetrical in quality and quantity from the right side of the body to the left.

- With the exception of the carotid arteries, pulse sites can be palpated bilaterally to make comparisons.

  ◊ **Carotid pulse** – on either side of the trachea, just medial to the sternocleidomastoid muscle on the neck

  ◊ **Radial pulse** – on the radial side of each wrist

  ◊ **Brachial pulse** – in the antecubital fossa above the elbow

  ◊ **Femoral pulse** – midway between the symphysis pubis and the anterosuperior iliac spine

  ◊ **Popliteal pulse** – behind the knee, deep in the popliteal fossa, just lateral to midline

◊ **Dorsalis pedis pulse** – on the top of the foot, along a line with the groove between the first toe and the extensor tendons of the great toe

◊ **Posterior tibial pulse** – behind and below the medial malleolus of the ankles

- **Skin color** of the extremities should be symmetrical and similar to the rest of the body.

  ◊ Brown pigmentation changes occur with venous insufficiency.

  ◊ **Shiny** and thin skin without hair on toes and foot is seen with **arterial insufficiency**.

- Inspect **peripheral veins** for varicosities, redness, and swelling. Evaluate for Homans' sign. The leg is supported and flexed slightly at the knee while the foot is dorsiflexed. A report of pain in the calf would be a positive Homans' sign and suspicious for **phlebitis** (inflammation of the vein) or deep vein thrombosis (DVT).

- Palpate **temperature** of the skin with the dorsal part of the hand; check for symmetry. The skin should feel warm. Slightly cooler temperatures of the hands or feet are acceptable. Changes may reflect circulation impairment or environmental temperature.

- **Nail beds** should be pink and symmetrical, and **capillary refill** should be brisk.

- **Edema** is the presence of fluid in the tissues causing swollen, tight, and shiny skin surfaces.

  ◊ Causes of edema include poor venous or lymphatic circulation, burns, or allergic reactions.

  ◊ Assess the swelling for discoloration, location, and tenderness. In the extremities, the circumference of the swollen body area should be measured and compared to the other side.

  ◊ Common clinical practice includes grading the level of pitting edema present. Use facility/agency grading scale. This grading is somewhat subjective, as findings may vary from examiner to examiner. Findings are most reliable when performed through a series of exams by the same examiner.

  ◊ Evaluate pitting edema by compressing the skin for at least 5 sec over a bony prominence (e.g., behind medial malleolus, dorsum of foot, or over shin) and assessing as follows:

Four-Point Scale	Degree	Response
1+	2 mm to trace	Rapid response
2+	4 mm to mild	10 to 15 sec
3+	6 mm to moderate	1 to 2 min
4+	8 mm to severe	2 to 5 min

Auscultation

Δ **Heart**

- **Positioning** the client in three different ways allows for optimal assessment of heart sounds, as some extra or abnormal sounds are accentuated by the various positions.

    ◊ **Sitting, leaning forward**

    ◊ **Lying supine**

    ◊ **Turned toward the left side** (best position for picking up extra heart sounds or murmurs)

- **Use both the diaphragm and the bell** of the stethoscope in a systematic manner to listen at all of the auscultatory sites.

Δ Assess the peripheral vascular system for the presence of **bruits**. Locations to assess for bruits include:

- **Carotid arteries** – over the carotid pulses.

- **Abdominal aorta** – just below the xiphoid process.

- **Renal arteries** – midclavicular lines above the umbilicus on the abdomen.

- **Iliac arteries** – midclavicular lines below the umbilicus on the abdomen.

- **Femoral arteries** – over the femoral pulses.

Sample Documentation

Heart rate is regular and 72/min. Blood pressure is 118/76 mm Hg. No thrills or heaves. PMI is approximately 1 cm at the fifth ICS left midclavicular line. S_1 is louder at the apex than S_2. S_2 is loudest in the pulmonary area on inspiration. No extra heart sounds, murmurs, or bruits were heard. JVP is 2 cm bilaterally. No edema noted. Peripheral pulses 2+ bilaterally. Negative Homans' sign bilaterally. Extremities are warm with no varicosities noted. Capillary refill is brisk.

Primary Reference:

Potter, P. A., & Perry, A. G. (2005). *Fundamentals of nursing* (6th ed.). St. Louis, MO: Mosby.

Additional Resources:

Bickley, L. S., & Szilagyi, P. G. (2003). *Bates' guide to physical examination and history taking* (8th ed.). Philadelphia: Lippincott Williams & Wilkins.

Jarvis, C. (2004). *Physical examination & health assessment.* (4th ed.). St. Louis, MO: Saunders.

NANDA International (2004). *NANDA nursing diagnoses: Definitions and classification 2005-2006*. Philadelphia: NANDA.

Chapter 36: Circulatory System

Application Exercises

1. Match the action within the heart/peripheral vascular system with the sound it produces.

____	Rapid ventricular filling	A. S_1
____	Closure of the mitral and tricuspid valves	B. S_2
____	Strong atrial contraction	C. Murmur
____	Obstructed blood flow in peripheral circulation	D. S_3
____	Impeded blood flow in the heart	E. S_4
____	Closure of the aortic and pulmonic valves	F. Bruits

2. Which of the following should be performed on a client following a total knee replacement to assess the peripheral vascular system of the affected extremity? (Select all that apply.)

_____ Range of motion

_____ Skin color

_____ Skin temperature

_____ Presence of skin lesions

_____ Capillary refill

_____ Edema

3. The proper placement of the stethoscope for auscultating the aortic valve is the

A. second ICS just right of the sternum.

B. second ICS just left of the sternum.

C. fourth ICS just left of the sternum.

D. fifth ICS at the left midclavicular line.

4. Correct assessment of the carotid arteries includes

A. assessing for bruits with the bell of the stethoscope.

B. palpating both arteries at the same time.

C. instructing the client to breathe deeply and rapidly.

D. measuring for jugular venous distention.

Chapter 36: Circulatory System

Application Exercises Answer Key

1. Match the action within the heart/peripheral vascular system with the sound it produces.

D Rapid ventricular filling   A. S_1

A Closure of the mitral and tricuspid valves   B. S_2

E Strong atrial contraction   C. Murmur

F Obstructed blood flow in peripheral circulation D. S_3

C Impeded blood flow in the heart   E. S_4

B Closure of the aortic and pulmonic valves   F. Bruits

2. Which of the following should be performed on a client following a total knee replacement to assess the peripheral vascular system of the affected extremity? (Select all that apply.)

        Range of motion

  X   **Skin color**

  X   **Skin temperature**

        Presence of skin lesions

  X   **Capillary refill**

  X   **Edema**

Assessment of the peripheral vascular system includes skin color, skin temperature, capillary refill, and edema. Determining range of motion will assess joint function. Assess for presence of skin lesions during the skin assessment.

3. The proper placement of the stethoscope for auscultating the aortic valve is the

    A. second ICS just right of the sternum.

    B. second ICS just left of the sternum.

    C. fourth ICS just left of the sternum.

    D. fifth ICS at the left midclavicular line.

Auscultate the aortic valve at the second ICS just right of the sternum. Auscultate the pulmonic valve at the second ICS just left of the sternum. Auscultate the tricuspid valve at the fourth ICS just left of the sternum. Auscultate the mitral valve at the fifth ICS at the left midclavicular line.

4. Correct assessment of the carotid arteries includes

   A. assessing for bruits with the bell of the stethoscope.

   B. palpating both arteries at the same time.

   C. instructing the client to breathe deeply and rapidly.

   D. measuring for jugular venous distention.

Bruits can best be heard with the bell of the stethoscope. Both arteries should not be assessed simultaneously to prevent total occlusion of blood flow to the brain. The client should breathe quietly or hold his breath. Jugular venous distention is assessed by measuring jugular venous pressure, not the carotid arteries.

Unit 2
Section:

Health Assessment
System-Specific Assessment

Chapter 37:   **Abdomen**
Contributor: Sally Swenson, MA, RN

 NCLEX® Connections:

Learning Objective: Review and apply knowledge within "**Abdomen**" in readiness for performance of the following nursing activities as outlined by the NCLEX® test plans:

Δ   Use effective communication to collect history assessment data related to the client's abdomen.

Δ   Perform the appropriate assessment of the client's abdomen, within the nursing role, including:

•   Preparing the client for the procedure.

•   Client teaching (before and following the procedure).

•   Using accurate technique based on the client's needs.

Δ   Assess/monitor the client's status by obtaining baseline data and comparing with subsequent findings.

Δ   Document baseline and subsequent findings according to facility/agency protocol.

Δ   Maintain confidentiality of all client information.

 Key Points

Δ   **Abdominal landmarks** are designated using the umbilicus. Imaginary vertical and horizontal lines through the umbilicus divide the abdomen into four quadrants:

•   Right upper quadrant (RUQ).

•   Left upper quadrant (LUQ).

•   Right lower quadrant (RLQ).

•   Left lower quadrant (LLQ).

Δ   **Age-related Changes**

- **There is more adipose** tissue in the lower abdomen.

- **Weaker abdominal muscles** create a potbelly appearance.

- **Diminished signs and symptoms** of peritoneal inflammation, such as less pain, guarding, fever, or rebound tenderness may alter the demonstration of typical clinical manifestations in the older adult client.

Key Procedural Points

Δ   Use the techniques of inspection, **auscultation**, percussion, and palpation. The **order** of assessment techniques **changes** to allow bowel sounds to be auscultated just after inspection. This change is done to allow the client's existing bowel sounds to be heard without being disturbed or distorted by percussion or palpation assessments.

Δ   Equipment

- Stethoscope

- Tape measure or ruler

- Marking pen

Δ   **Preparing and positioning the client** includes having the client void prior to the abdominal exam. Then, position the client lying supine with his arms at his sides and with his knees slightly bent.

Health History – Review of Systems

Δ   Questions the nurse should ask include:

- Do you ever experience nausea, vomiting?

- Have you experienced any change in your appetite? Do you have any food intolerances? Any recent weight changes?

- Do you have any problems with your bowels? Do you experience diarrhea? Constipation? When was your last bowel movement?

- Do you ever experience heartburn? When? How often?

- What is your typical day's intake of food and fluid?

- Do you have any dietary restrictions or special practices?

Inspection

Δ   **Skin** is assessed for:

- **Lesions** – note any bruising, rashes, or other primary lesions.

- **Scars** – note the location and length.

- **Striae** or stretch marks that are silver in color. These are considered expected findings.

- **Dilated** veins – an unexpected finding associated with cirrhosis or inferior vena cava obstruction.

Δ **Shape or contour** can be described as:

- Flat – lies in a horizontal line from the chest to the symphysis pubis.

- Convex – rounded.

- Concave – has a sunken appearance.

- Distended – a large protrusion of the abdomen caused by fat, fluid, or flatus that can be differentiated as follows:

  ◊ Fat – the client has rolls of fat tissue along her sides, and the skin does not look taut.

  ◊ Fluid – the flanks also protrude, and when the client turns onto her side, the protrusion moves to the dependent side.

  ◊ Flatus – the protrusion is mainly midline, and the flanks are unchanged.

Δ **Movement** of the abdominal wall may be observed as:

- **Peristalsis** – Wave-like movements are visible in thin adults or in clients with intestinal obstructions.

- **Pulsations** – Regular beats of movement seen midline above the umbilicus are expected findings in thin adults, but a pulsating mass would be unexpected.

Δ **Umbilicus** should be inspected for position, shape, color, inflammation, discharge, or masses. No discharge, inflammation, or masses should be noted.

Auscultation

Δ **Bowel sounds** are produced by the movement of air and fluid in the intestines.

- **Technique** – Listen with the diaphragm of the stethoscope in all four quadrants.

- **Expected sounds** – High-pitched clicks and gurgles are heard 5 to 30 times/min. To make the determination of absent bowel sounds, the examiner needs to listen for a **full 5 min** without hearing anything.

Δ **Friction rubs are abnormal sounds** caused by the rubbing together of inflamed layers of the peritoneum. The technique is as follows:

- Listen with the diaphragm over the liver and spleen.

- Ask the client to take a deep breath while you listen for any grating sounds (like sandpaper rubbing together).

Δ **Vascular Sounds (Bruits)**

- **Abdominal aorta** – just below the xiphoid process
- **Renal arteries** – midclavicular lines above the umbilicus on the abdomen
- **Iliac arteries** – midclavicular lines below the umbilicus on the abdomen
- **Femoral arteries** – over the femoral pulses

Percussion

Δ **Tympany** is the expected percussion sound heard over the majority of the abdomen. A lower-pitch tympany over the gastric bubble in the left upper quadrant may be heard.

Δ **Dullness** over the liver or a distended bladder may be heard.

Δ **Liver span** is a measurement of liver size taken at the right midclavicular line and can be determined using percussion techniques.

- Establish the lower border of the liver by percussing upward from below the umbilicus at the right midclavicular line until tympany turns to dullness.
- Make a mark.
- Establish the upper border by percussing downward, starting at the right midclavicular line over the lung until resonance turns to dullness.
- Make a mark.
- Measure the distance between the two markings for the size of the liver span.
- The expected finding is 6 to 12 cm.

Δ **Kidney** tenderness is assessed by fist percussion over the costovertebral angles at the scapular lines on the back. The expected finding is no tenderness.

Palpation

Δ **Tender areas** should be palpated last.

Δ **Light**

- Use finger pads on one hand to palpate to a depth of 1 cm.
- Expected findings include consistency of softness, no nodules, and no guarding.

Δ **Deep**

- Two-handed approach – Top hand depresses bottom hand 3 to 4 cm in depth. The bottom hand assesses for organ enlargement or masses. Location, consistency, shape, and size of any mass should be documented.

- Expected findings can include:
  - ◊ Bladder may be palpated if full; otherwise, it is nonpalpable.
  - ◊ Stool may be palpated in the descending colon.

Δ **Rebound tenderness (Blumberg's sign)** is an indication of irritation or inflammation somewhere in the abdominal cavity. The following technique should be done in all four quadrants.

- Apply firm pressure for 4 sec with the hand at a 90° angle and with fingers extended.

- After releasing the pressure, observe the client's response to see if pain was elicited once the pressure was released.

- Ask about pain/tenderness.

NANDA Nursing Diagnoses

Δ Acute pain

Δ Imbalanced nutrition: less than body requirements

Sample Documentation

Abdomen is flat with active bowel sounds heard every 10 to 20 sec in all four quadrants. No bruits or friction rubs heard. Abdomen is soft, nontender, and without masses or enlargement of spleen or liver. Liver span is 8 cm. No rebound or costovertebral tenderness noted. Bladder is not palpable.

Primary Reference:

Potter, P. A., & Perry, A. G. (2005). *Fundamentals of nursing* (6th ed.). St. Louis, MO: Mosby.

Additional Resources:

Bickley, L. S., & Szilagyi, P. G. (2003). *Bates' guide to physical examination and history taking* (8th ed.). Philadelphia: Lippincott Williams & Wilkins.

Jarvis, C. (2004). *Physical examination & health assessment.* (4th ed.). St. Louis, MO: Saunders.

NANDA International (2004). *NANDA nursing diagnoses: Definitions and classification 2005-2006.* Philadelphia: NANDA.

Chapter 37: Abdomen

Application Exercises

1. A nurse should perform the abdominal assessment using which of the following sequences?

    A. Inspection, palpation, percussion, and auscultation

    B. Auscultation, inspection, palpation, and percussion

    C. Percussion, inspection, auscultation, and palpation

    D. Inspection, auscultation, percussion, and palpation

2. Which of the following are assessed during inspection of the abdomen? (Select all that apply.)

    _____ Bowel sounds

    _____ Shape

    _____ Skin lesions

    _____ Tenderness

    _____ Pulsations

3. True or False: Bowel sounds should be heard every 1 to 2 min.

4. A client presents to the emergency department reporting vomiting and abdominal pain for the last 12 hr. To assess the client's abdominal pain, the nurse applies firm pressure to the client's abdomen for 4 sec with her hand at a 90° angle and her fingers extended. After the nurse releases the pressure, the client reports pain at the pressure site, which indicates

    A. localized pain.

    B. rebound tenderness.

    C. positive Homans' sign.

    D. CVA tenderness.

5. When performing percussion, which of the following sounds should be heard over the majority of the abdomen?

    A. Dullness

    B. Tympany

    C. Grating

    D. Gurgling

Chapter 37: Abdomen

Application Exercises Answer Key

1. A nurse should perform the abdominal assessment using which of the following sequences?

        A. Inspection, palpation, percussion, and auscultation

        B. Auscultation, inspection, palpation, and percussion

        C. Percussion, inspection, auscultation, and palpation

        D. Inspection, auscultation, percussion, and palpation

This sequence allows the client's existing bowel sounds to be heard without being disturbed or distorted by percussion or palpation assessments.

2. Which of the following are assessed during inspection of the abdomen? (Select all that apply.)

        _____ Bowel sounds

        __X__ **Shape**

        __X__ **Skin lesions**

        _____ Tenderness

        __X__ **Pulsations**

The shape of the abdomen, presence of lesions, and visualization of pulsations can all be assessed during inspection of the abdomen. Bowel sounds are assessed by auscultation. Tenderness is assessed by palpation.

3. True or False: Bowel sounds should be heard every 1 to 2 min.

False: Bowel sounds are soft clicks and gurgles that should be heard 5 to 30 times per min.

4. A client presents to the emergency department reporting vomiting and abdominal pain for the last 12 hr. To assess the client's abdominal pain, the nurse applies firm pressure to the client's abdomen for 4 sec with her hand at a 90° angle and her fingers extended. After the nurse releases the pressure, the client reports pain at the pressure site, which indicates

> A. localized pain.
>
> **B. rebound tenderness.**
>
> C. positive Homans' sign.
>
> D. CVA tenderness.

Rebound tenderness is elicited by applying firm pressure for 4 sec and then releasing the pressure. Localized pain is usually constant and may not need to be elicited by pressure. A positive Homans' sign is elicited when the client's foot is dorsiflexed and pain is felt in the calf. CVA tenderness is elicited by applying fist percussion to the kidneys.

5. When performing percussion, which of the following sounds should be heard over the majority of the abdomen?

> A. Dullness
>
> **B. Tympany**
>
> C. Grating
>
> D. Gurgling

The abdomen is primarily filled with air, and tympany is the sound that will predominate. Dullness is heard over the liver or a distended bladder. A grating sound may indicate a friction rub. Gurgling sounds are heard through a stethoscope and indicate peristalsis.

Unit 2   Health Assessment
Section: System-Specific Assessment

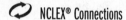

Chapter 38:   Musculoskeletal System
                Contributor: Sally Swenson, MA, RN

NCLEX® Connections

> **Learning Objective**: Review and apply knowledge within "**Musculoskeletal System**" in readiness for performance of the following nursing activities as outlined by the NCLEX® test plans:
>
> Δ   Use effective communication to collect history assessment data related to the client's musculoskeletal system.
>
> Δ   Perform the appropriate assessment of the client's musculoskeletal system, within the nursing role, including:
>
>   •   Preparing the client for the procedure.
>
>   •   Client teaching (before and following the procedure).
>
>   •   Using accurate technique based on the client's needs.
>
> Δ   Assess/monitor the client's status by obtaining baseline data and comparing with subsequent findings.
>
> Δ   Document baseline and subsequent findings according to facility/agency protocol.
>
> Δ   Maintain confidentiality of all client information.

Key Points

Δ   Assess the structure and function of the musculoskeletal system.

Δ   Assess each joint/muscle and the surrounding tissues, and compare symmetrical parts.

Δ   Assess

   •   Alignment

   •   Symmetry and muscle mass

   •   Muscle tone

- Range of motion (ROM)

- Any involuntary movements

- Signs of inflammation (e.g., redness, swelling, warmth, tenderness, loss of function)

- Gross deformities

Δ **Age-related Changes**

- Height loss is due to thinner intervertebral discs, osteoporosis, or kyphosis.

- Skeletal muscles decrease in size.

- Range of motion decreases.

- Posture changes are a result of a wider stance.

- Flexion of the hips, knees, and elbows is typical.

Key Procedural Points

Δ Use the techniques of inspection and palpation to assess the musculoskeletal system.

Δ Equipment – A tape measure may be needed to measure joint or limb enlargements and to make bilateral comparisons.

Δ **Range of Motion** of Joint Movement

- Flexion – to decrease the angle

- Extension – to extend the angle

- Hyperextension – extreme extension

- Supination – ventral surface facing up

- Pronation – ventral surface facing down

- Abduction – to move extremity away from midline

- Adduction – to move extremity toward the midline

- Dorsiflexion – movement toward the dorsum (or top of the wrist or foot)

- Plantar flexion – movement toward the plantar surface (or bottom of the foot)

- Eversion – to turn body part away from midline

- Inversion – to turn body part toward the midline

Health History – Review of Systems

Δ Questions the nurse should ask include:

- Do you have any pain in your joints or muscles?

- Do you have any stiffness, weakness, or twitching?

- Have you experienced any recent falls? Are you able to care for yourself?

- Is your activity limited by any physical factors?

- How would you describe your physical activity? Do you exercise on a regular basis?

Inspection

Δ **Height** – Measure for comparison over time; gradual height loss is a common finding as a person ages.

Δ **Posture** – Observe when the client is unaware he is being assessed. Expected finding: the client is standing with head erect. Both shoulders and both hips should be at the same height bilaterally.

Δ **Spine** – Inspect from the side. The following curvatures may be noted:

- Normal curvatures.

  ◊ Concave cervical spine

  ◊ Convex thoracic spine

  ◊ Concave lumbar spine

- Common abnormalities.

  ◊ **Kyphosis** – exaggerated curvature of the thoracic spine

  ◊ **Lordosis** – exaggerated curvature of the lumbar spine (common during the toddler years and pregnancy)

Inspection and Palpation

Δ **Range of motion (ROM)** should be equal in the joints bilaterally.

- Assess **passive ROM** by moving the client's joints through their full range of movements. Do not move a joint past a point of pain or resistance.

- Assess **active ROM** by having the client repeat the movements demonstrated by the nurse.

- Assess **joints** for abnormalities such as warmth, inflammation, crepitus, deformities, tenderness, limitations, or instability. The joints to be assessed include:

  ◊ Temporomandibular joint (TMJ).

  ◊ Shoulders.

  ◊ Elbows.

  ◊ Wrists and hands.

  ◊ Spine scoliosis.

  ◊ Hips.

  ◊ Knees.

  ◊ Ankles and feet.

Δ **Muscles** should be symmetrical in size and strength. The dominant side is usually slightly larger with a < 1 cm difference not being significant.

- Size variations include:

  ◊ **Hypertrophy** – an enlargement of muscle due to strengthening.

  ◊ **Atrophy** – a decrease in muscle size due to disuse.

- Assess **tone** during ROM. Tone is determined by the presence of slight resistance of the muscles during relaxation.

- Assess **strength** of muscle groups by asking the client to push or pull against resistance. Expected finding: strength should be equal or slightly stronger on the dominant side of the body.

Δ Inspect and palpate the **spine** from the back for any lateral deviations or **scoliosis.**

- Instruct the client to bend at the waist with arms reaching for the toes.

- Inspect and palpate down the spine using thumb and forefinger.

- Inspect and palpate the spine again with the client standing.

- Expected findings: there is no tenderness with spinal vertebrae that are midline.

NANDA Nursing Diagnoses

Δ Impaired physical mobility

Δ Risk for disuse syndrome

Sample Documentation

Full range of motion without pain in all joints and spine. No joint deformities, warmth, or swelling. Posture is erect. Spine is midline with expected cervical, thoracic, and lumbar curvatures. No scoliosis noted. Muscle strength is equal and strong bilaterally.

Primary Reference:

Potter, P. A., & Perry, A. G. (2005). *Fundamentals of nursing* (6th ed.). St. Louis, MO: Mosby.

Additional Resources:

Bickley, L. S., & Szilagyi, P. G. (2003). *Bates' guide to physical examination and history taking* (8th ed.). Philadelphia: Lippincott Williams & Wilkins.

Jarvis, C. (2004). *Physical examination & health assessment.* (4th ed.). St. Louis, MO: Saunders.

NANDA International (2004). *NANDA nursing diagnoses: Definitions and classification 2005-2006.* Philadelphia: NANDA.

Chapter 38: Musculoskeletal System

Application Exercises

1. Which of the following are normal aging changes of the musculoskeletal system? (Select all that apply.)

　　_____　Wider stance resulting in posture changes
　　_____　Loss of height
　　_____　Increased range of motion
　　_____　Increased muscle bulk
　　_____　Flexion of hips, knees, and elbows

2. Assessment of the musculoskeletal system should start with

　　A. measuring limb length.
　　B. testing range of motion.
　　C. inspection for symmetry and posture.
　　D. assessment of muscle strength.

3. During an assessment, the client reports pain on internal rotation of her right shoulder. This will most likely affect which of the following activities?

　　A. Brushing the back of her hair
　　B. Fastening her bra behind her back
　　C. Reaching for something in a cabinet above the sink
　　D. Mopping the floor

4. Unilateral hypertrophy of the arm muscles is most likely seen in an individual who regularly

　　A. lifts weights.
　　B. plays soccer.
　　C. moves furniture.
　　D. plays tennis.

5. Dorsiflexion of the feet is assessed by instructing the client to

　　A. point the toes toward the head.
　　B. point the toes toward the floor.
　　C. turn the soles of the feet outward.
　　D. turn the soles of the feet inward.

Chapter 38: Musculoskeletal System

Application Exercises Answer Key

1. Which of the following are normal aging changes of the musculoskeletal system? (Select all that apply.)

   __X__ Wider stance resulting in posture changes

   __X__ Loss of height

   _____ Increased range of motion

   _____ Increased muscle bulk

   __X__ Flexion of hips, knees, and elbows

   Normal aging changes of the musculoskeletal system include posture changes, loss of height, and flexion of the hips, knees, and elbows. Range of motion and muscle size also decrease.

2. Assessment of the musculoskeletal system should start with

   A. measuring limb length.

   B. testing range of motion.

   C. inspection for symmetry and posture.

   D. assessment of muscle strength.

   Assessment of the musculoskeletal system should start with inspection of the skeleton. Measuring limb length and testing range of motion and muscle strength are performed after inspection.

3. During an assessment, the client reports pain on internal rotation of her right shoulder. This will most likely affect which of the following activities?

   A. Brushing the back of her hair

   B. Fastening her bra behind her back

   C. Reaching for something in a cabinet above the sink

   D. Mopping the floor

   Fastening a bra from behind requires internal rotation of the shoulder. Brushing the back of the hair and reaching for something up high require external rotation of the shoulder. Mopping the floor requires flexion and extension of the shoulder.

4. Unilateral hypertrophy of the arm muscles is most likely seen in an individual who regularly

    A. lifts weights.

    B. plays soccer.

    C. moves furniture.

    D. plays tennis.

A tennis player will use one arm primarily, and unilateral hypertrophy will most likely result. Lifting weights, moving furniture, and playing soccer will most likely result in bilateral muscle hypertrophy.

5. Dorsiflexion of the feet is assessed by instructing the client to

    A. point the toes toward the head.

    B. point the toes toward the floor.

    C. turn the soles of the feet outward.

    D. turn the soles of the feet inward.

Pointing the toes toward the head results in dorsiflexion. Pointing the toes toward the floor results in plantar flexion. Turning the soles of the feet outward results in eversion, and turning the soles of the feet inward results in inversion.

Unit 2   Health Assessment
Section: System-Specific Assessment

Chapter 39:	Neurological System

Contributor: Sally Swenson, MA, RN

 NCLEX® Connections:

Learning Objective: Review and apply knowledge within "**Neurological System**" in readiness for performance of the following nursing activities as outlined by the NCLEX® test plans:

Use effective communication to collect history assessment data related to the client's neurological system.

Perform the appropriate assessment of the client's neurological system, within the nursing role, including:

Δ   Preparing the client for the procedure.

Δ   Client teaching (before and following the procedure).

Δ   Using accurate technique based on the client's needs.

Δ   Assess/monitor the client's status by obtaining baseline data and comparing with subsequent findings.

Δ   Document baseline and subsequent findings according to facility/agency protocol.

Δ   Maintain confidentiality of all client information.

 Key Points

Δ   A neurological screening exam can evaluate the major indicators of neurological function and assist with recognition of areas of dysfunction.

Δ   **Integration** of the neurological system with other assessments is recommended.

Δ   **Extent** of the exam is based on the client's level of consciousness and general state of health.

Δ   **Age-related changes include**:

- Decline in mental function may result from the decrease in mental stimulation and increase in loneliness that occurs with the loss of employment, relatives, and friends.

- Brain volume and brain cells decrease with aging.

- Motor responses are typically slow.

- Vibration, position, sense, and some reflexes may be diminished or absent.

- The processing of and learning of new material occurs at a slower rate.

- Delirium is a more common characteristic of infection than an elevated temperature.

- Depression becomes more prevalent.

Key Procedural Points

Δ   A neurological screening exam includes:

- Mental status exam to test cerebral function.

- Assessment of cranial nerves.

- Motor function to test cerebellar function.

- Sensory function.

- Reflexes.

Δ   Equipment

- Snellen and Rosenbaum eye charts

- Aromatic substances

- Tongue blades

- Penlight

- Sugar and salt

- Tuning fork

- Reflex hammer

- Cotton balls

Δ   Two test tubes filled with water (one cold, one warm)

Δ   Pencil

Health History - Review of Systems

Δ   Questions the nurse should ask include

- Do you have any problems with dizziness or headaches? Do you ever have seizures?

- Do you have a history of head trauma, any loss of consciousness?

- Have you noticed any change in your speech, ability to think clearly, loss of or change in memory?

- Do you have any weakness, numbness, tremors or tingling? If so, where?

Mental Status

Δ   **Levels of consciousness** should be described as follows:

- **Alert** – The client is responsive and able to fully respond by opening eyes and attending to a normal tone of voice and speech.

- **Lethargy** – The client is able to open eyes and respond, but is drowsy and falls asleep readily.

- **Obtundation** – The client needs to be lightly shaken to respond, but may be confused and slow to respond.

- **Stupor** – The client requires painful stimuli (e.g., pinching a tendon or rubbing the sternum) to achieve a brief response. The client may not be able to respond verbally.

- **Coma** – There is no response to repeated painful stimuli. Abnormal posturing in the comatose client:

  ◊   Decorticate rigidity – flexion and internal rotation of upper extremity joints and legs

  ◊   Decerebrate rigidity – neck and elbow extension, wrists and fingers flexed

Δ   **Altered levels of consciousness** can be measured more objectively using the Glasgow Coma Scale.

Expected action	Best response	Score
Eyes open	Spontaneously	4
	To speech	3
	To pain	2
	None	1
Best verbal response	Oriented	5
	Confused	4
	Inappropriate words	3
	Incomprehensible sounds	2
	None	1
Best motor response	Obeys commands	6
	Localized pain	5
	Flexion withdrawal	4
	Abnormal flexion	3
	Abnormal extension	2
	Flaccid	1
	TOTAL SCORE	15

Δ   **Appearance** assessment includes hygiene, grooming, and clothing choice. Expected findings: the client is well-kept, clean, and dressed appropriately for the environment or situation.

Δ   Assess **mood** by inspecting the mannerisms and actions during interactions with the client. Expected findings: the client makes eye contact, and emotions correspond to the conversation and situation.

Δ   Assess **cognitive processes**:

  •   **Memory,** both recent and remote, should be assessed.

      ◊   Recent – Ask the client to repeat a series of numbers or a list of objects.

      ◊   Remote – Ask the client to state birth date or mother's maiden name (verifiable).

  •   **Knowledge** – Ask the client what he knows about his current hospitalization or illness.

  •   **Abstract thinking** – Ask the client the interpretation of a cliché such as "A bird in the hand is worth two in the bush" This would demonstrate a higher level of thought processes.

- **Association** – Ask the client to explain how various concepts are related, such as a creek and a river.

- **Judgment** – Ask the client about the solution to a specific dilemma (e.g., "What would you do if you locked your keys in your car?"). The response should be logical.

Δ **Speech and language** should be articulate and responses meaningful and appropriate.

Δ Use the **Mini-Mental State Examination** (MME) to objectively assess cognitive status. The tool evaluates:

- **Orientation** to time and place.

- **Attention and calculation** of counting backward by 7s.

- **Registration and recalling** of objects.

- **Language,** including naming of objects, following of commands, and ability to write.

Cranial Nerve Function

Cranial nerve (CN)	Function of the nerve	System
I (Olfactory)	• Sensory - smell	Ears, nose, mouth, and throat
II (Optic)	• Sensory –visual acuity, visual fields.	Eyes
III (Oculomotor), IV (Trochlear, and VI (Abducens)	• Sensory – PERRLA, six cardinal positions of gaze	Eyes
V (Trigeminal)	• Sensory – light touch sensation to face (forehead, cheek, jaw) • Motor – jaw opening, clenching, chewing	Head and neck
VII (Facial)	• Sensory – taste (salt/sweet) on anterior 2/3's of tongue • Motor – facial movements	Head and neck
VIII (Auditory)	• Sensory—hearing and balance	Ears, nose, mouth, and throat
IX (Glossopharyngeal)	• Sensory – taste (sour/bitter) on posterior 1/3 of tongue • Motor – swallowing, speech sounds and gag reflex	Ears, nose, mouth, throat, neurological

Cranial nerve (CN)	Function of the nerve	System
X (Vagus)	• Motor – swallowing, speech sounds and gag reflex	Ears, nose, mouth, and throat
XI (Spinal accessory)	• Motor – turn head, shrug shoulders	Head and neck
XII (Hypoglossal)	• Motor – tongue movement	Ears, nose, mouth, and throat

Motor Function

Δ   Assess **coordination** by asking the client to extend arms and rapidly touch his finger to his nose, alternating hands and then doing the technique with his eyes closed. Expected findings include smooth, coordinated movements.

Δ   Assess **gait** when the client is unaware of being assessed. Expected finding: gait is steady, smooth, and coordinated.

Δ   Assess **balance** using the following tests:

- Romberg test – Ask the client to stand with feet at a comfortable distance apart, arms at sides, and eyes closed. Expected finding: the client should be able to stand with minimal swaying for at least 5 sec.

- Heel-to-toe walk – Ask the client to place the heel of one foot in front of the toes of the other foot as he walks in a straight line. Expected finding: the client is able to walk in a straight line without losing his balance.

Δ   **Muscle strength**

- Assess **strength** of muscle groups by asking the client to push or pull against resistance. Expected finding: strength should be equal or slightly stronger on the dominant side of the body.

Δ   **Sensory function** tests are performed on all four extremities with the client's eyes closed.

- Assess **pain** sensation by alternating sharp and dull objects on the skin and asking the client to report what he feels.

- Assess **temperature** by using two test tubes filled with water (one warm and one cold), asking the client to identify which he feels (usually deferred).

- Assess **light touch** by asking the client to report when and where he feels a cotton ball touching his skin.

- Assess **vibration** by having the client report when and where he feels the handle of the vibrating tuning fork on his skin.

- Assess **position** by repositioning the client's appendages and asking him to report whether it is positioned up or down.

- Assess **discrimination** by using one of the following:

  ◊ **Two-point discrimination** – Use open paper clips to determine the distance at which the two points are felt as one. Compare bilaterally. Minimal distance will vary depending on the body part being evaluated.

  ◊ **Stereognosis** – Use a familiar object (e.g., key, cotton ball) placed in the client's hand, and ask him to identify it.

  ◊ **Graphesthesia** – Ask the client to identify a number drawn on his palm with the blunt end of a pencil.

Deep tendon reflexes (DTR)

Δ Using a reflex hammer, assess **DTRs** bilaterally and compare results for symmetry as follows:

DTR –spinal cord innervation	Technique	Expected response
Biceps – C_5 and C_6	• Flex arm 45°. • Place thumb on tendon in antecubital fossa. • Strike thumb with a reflex hammer.	Flexion of elbow
Brachioradialis – C_5 and C_6	• Forearm rests on examiner's forearm with the wrist slightly pronated. • Strike the tendon 2.5 to 5 cm above the wrist.	Pronation of forearm and flexion of elbow
Triceps – C_6, C_7, and C_8	• Support upper arm with the forearm hanging at a 90°. • Strike the tendon above the elbow.	Extension of elbow
Patellar – L_2, L_3, and L_4	• With upper leg supported and lower leg dangling freely, strike the tendon below the knee.	Extension of lower leg
Achilles – S_1 and S_2	• Flex knee, dorsiflex foot, and strike the tendon above heel.	Plantar flexion of foot

Δ Grading of DTR responses are done on a scale of 0 to 4.

- **4+** = Very brisk with clonus

- **3+** = More brisk than average

- **2+** = Expected

- **1+** = Diminished

- **0** = No response

NANDA Nursing Diagnoses

Δ   Impaired memory

Δ   Impaired physical mobility

Δ   Altered thought processes

Sample Documentation

Alert and oriented to person, place, and time. Client is pleasant and cooperative. Recent and remote memories are intact. Speech is clear and articulate. Cranial nerves I to XII are intact. Able to rapidly alternate arm movements with accuracy. Gait is steady. Ambulating without assistance. Hand grips are strong and equal. Romberg – minimal swaying noted. Pain, light touch, stereognosis are intact. DTRs are 2+ and symmetrical.

Primary Reference:

Potter, P. A., & Perry, A. G. (2005). *Fundamentals of nursing* (6th ed.). St. Louis, MO: Mosby.

Additional Resources:

Bickley, L.S., & Szilagyi, P.G. (2003). *Bates' guide to physical examination and history taking* (8th ed.). Philadelphia: Lippincott Williams & Wilkins.

Jarvis, C. (2004). *Physical examination & health assessment.* (4th ed.). St. Louis, MO: Saunders.

NANDA International (2004). *NANDA nursing diagnoses: Definitions and classification 2005-2006.* Philadelphia: NANDA.

Chapter 39: Neurological System

Application Exercises

1. Match the following cranial nerves with the appropriate assessment technique.

_____ Olfactory (CN I)

_____ Optic (CN II)

_____ Oculomotor (CN III), Trochlear (CN IV)

Abducens (CN VI)

_____ Facial (CN VII)

_____ Acoustic (CN VIII)

_____ Spinal Accessory (CN XI)

_____ Hypoglossal (CN XII)

A. Snellen chart

B. Six cardinal positions of gaze

C. Identification of a familiar smell with eyes closed

D. Smiling, frowning, and raising the eyebrows

E. Shrugging the shoulders against resistance

F. Moving the tongue up, down, and side to side

2. Which of the following questions should be asked during a health history to assess the client's cerebral function?

   A. "Do your fingers ever feel numb and tingly?"

   B. "Do you have difficulty remembering things?"

   C. "Do you have any problems keeping your balance?"

   D. "Do you have any difficulties with your sense of taste?"

3. When the triceps tendon is hit with a reflex hammer, the expected response is for the elbow t

   A. flex.

   B. extend.

   C. internally rotate.

   D. pronate.

4. To evaluate stereognosis, the nurse should ask the client to close his eyes and to identify

   A. a number drawn in the palm of his hand.

   B. a word whispered 30 cm from his ear.

   C. a familiar object placed in his hand.

   D. the vibration of a tuning fork placed on his foot.

5. Which of the following is included in the assessment of the client's cognitive processes? (Select all that apply.)

_____ Level of consciousness

_____ Mood

_____ Appearance

_____ Knowledge

_____ Judgment

Chapter 39: Neurological System

Application Exercises Answer Key

1. Match the following cranial nerves with the appropriate assessment technique.

__C__	Olfactory (CN I)	A. Snellen chart
__A__	Optic (CN II)	B. Six cardinal positions of gaze
__B__	Oculomotor (CN III), Trochlear (CN IV) Abducens (CN VI)	C. Identification of a familiar smell with eyes closed
__D__	Facial (CN VII)	D. Smiling, frowning, and raising the eyebrows
__G__	Acoustic (CN VIII)	E. Shrugging the shoulders against resistance
__E__	Spinal Accessory (CN XI)	F. Moving the tongue up, down, and side to side
__F__	Hypoglossal (CN XII)	

2. Which of the following questions should be asked during a health history to assess the client's cerebral function?

    A. "Do your fingers ever feel numb and tingly?"

    B. "Do you have difficulty remembering things?"

    C. "Do you have any problems keeping your balance?"

    D. "Do you have any difficulties with your sense of taste?"

Memory is tested during the mental status exam, which evaluates cerebral function. Numbness and tingling are abnormal findings of the sensory system. Balance is a test for muscle function, and the sense of taste is controlled by cranial nerves VII and IX.

3. When the triceps tendon is hit with a reflex hammer, the expected response is for the elbow t

    A. flex.

    B. extend.

    C. internally rotate.

    D. pronate.

4. To evaluate stereognosis, the nurse should ask the client to close his eyes and to identify

     A. a number drawn in the palm of his hand.

     B. a word whispered 30 cm from his ear.

     C. a familiar object placed in his hand.

     D. the vibration of a tuning fork placed on his foot.

Identifying a familiar object placed in the hand assesses for stereognosis. Graphesthesia is identifying a number drawn in the palm of the hand. Hearing whispered words tests CN VIII. Identifying a vibrating tuning fork tests the vibratory sense.

5. Which of the following is included in the assessment of the client's cognitive processes? (Select all that apply.)

     _____ Level of consciousness

     _____ Mood

     _____ Appearance

     _X_ Knowledge

     _X_ Judgment

All are components of a mental status examination. Assessment of knowledge and judgment are included in cognitive processes.

Unit 2   Health Assessment
Section: System-Specific Assessment

Chapter 40:	Genitalia and Rectum

Contributor: Sally Swenson, MA, RN

 NCLEX® Connections:

Learning Objective: Review and apply knowledge within "**Genitalia and Rectum**" in readiness for performance of the following nursing activities as outlined by the NCLEX® test plans:

Δ   Use effective communication to collect history assessment data related to the client's genitalia and rectum.

Δ   Perform the appropriate assessment of the client's genitalia and rectum, within the nursing role, including:

  •   Preparing the client for the procedure.

  •   Client teaching (before and following the procedure).

  •   Using accurate technique based on the client's needs.

Δ   Assess/monitor the client's status by obtaining baseline data and comparing with subsequent findings.

Δ   Document baseline and subsequent findings according to facility/agency protocol.

Δ   Maintain confidentiality of all client information.

 Key Points

Δ   **Age-related Changes**

  •   **Female**

    ◊   There is a decrease in ovarian function. Ovaries may not be palpable 3 to 5 years after menopause.

    ◊   Menstruation ceases.

    ◊   Pubic hair becomes sparse and grays.

    ◊   Labia, clitoris, uterus, and vagina atrophy.

- **Male**
  - ◊ Decreased testosterone levels lead to a decline in sexual function.
  - ◊ Pubic hair becomes sparse and grays.
  - ◊ Prostate gland enlarges in males as they age.

Key Procedural Points

Δ Use the techniques of inspection and palpation.

Δ Equipment

- Gloves and lubricant
- Speculum
- Exam table with stirrups
- Light source
- Pap smear equipment (cervical scrape, endocervical brush, slides, fixative)

Health History – Review of Systems

Δ Questions the nurse should ask include:

- Do you have any difficulties voiding? Do you ever experience burning, urgency, frequency, hesitancy?
- Do you ever experience incontinence? When does it happen?
- Have you had any change in bladder or bowel patterns? Do you ever notice blood in your urine or stool?
- Do you have any discharge from your vagina/penis? Do you experience any itching?
- Are you sexually active? What form of birth control do you use?
- Female clients – When was your last menstrual period? Are your menstrual cycles regular? Have you noticed any changes in the bleeding pattern? Ask obstetrical history.

Inspection and Palpation – Female Genitalia

Δ **Positioning the Client**

- Ask the client to **empty her bladder**.
- Ask the client to **lie supine** on the exam table.
- Place feet in the **stirrups**.
- Ask the client to move down so that her buttocks are at the edge of the exam table.

- A side-lying position can be used as an alternative for clients unable to assume the above position.

Δ **External Exam**

	Expected Findings
Pubic region	• Female hair distribution pattern in a downward triangle • No parasites • No lesions
Labia are separated and palpated using thumb and index finger.	• Symmetrical with the possibility of one side being slightly larger • Without lesions or edema • Labia minora thinner than labia majora • Soft and nontender
Clitoris	• 2 cm or less in length • 0.5 cm wide • Pink in color • Without lesions or adhesions
Urethral meatus	• Slit-like opening anterior to the vaginal opening • Without erythema or nodules • No discharge
Skene's glands are at the 4 and 8 o'clock position of the urethral meatus.	• The nurse inserts a gloved finger into the vaginal introitus. • With upward pressure the glands are milked to check for discharge • No discharge should be noted.
Introitus or vaginal opening	• Tensing of the vaginal walls • No lesions • No protrusions of the bladder or rectum palpated • Clear to whitish discharge with bloody discharge expected during menses
Bartholin's glands are at the 4 and 8 o'clock position of the introitus.	• The nurse inserts a gloved finger into the vaginal introitus. • With the index finger and thumb the labia majora is palpated for enlargement or tenderness. • The glands should not be palpable.
Perineum	Intact without lesions

Δ **Internal Exam**

- Perform **speculum exam** using an adjustable light source in order to obtain specimens and visualize structures.

◊ **Insertion of the speculum** is explained to the client and should be done in the following manner:

  ° With the blades closed, the handle is obliquely positioned.

  ° Place two fingers in the introitus and exert downward pressure.

  ° Insert the speculum over the fingers at a downward 45° angle.

  ° Turn handle downward once the blades clear the introitus.

  ° Open the blades, and when the cervix is visible, the blades may be locked into place.

◊ **Inspect the cervix** for color, lesions, size, position, appearance of the os, and discharge. Expected findings: the cervix is pink, 2.5 to 3 cm in diameter, midline, without lesions or discharge, and round os in a nulliparous client/slit-like os in a parous client.

◊ Obtain **Pap smear** specimens and fix onto slides from two locations:

  ° Obtain **ectocervical** specimens by rotating a spatula around the os and placing the sample on a slide.

  ° Obtain **endocervical** specimens by rotating a cervical brush 180° inside the os and placing the sample on a slide.

◊ Inspect the **vagina** as the speculum is slowly withdrawn and the blades are allowed to close. Expected findings: vagina is rugose, pink, and without lesions or masses.

• Perform **bimanual exam** by inserting lubricated gloved fingers into the vagina to palpate the cervix. With the other hand on the abdomen and the fingers remaining on the cervix, the nurse palpates the uterus and ovaries through the abdominal wall. Expected findings:

◊ **Cervix** is slightly mobile and firm.

◊ **Uterus** – nonpregnant uterus is 7.5 cm long, pear-shaped, smooth, firm, and slightly mobile.

◊ **Ovaries** are slightly tender, 4 cm long by 2 cm wide by 8 mm thick.

Inspection and Palpation – Male Genitalia

Δ **Positioning the client** – The exam may be performed with the client in a lying or standing position, except for the examination for hernias, which needs to be done with the client standing.

Δ Assess **the pubic region** for the following expected findings:

• Hair is in a triangular pattern.

• There are no parasites.

• There are no lesions.

Δ   Assess **the penis** for the following expected findings:

- Skin is intact and without lesions.

- Prepuce, if present, is easily retracted; smegma may be present.

- Glans is without erythema or lesions.

Δ   **Urethral meatus** should be at the tip of the penis with no discharge noted.

Δ   **Scrotum** is a two-compartment pouch of wrinkled, loose skin that should be without lesions, edema, or erythema. Each compartment should contain a testicle.

Δ   **Palpate the testes** gently for the following expected findings:

- Each testicle is ovoid and approximately **2 to 4 cm** in length.

- One testicle hangs lower in the scrotum than the other (usually left lower than right).

- The testes are rubbery in consistency.

- The testes are without nodules.

Δ   **Teach testicular self-examination** to the client while performing the genitalia exam.

Δ   **Epididymis** is comma-shaped and is superior, posterior, and lateral on each testicle and should be without tenderness or edema.

Δ   **Hernias** are loops of bowel that have left the abdominal cavity and are abnormal findings.

- Assess as follows:

  ◊   **Inspect** for any bulges in the inguinal or femoral areas.

  ◊   Starting low in the scrotal sac, use one finger to follow the spermatic cord to the inguinal ring.

  ◊   Ask the client to bear down or cough.

  ◊   Note any mass that comes in contact with your fingers.

  ○   **Direct inguinal hernias** occur between the posterior inguinal canal wall and the inguinal ligament.

  ○   **Indirect inguinal hernias** occur in the inguinal canal.

  ○   **Femoral hernias** occur where the femoral artery leaves the abdomen in the groin. Femoral hernias may be palpated by asking the client to cough again while feeling for bulges over the femoral canal.

Inspection and Palpation – Rectal Exam (Female and Male)

Δ **Positioning** for this exam includes:

- **Lying on the left side (Sims' position).**

- Standing with the upper body supported on the exam table.

- **Women – while in the stirrups for the genitalia exam.**

Δ **Inspect the skin of the perirectal area** for lesions, inflammation, scarring, or the presence of external hemorrhoids or fissures.

- Ask the client to bear down, and then the anus is inspected for any protrusions such as internal hemorrhoids, prolapses, or polyps.

- Expected findings: the skin is smooth and intact; skin around the anus is darker pigmented; no hemorrhoids or fissures noted.

Δ **External sphincter** – waiting for the external sphincter to relax, the examiner inserts his lubricated, gloved finger into the rectum.

- Expected findings: The sphincter should feel tight all the way around the finger.

Δ Palpate the **rectal walls** for nodules, polyps, tenderness, and the presence of stool.

- Expected findings: smooth, firm walls without nodules or tenderness. If stool is present, it should be soft.

Δ **Stool** may be noticed on the glove once the finger is withdrawn. Note the color of the stool and, if necessary, check for the presence of blood using fecal occult blood testing (FOBT) or guaiac testing. Follow manufacturer's directions for performing test.

Males

Δ **Prostate gland** is bilobed and approximately 2.5 to 4 cm in diameter. With lubricated, gloved finger in the rectum, palpate the prostate gland in a systematic manner by indenting the finger into the gland. The prostate should be without nodules and should not protrude more than 1 cm into the anterior rectal wall. For protrusions greater than 1 cm, the enlargement should be described as:

- **Grade I**: 1 to 2 cm.

- **Grade II**: 2 to 3 cm.

- **Grade III**: 3 to 4 cm.

- **Grade IV**: greater than 4 cm.

Sample Documentation

Female Genitalia: Symmetrical female hair distribution pattern noted without parasites. No lesions, erythema, or edema of the clitoris or labia is noted. No discharge from urethral meatus or introitus. Vaginal walls are intact, rugose, and pink. Cervix is pink with a round os. Uterus is firm and midline. Perineum is intact. Pap smear collected. Skin of perirectal area is intact. No lesions, erythema, or discharge noted. Good sphincter tone at rest and with bearing down. Stool palpable in the rectum, no masses noted. Stool is brown in color and negative for blood.

Male Genitalia: Male hair distribution pattern is symmetrical and without parasites. Circumcised, with no lesions or discharge noted. Urethral meatus is at the tip of the penis. Scrotum is without lesions or swelling. Testes are palpable bilaterally, smooth, and without nodules. Epididymis is nontender. No hernias noted. Skin of perirectal area is intact. No lesions, erythema, or discharge noted. Good sphincter tone at rest and with bearing down. Stool palpable in the rectum, no masses noted. Prostate is Grade I; no nodules noted. Stool is brown in color and negative for blood.

Primary Reference:

Potter, P. A., & Perry, A. G. (2005). *Fundamentals of nursing* (6th ed.). St. Louis, MO: Mosby.

Additional Resources:

Bickley, L. S., & Szilagyi, P. G. (2003). *Bates' guide to physical examination and history taking* (8th ed.). Philadelphia: Lippincott Williams & Wilkins.

NANDA International (2004). *NANDA nursing diagnoses: Definitions and classification 2005-2006*. Philadelphia: NANDA.

Chapter 40: Genitalia and Rectum

Application Exercises

1. The optimal time for a nurse to provide or reinforce client teaching regarding testicular self-examination is

     A. before performance of the genitalia exam.

     B. during performance of the genitalia exam.

     C. following performance of the genitalia exam.

     D. on a follow-up exam.

2. It is recommended that a digital rectal examination be performed annually on men over the age of 50 to assess for the presence of

     A. indirect or direct inguinal hernias.

     B. stool in the rectal vault.

     C. occult blood in stool

     D. prostate enlargement or nodules.

3. When preparing for a female genitalia inspection, the nurse should

     A. instruct the client to empty her bladder.

     B. cleanse the client's perineal area.

     C. promote comfort by having the client hold her breath.

     D. inquire about any sexually transmitted infections.

4. Which of the following are normal female genitalia age-related changes following menopause? (Select all that apply.)

     _____ Irregular menses

     _____ Sparse pubic hair

     _____ Increased vaginal lubrication

     _____ Nonpalpable ovaries

     _____ Vaginal atrophy

     _____ Clitoral atrophy

Chapter 40: Genitalia and Rectum

Application Exercises Answer Key

1. The optimal time for a nurse to provide or reinforce client teaching regarding testicular self-examination is

   A. before performance of the genitalia exam.

   B. during performance of the genitalia exam.

   C. following performance of the genitalia exam.

   D. on a follow-up exam.

   The optimal time for providing or reinforcing client teaching regarding testicular self-examination is during the performance of the examination. During the examination, the nurse is able to describe the process as it is being performed, which will provide a better learning opportunity for the client than before or following the genitalia exam. Client teaching on a follow-up visit regarding the exam is too long after the exam performance, and the client may not remember how the exam was performed.

2. It is recommended that a digital rectal examination be performed annually on men over the age of 50 to assess for the presence of

   A. indirect or direct inguinal hernias.

   B. stool in the rectal vault.

   C. occult blood in stool

   D. prostate enlargement or nodules.

   The American Cancer Society recommends that a digital rectal exam, as well as a prostatic-specific antigen (PSA) blood test, be performed annually on male clients over the age of 50 to screen for prostate cancer. A digital rectal exam assesses for size, shape, and consistency of the prostate to determine the presence of enlargement or nodules. Hernias are the protrusion of abdominal organs through abdominal musculature and are not palpated in the rectal area. Although stool can be obtained following a digital rectal exam, it is not necessary to perform a digital rectal exam to obtain stool for fecal occult blood testing. Determination of the presence of stool in the rectal vault, or digital removal of a fecal impaction may be indicated for a client with constipation, but this is not indicated as part of an annually scheduled assessment.

3. When preparing for a female genitalia inspection, the nurse should

    A. instruct the client to empty her bladder.

    B. cleanse the client's perineal area.

    C. promote comfort by having the client hold her breath.

    D. inquire about any sexually transmitted infections.

The client is asked to empty her bladder prior to the genitalia examination to promote comfort and prevent the accidental leakage of urine during the procedure. It is not necessary for the nurse to cleanse the client's perineal area prior to examination. Observation is made for the presence of parasites, lesions, and discharge. Having the client hold her breath will not promote comfort, but instead increase discomfort. It is important to inquire about any history of sexually transmitted infections, but this should be done when obtaining a history, not in preparation for a genitalia exam.

4. Which of the following are normal female genitalia age-related changes following menopause? (Select all that apply.)

    _____ Irregular menses

    __X__ **Sparse pubic hair**

    _____ Increased vaginal lubrication

    __X__ **Nonpalpable ovaries**

    __X__ **Vaginal atrophy**

    __X__ **Clitoral atrophy**

Age-related female changes that occur following menopause are generally the result of a decrease in ovarian function. This can cause the ovaries to be nonpalpable 3 to 5 years following menopause. The labia, clitoris, uterus, and vagina atrophy, and pubic hair becomes sparse following menopause. Menstruation ceases after menopause and vaginal lubrication decreases.

Unit 3 Basic Nursing Care
Section: Admission, Transfer, and Discharge Processes

Chapter 41: Admission Process
Contributor: Wendy Buenzli, MN, RN

 NCLEX® Connections:

Learning Objective: Review and apply knowledge within **"Admission Process"** in readiness for performance of the following nursing activities as outlined by the NCLEX® test plans:

Δ Perform a thorough assessment of the client's current health status.

Δ Obtain assessment data that is used as the baseline information to compare any future changes in client status.

Δ Collect assessment data that is accurate, factual, timely, and without bias.

Δ Provide for client privacy throughout the admission process.

Δ Plan and/or provide the client with an orientation to the facility/agency and the room.

Δ Safeguard the client's valuables and/or medications according to hospital policy.

 Key Points

Δ The admission assessment will provide baseline data to use in the development of the nursing care plan. Baseline data can be compared with future assessments to monitor client status and response to treatment.

Key Procedural Points

Δ Establish ability of the client to participate in the admission assessment. The client in distress or with mental status changes may need to have a family member provide necessary information.

Δ The nurse begins establishing the therapeutic relationship with the client and family during the admission process.

Nursing Interventions

Δ   Equipment

•   Prior to arrival of the client, take necessary equipment into the room. This should include appropriate documentation forms, equipment to obtain vital signs, pulse oximeter, and hospital attire for the client.

Δ   Procedure

•   Introduce self to the client.

•   Provide hospital attire and assist the client as necessary.

•   Position the client comfortably.

•   Apply client identification bracelet and allergy band, if needed.

•   Assess/collect the following data:

◊   Baseline data: vital signs, height, weight, allergy status, home medications.

◊   Biographical information on the client.

◊   Client's reason for seeking health care.

◊   Present illness and symptoms.

◊   Health history of:

°   Current illness

°   Current medications (prescription and over-the-counter)

°   Prior illnesses, chronic diseases

°   Surgeries

°   Previous hospitalizations

°   Other relevant data

◊   Family history (e.g., hypertension, cancer, heart disease, diabetes)

◊   Psychosocial assessment

°   Alcohol, tobacco, drug, and caffeine use

°   History of mental illness

°   History of abuse or homelessness

°   Home situation/significant others

◊   Nutrition

°   Current diet, any chewing or swallowing problems

°   Recent weight gain/loss

◊ Spiritual health/quality-of-life concerns:

    ° Religion

    ° Advance directive/living will

◊ Review of systems (*Refer to chapter 27, Health History.*)

◊ Safety assessments:

    ° History of falls

    ° Sensory impairments (e.g., vision, hearing)

    ° Use of assistive devices (e.g., walker, cane, crutches, or wheelchair)

◊ Discharge information

    ° Family members in the home

    ° Transportation for discharge

    ° Any relevant phone numbers

    ° Medical equipment needs at home

- Inventory any personal items brought by the client to the facility.

  ◊ Items to be inventoried usually include clothing, jewelry, money, assistive devices (e.g., hearing aids, cane, dentures), medications, and religious articles.

  ◊ Document how items are disposed of to include leaving items at the bedside, storing items in the client's room closet, sending items home with family members, and locking up valuables in the facility's safe. The client should be discouraged from keeping valuables at the bedside.

- Orient the client and family to the room/facility. Share information with the client, which includes:

  ◊ Call light operation.

  ◊ Electric bed operation.

  ◊ Telephone services/television controls.

  ◊ Overhead lighting operation.

  ◊ Smoking policy.

  ◊ Restroom locations.

  ◊ Waiting areas.

  ◊ Dining/vending services.

  ◊ Visiting policies.

Primary Reference:

Potter, P. A., & Perry, A. G. (2005). *Fundamentals of nursing* (6th ed.). St. Louis, MO: Mosby.

Additional Resources:

DeLaune, S, & Ladner, P. (2006). *Fundamentals of nursing* (3rd ed.). Clifton Park: Thomson Delmar.

NANDA International (2004). *NANDA nursing diagnoses: Definitions and classification 2005-2006*. Philadelphia: NANDA.

Chapter 41: Admission Process

Application Exercises

1. Which of the following is the best source for client data during the admission process?

> A. The client
>
> B. The family
>
> C. The emergency department staff
>
> D. The primary care provider

2. After gathering the assessment data and performing the review of systems, which of the following actions is a priority for the nurse?

> A. Orient the client to his room.
>
> B. Conduct a client care conference.
>
> C. Contact the primary care provider to notify her of the completed admission.
>
> D. Develop a plan of care.

3. What is the importance of performing a thorough and accurate admission assessment?

4. True or False: Clients should be advised to send jewelry and money home with family members.

5. True or False: The primary care provider is responsible for documenting an inventory of a client's personal items.

Chapter 41: Admission Process

Application Exercises Answer Key

1. Which of the following is the best source for client data during the admission process?

    A. The client
    B. The family
    C. The emergency department staff
    D. The primary care provider

    If capable, the client is the best source of information. A family member is acceptable, if the client is having difficulties communicating or is in distress. The emergency department staff and the primary care provider will have valuable information to contribute, but the client will provide the most comprehensive information.

2. After gathering the assessment data and performing the review of systems, which of the following actions is a priority for the nurse?

    A. Orient the client to his room.
    B. Conduct a client care conference.
    C. Contact the primary care provider to notify her of the completed admission.
    D. Develop a plan of care.

    Before the nurse leaves the room, the client should know how to use the call light and other equipment at the bedside. A client care conference is not typically done until more is known about the client following diagnostic tests, or determining how the client responds to treatment. The nurse does not usually contact the primary care provider regarding completion of admission assessment unless specifically requested by the provider. Developing a plan of care can be completed once the orientation is done.

3. What is the importance of performing a thorough and accurate admission assessment?

    It is important for the nurse to perform a thorough and accurate admission assessment in order to have a baseline for comparison with future client assessments and to be able to develop an effective nursing care plan.

4. True or False: Clients should be advised to send jewelry and money home with family members.

True: Clients are advised to send valuables home with family members to prevent theft and loss.

5. True or False: The primary care provider is responsible for documenting an inventory of a client's personal items.

False: The nurse is responsible for conducting an inventory of personal items as part of the admission process.

Unit 3   Basic Nursing Care
Section: Admission, Transfer, and Discharge Processes

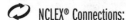

Chapter 42:   Transfer and Discharge Process
Contributor: Wendy Buenzli MN, RN

NCLEX® Connections:

Learning Objective: Review and apply knowledge within **"Transfer and Discharge Process"** in readiness for performance of the following nursing activities as outlined by the NCLEX® test plans:

Δ   Communicate and document pertinent information to the health care provider receiving the client in transfer.

Δ   Identify the documentation accompanying a client who is being transferred.

Δ   Plan and/or provide for the client's needs while being transitioned from one setting to another.

Δ   Assess the client on admission for potential discharge needs.

Δ   Plan and/or provide for the client's needs to be met after discharge.

Δ   Communicate/coordinate with health care providers caring for the client after discharge.

Δ   Complete and discuss discharge instructions with the client and/or family.

Key Points

Δ   Ensure continuity of care when transferring a client from one setting to another.

Δ   Keep information organized and in a logical order for easy dissemination between the nurse transferring, and the nurse receiving, the client.

Δ   Promote professional communication between health care providers.

Δ   Perform discharge planning as an interdisciplinary process that is started by the nurse at admission.

Δ   Use the nursing process as a guide to plan teaching and interventions for the client during discharge.

Δ   Conduct discharge planning with both the client and client's family for optimal results.

Key Procedural Points

△ Indications for Transfer and Discharge

- The client's level of care has changed. For example, health status has improved so that intensive care is no longer needed.

- Another setting is required to provide necessary care for the client. For example, the client is transferred from the medical unit to the operating room.

- The facility does not offer the type of care the client now requires. For example, after the acute phase of a stroke, the client now requires care in a skilled facility.

- The client no longer needs inpatient care and is ready to return home.

△ Discharge Planning

- This should begin when the client is admitted to the facility, unless the facility is to be the client's permanent residence (e.g., long-term care).

- Assess whether or not the client will be able to return to his previous residence.

- Determine whether or not the client will need and/or have someone to assist him at home.

- Assess the residence to see if adaptations are required to accommodate the client prior to discharge.

- Make a referral to the social worker to arrange for community services required by the client at discharge.

- Communicate client health status and needs to community service providers.

△ Discharge Education

- Discharge instructions are discussed with the client and written down for the client to have a copy at home.

- Instructions should use clear, concise language that the client will understand.

- Standards for discharge education include:

  ◊ Identifying safety concerns for the client at home.

  ◊ Reviewing signs and symptoms of potential complications and when to contact either emergency care or the primary care provider.

  ◊ Providing the phone number of the primary care provider.

  ◊ Providing names and phone numbers of community resources that will give care at the client's residence.

  ◊ Step-by-step instructions for performing continuing treatments, such as dressing changes.

◊ Dietary restrictions and guidelines, including those that pertain to medication administration.

◊ Amount and frequency of therapies the client is to perform to support continued independence at home.

◊ Directions on how to take medications and explanations for why each one is being prescribed.

Nursing Interventions

Δ Equipment

• Items to be transferred/discharged with the client include:

◊ The client's personal belongings at the bedside (e.g., flowers, books, clothing, personal care items).

◊ Valuables from the safe (if leaving the facility).

◊ Medications (especially those belonging to the client or those that cannot be returned to the pharmacy for credit).

◊ Assistive devices.

◊ Medical records or a transfer form.

Δ Procedure

• Responsibilities of the nurse include:

Transferring/Discharging the Client	Receiving the Transferred Client
• On the day/time of transfer, confirm that the receiving facility/unit is expecting the client and that the room/bed is available. • Communicate the time the client will transfer to the receiving facility/unit. • Complete documentation (e.g., medical records, transfer form). • Give a verbal transfer report in person or via telephone. • Confirm the mode of transportation the client will be using to complete the transfer/discharge (e.g., cart, wheelchair, ambulance). • Make sure the client is dressed appropriately if going outside the facility. • Account for all of the client's valuables.	• Have any specialized equipment ready. • If appropriate, inform the client's roommate of the impending admission/transfer. • Inform other health care team members of the client's arrival and needs. • Meet with the client and family on arrival to complete the admission process and orient the client/family to the new facility/unit. • Assess how the client tolerates the transfer. • Review transfer documentation. • Implement appropriate nursing interventions in a timely manner.

- **Transfer documentation** – Transfers within a facility usually require that the chart and other documentation accompany the client. Information should include:

  ◊ Client medical diagnosis.

  ◊ Client demographic information.

  ◊ Summary of progress up to transfer.

  ◊ Current health status, both physical and psychosocial.

  ◊ Critical assessments or interventions to be completed immediately.

  ◊ Current nursing care plan, including nursing diagnoses, plan, and interventions.

  ◊ Medications currently taken and last dose administered.

  ◊ Allergies.

  ◊ Diet and activity orders.

  ◊ Advance directives.

  ◊ Family support system.

  ◊ Special equipment needed (e.g., oxygen, suction, wheelchair).

- **Discharge summary documentation** – Each client record should be closed with a discharge summary to include discharge instructions. Nursing documentation at discharge includes:

  ◊ Type of discharge (e.g., ordered by primary care provider, against medical advice [AMA]).

  ◊ Actual date and time of discharge, who went with the client, and how the client was transported (e.g., wheelchair to a private car, stretcher to an ambulance).

  ◊ Where the client was discharged to (e.g., home, long-term care facility).

  ◊ A summary of the client's condition at discharge (e.g., steady gait, ambulating independently, in no apparent distress).

  ◊ A description of any unresolved difficulties and procedures for follow-up.

  ◊ Disposition of valuables, client's medications brought from home, and/or prescriptions.

  ◊ A copy of the client's discharge instructions.

Primary Reference:

Potter, P. A., & Perry, A. G. (2005). *Fundamentals of nursing* (6th ed.). St. Louis, MO: Mosby.

Additional Resources:

NANDA International (2004). *NANDA nursing diagnoses: Definitions and classification 2005-2006*. Philadelphia: NANDA.

Chapter 42: Transfer and Discharge Process

Application Exercises

1. When transferring a client with a fractured radius from the emergency department to the orthopedic unit, which of the following information is the most important for the nurse to include in the transfer report?

  A. The name of the client's partner

  B. Where the client was when the fracture occurred

  C. Information regarding the pain medication recently administered

  D. The client's occupation

2. Which of the following information should be included in a transfer report? (Select all that apply.)

  _____ The client is alert and oriented.

  _____ The client does not like spinach.

  _____ The client has an allergy to shellfish.

  _____ The client needs morphine every 4 hr.

  _____ The client has two cats at home.

3. Who is responsible for making sure all documentation is finished prior to transfer of a client to a new health care facility/agency?

  A. Primary care provider

  B. Certified nursing assistant

  C. Nurse transferring the client

  D. Social worker who set up the transfer

4. When does discharge planning begin in an acute care facility/agency?

  A. Two days from discharge

  B. The day of discharge

  C. When the nurse gets the order for discharge

  D. When the client is admitted

5. A client with a new diagnosis of type 2 diabetes is being discharged home. Which of the following should be included in the client's discharge teaching? (Select all that apply.)

_____ Proper use of a glucometer

_____ Foot care

_____ Signs and symptoms of hyper/hypoglycemia

_____ Measurement of input and output

_____ Management of sick days

_____ Date of follow-up appointment

6. What data should be included in a client's discharge summary? (Select all that apply.)

_____ Interventions performed by the physical therapist 2 days ago

_____ Where the client needs to go for follow-up care

_____ Instructions given on medication and treatments

_____ Summary of the client's condition at time of discharge

_____ The phone number of the home health agency that will be making home visits

Chapter 42: Transfer and Discharge Process

Application Exercises Answer Key

1. When transferring a client with a fractured radius from the emergency department to the orthopedic unit, which of the following information is the most important for the nurse to include in the transfer report?

> A. The name of the client's partner
>
> B. Where the client was when the fracture occurred
>
> **C. Information regarding the pain medication recently administered**
>
> D. The client's occupation

It is most important for the receiving nurse to know how much and when the client last received pain medication. This will assist the nurse to plan and implement further care for the client. Knowing the name of the client's partner, where the fracture occurred, and the client's occupation may have an impact on the client's overall care, but information regarding pain medication the client received is more important.

2. Which of the following information should be included in a transfer report? (Select all that apply.)

> **__X__ The client is alert and oriented.**
>
> _____ The client does not like spinach.
>
> **__X__ The client has an allergy to shellfish.**
>
> **__X__ The client needs morphine every 4 hr.**
>
> _____ The client has two cats at home.

Personal preferences, such as the client not liking spinach and keeping cats as pets, may sometimes be helpful, but neither are clinically significant for a transfer report. The client's level of consciousness, allergies, and need for pain medication are relevant to evaluating the client's health status and maintaining safety and comfort.

3. Who is responsible for making sure all documentation is finished prior to transfer of a client to a new health care facility/agency?

> A. Primary care provider
>
> B. Certified nursing assistant
>
> **C. Nurse transferring the client**
>
> D. Social worker who set up the transfer

The nurse who is transferring the client needs to complete the required documentation. The primary care provider may write transfer orders for the client at the new facility/ agency. The certified nursing assistant can assist with the physical transfer of the client or belongings, but she cannot complete the transfer documentation. The social worker may assist in finding placement for the client, but the forms need to be completed by the nurse.

4. When does discharge planning begin in an acute care facility/agency?

> A. Two days from discharge
>
> B. The day of discharge
>
> C. When the nurse gets the order for discharge
>
> **D. When the client is admitted**

Discharge planning needs to begin when the client is admitted. Due to short hospital stays, this will allow for the maximum amount of time available to make all necessary arrangements and provide any necessary teaching.

5. A client with a new diagnosis of type 2 diabetes is being discharged home. Which of the following should be included in the client's discharge teaching? (Select all that apply.)

> __X__ **Proper use of a glucometer**
>
> __X__ **Foot care**
>
> __X__ **Signs and symptoms of hyper/hypoglycemia**
>
> _____ Measurement of input and output
>
> __X__ **Management of sick days**
>
> __X__ **Date of follow-up appointment**

Proper use of a glucometer, foot care, signs and symptoms of hyper/hypoglycemia, management of sick days, and follow-up care are all important for the client with a new diagnosis of diabetes. The client should be aware of the increased need for fluids and the resulting increased urination, but it is not necessary for him to measure input and output on a regular basis.

6. What data should be included in a client's discharge summary? (Select all that apply.)

_____ Interventions performed by the physical therapist 2 days ago

__X__ **Where the client needs to go for follow-up care**

__X__ **Instructions given on medication and treatments**

__X__ **Summary of the client's condition at time of discharge**

__X__ **The phone number of the home health agency that will be making home visits**

All of the above information, with the exception of interventions performed by the physical therapist 2 days ago, is pertinent information that should be included in the discharge summary. The physical therapist should have written a progress note on the day of care.

Unit 3   Basic Nursing Care
Section: Medication Administration and Error Prevention

Chapter 43:   **Basic Principles of Medication Administration**
                Contributors: Wendy Buenzli MN, RN
                              Judith A. Harris, MSN, RNC

 NCLEX® Connections:

Learning Objective: Review and apply knowledge within **"Basic Principles of Medication Administration"** in readiness for performance of the following nursing activities as outlined by the NCLEX® test plans:

Δ   Identify various medication classifications and implications for nursing practice.

Δ   Plan/provide care to clients receiving medications through various routes.

Δ   Use appropriate technique to prepare medications for administration.

Δ   Demonstrate safe administration of different routes of medications (e.g., oral, topical, subcutaneous, intradermal, intravenous, and epidural).

 Key Points

Δ   **Pharmacokinetics** refers to how medication travels through the body. The medication is subjected to a variety of biochemical and physiochemical processes that result in absorption, distribution, metabolism, and excretion of the medication.

•   **Absorption** is the movement of a medication from its site of administration (e.g., GI tract, muscle, skin, or subcutaneous tissue) to the bloodstream. The most common routes of administration are enteral (through the GI tract) and parenteral (by injection). Each of these routes will have a unique pattern of absorption.

•   **Distribution** is the transportation of a medication to its site of action by bodily fluids. Distribution may be influenced by circulation to site of action, number of plasma protein binding sites, and barriers such as the blood brain barrier.

•   **Metabolism** (**biotransformation**) changes a medication into a less active form or an inactive form by the action of enzymes. This occurs primarily in the liver, but also takes place in the kidneys, lungs, bowel, and blood.

- **Excretion** is the elimination of a medication from the body primarily through the kidneys. Elimination also takes place through the liver, lungs, bowel, and exocrine glands.

Δ **Pharmacodynamics** describes the interactions between medications and target cells, body systems, and organs to produce pharmacological effects. These interactions result in functional changes that are considered the mechanism of action of the medication.

Δ Medication Category and Classification

- **Prescription medications** are administered under the supervision of primary care providers. These medications may be habit-forming, have potential harmful effects, and require supervision.

  - ◊ **Uncontrolled substances** – medications that require monitoring by a primary care provider, but do not pose risk of abuse and/or addiction. Antibiotics, nonsteroidal anti-inflammatory (NSAIDs) agents, and insulin are examples of uncontrolled substances.

  - ◊ **Controlled substances** – Medications that have a potential for abuse and dependence are categorized into schedules. Heroin is a drug in Schedule I and has no medical use in the United States. Medications categorized in Schedules II through V all have approved applications. Each level has decreasing risk of abuse and dependence. Codeine, phenobarbital, and methylphenidate (Ritalin) are examples of controlled substances.

- **FDA pregnancy risk category** (A, B, C, D, X) categorizes medications in terms of their potential harm during pregnancy, with Category A being the safest and Category X the most dangerous. Teratogenesis is most likely to occur during the first trimester. Before giving any medication to a woman who is pregnant (or to one who could be pregnant), determine whether or not it is safe for administration during pregnancy.

Key Procedural Points

Δ   Routes of Administration

Oral or enteral (tablets, capsules, liquids, suspensions, and elixirs)	• The client should be sitting, in semi-Fowler's, or Fowler's, position. • Contraindications for oral medication administration include vomiting, absence of gag reflex, difficulty swallowing, and decreased level of consciousness. • Do not mix with large amounts of food or beverages. • Avoid administration with contraindicated foods or beverages such as grapefruit juice. • Enteric-coated or time-release medications must be swallowed whole. • Administer irritating medications with small amounts of food. • In general, administer oral medications on an empty stomach (1 hr before meals, 2 hr after meals).
Sublingual (under tongue) and **buccal** (between cheek and gum)	• Instruct the client to have medication remain in place until absorbed. • The client should not eat or drink while the tablet is in place.
Liquids, suspensions, and elixirs	• Determine whether shaking or dilution is required. • When administering the medication, the meniscus (lowest fluid line) is at the level of the desired dose.
Transdermal – medication stored in a skin patch and absorbed through the skin producing systemic effects	• In general, to prevent underdosing or overdosing, patches should not be cut. • Instruct the client to place the patch on a hairless area of the skin and to rotate sites to prevent skin irritation. • Wash skin with soap and water, and dry thoroughly before applying a new patch.
Topical	• Apply with a glove, tongue blade, or cotton-tipped applicator. • Never apply with bare hand.

Instillation (drops, ointments, and sprays) – generally used for eyes, ears, and nose	• **Eyes** • Use a surgical aseptic technique when instilling medications in the eyes. • The client should be sitting or supine with the head tilted slightly back. Have the client look up at the ceiling. • Rest the dominant hand on the client's forehead. Holding the dropper above the conjunctival sac approximately 1 to 2 cm, drop medication into the center of the sac and have the client close the eye gently. • Apply gentle pressure with the finger and a clean tissue on the nasolacrimal duct for 30 to 60 sec to prevent systemic absorption of medication. • **Ears** • Use medical aseptic technique when administering medications into ears and nose. • Ear drops can be administered with the client sitting up or in a side-lying position, with the ear receiving the medication facing up. • The ear canal should be straightened by pulling the auricle upward and outward for adults, or down and back for children. • Hold the dropper 1 cm above the ear canal, instill medication, and then gently apply pressure with the finger to the tragus of the ear. • **Nose** • The client should be supine with his head positioned to allow the medication to enter the appropriate nasal passage. • Use the dominant hand to instill drops supporting the client's head with the nondominant hand. • Instruct the client to breathe through the mouth, stay in a supine position, and not blow his nose for 5 min after drop insertion.
Inhalation – medications usually administered through metered dose inhalers (MDI) or dry powder inhalers (DPI)	• For both types of devices, the client should exhale, and then inhale the medication deeply through the mouth for 3 to 5 sec, and then hold the breath for 5 to 10 sec. • The client should wait for a 1-min interval between puffs if taking 2 puffs of the same medication. • Instruct the client taking MDI medications to: ◊ Shake the medication vigorously 5 to 6 times prior to use. ◊ Place the mouthpiece between his lips or 2 to 4 cm in front of the mouth. ◊ Depress the canister to deliver the medication. ◊ Use a spacer to keep the medication in the device longer, thereby facilitating delivery of the medication to the lungs and decreasing the amount of the medication deposited into the oropharynx. • Instruct the client taking DPI medications to: ◊ Not shake the medication. ◊ Place the mouthpiece between his lips.

Nasogastric and gastrostomy tubes	<ul><li>Check for proper tube placement.</li><li>Use a syringe without a plunger or bulb, and allow the medication to flow in by gravity.</li><li>General guidelines<ul><li>Liquid forms of medications must be used.</li><li>Sublingual medications should not be given.</li><li>Do not crush specially prepared oral medications (e.g., extended/time-release, fluid-filled, enteric coated).</li><li>Check the compatibility of medications before mixing.</li><li>Do not mix medications with enteral feedings.</li><li>To prevent clogging, flush the tubing before and after each medication with 5 to 10 mL of water.</li></ul></li></ul>
Suppositories	<ul><li>Follow the manufacturer's directions for storage.</li><li>Wear gloves for the procedure.</li><li>Remove foil wrapper, and lubricate the suppository if necessary.</li><li>Rectal suppositories<ul><li>Position the client in left lateral position.</li><li>Insert just beyond the internal sphincter.</li><li>Instruct the client to retain the medication 20 to 30 min for stimulation of defecation and 60 min for systemic absorption.</li></ul></li><li>Vaginal suppositories<ul><li>Position the client supine with knees bent, feet flat on the bed and close to hips (modified lithotomy position).</li><li>Vaginal suppositories are generally inserted with an applicator.</li><li>Instruct the client to remain in the position for a specified amount of time (will vary).</li></ul></li></ul>

Δ   General considerations for parenteral medications include:

- Discarding all sharps (broken ampule bottles, needles) in designated containers according to facility/agency protocol. Containers are usually leak and puncture proof.

- Using the vastus lateralis site for infants and children < 2 years of age. After age 2, the ventral gluteal site can be used. Both of these sites can accommodate fluid up to 2 mL. The deltoid site has a smaller muscle mass and can only accommodate up to 1 mL of fluid.

- Using a needle gauge and length appropriate to the type of injection and client size.

  ◊   The gauge of the needle is the size of the diameter of the needle.

  ◊   The larger the gauge, the smaller the diameter of the needle. For example, a 25-gauge needle has a smaller diameter than a 20-gauge needle.

- Using a tuberculin syringe for solution volume < 0.5 mL. Syringe size should approximate volume of medication.

- Rotating injection sites to enhance medication absorption, and documenting each site used.

- Washing site with alcohol and allowing to dry. Using soap and water for insulin injections.

- Avoiding the use of injection sites that are edematous, inflamed, or those sites that have moles, birthmarks, or scars.

Type of Injection	Uses	Equipment	Sites/Technique
Intradermal	• Usually used for tuberculin testing or checking for medication/allergy sensitivities • May be used for some cancer immunotherapy	• Use small amounts of solution (0.01 to 0.1 mL) in a tuberculin syringe with a fine-gauge needle (26 to 27).	• Lightly pigmented, thin-skinned, hairless sites (e.g., inner surface mid-forearm or scapular area of back) at a 10 to 15° angle.
Subcutaneous	• Appropriate for small doses of nonirritating, water-soluble medications • Commonly used for insulin and heparin	• Use a short, fine-gauge needle (3/8- to 5/8-inch, 25- to 27-gauge). • Inject no more than 1.5 mL solution. • Insulin syringes can be 26- to 29-gauge.	• Sites are selected for adequate fat-pad size (e.g., abdomen, upper hips, lateral upper arms, thighs). • Use 3/8-inch, 25-gauge needle at a 45° angle, or use 1/2-in, 25-gauge needle at a 90° angle. • Follow facility/agency protocol for aspiration.

Type of Injection	Uses	Equipment	Sites/Technique
Intramuscular	• Used for irritating medications, solutions in oils, and aqueous suspensions	• Use needle size 18 to 27 (usually 20- to 25-gauge) 1 to 1 ½ inch long. • Volume injected is usually 1 to 3 mL. If a greater amount is required, it should be divided into two syringes, and two different sites should be used.	• Most common sites include ventrogluteal, dorsogluteal, deltoid, and vastus lateralis (pediatric). • Aspirate prior to medication injection. If there is blood return, discard the needle and syringe and prepare new medication. • Z-track technique can be used to prevent medication from leaking back into subcutaneous tissue. • It is often used for medications that cause visible and/or permanent skin stains such as certain iron preparations.
Intravenous	• Administration of medications, fluid, and blood products	• Vascular access devices can be for short-term use (catheters) or long-term use (infusion ports). • Use 16-gauge for trauma clients, 18-gauge for surgical clients, and 22- to 24-gauge for children, older adults, medical clients, and stable postoperative clients.	• Preferred sites are peripheral veins in the arm or hand. • In newborns, veins of the head, lower legs, and feet may be used.

Type of Injection	Uses	Equipment	Sites/Technique
Epidural	• Administration of intravenous opioid analgesia (e.g., morphine [Duramorph] or fentanyl [Sublimaze])	• Infusion pumps are necessary to administer medication.	• Catheter is advanced through the needle that is inserted into the epidural space at the level of the fourth of fifth vertebrae.

Δ   **Advantages and Disadvantages of Different Routes**

Route	Advantages	Disadvantages
Oral	• Safe • Inexpensive • Easy and convenient	• Oral medications have a highly variable absorption. • Inactivation can occur by GI tract or first-pass effect. • The client must be cooperative and conscious. • Contraindications include nausea and vomiting.
Intramuscular (subcutaneous – almost identical)	• Use for poorly-soluble medications. • This route is appropriate for preparing medications that are absorbed slowly for an extended period of time (depot preparations).	• Intramuscular (IM) injections are associated with a higher cost. • IM injections are inconvenient. • There can be pain with the risk for local tissue damage and nerve damage. • There is a risk for infection at the injection site.
Intravenous	• Onset is rapid, and absorption of the medication into the blood is immediate, which provides an immediate response. • This route allows control over the precise amount of medication given. • This route allows for administration of large volumes of fluid. • Irritating medications can be given with free-flowing IV.	• Intravenous (IV) injections are associated with an even higher cost. • IV injections are more inconvenient. • Absorption of the medication into the blood is immediate. This can be potentially dangerous if the wrong amount, or the wrong medication, is given. • There is an increased risk for infection or embolism with IV injections.

Nursing Interventions

Δ **Crushing/dissolving Tablets or Capsules**

- Most tablets are scored and can be readily broken in half. Tablets may also be crushed or dissolved according to the manufacturer's instructions.

- Capsules are gelatin shells containing powder or time-release beads. Capsules containing powder may be broken apart, and powdered medication dissolved according to manufacturer's instructions. Time-release capsules should not be crushed or diluted, as medication will be absorbed at a faster rate than recommended. As a safety measure, try to use a liquid form of the medication instead of crushing the tablets or diluting the powder from capsules. Enteric-coated (hard shell) tablets must not be crushed because of the potential for irritation to gastric mucosa.

Δ An **ampule** is a glass container holding medication in a solution. Preparation of medications from an ampule requires a syringe, filter needle for withdrawing the medication into the syringe, and a needle for injection into the client.

- Place filter needle on syringe.

- Rotate ampule to place all liquid in bottom of container

- Break glass top by holding the top with 2 inch x 2 inch gauze and quickly snapping the glass away from the body.

- Insert the needle into the opening of the ampule, and withdraw the medication by pulling back on the plunger.

- Replace the filter needle with the appropriate size/gauge needle for injection.

- Expel excess medication and air bubbles to obtain the correct dose.

Δ A **vial** is a single- or multiple-dose closed system glass container. Medication may be in liquid form or powder form. Follow directions when reconstituting medication.

- If the vial is new, remove its lid and wipe the top with alcohol. If it is a multiple-dose vial, wipe the top with alcohol or follow facility/agency policy.

- Draw air into a syringe equal to the amount of solution to be withdrawn from the vial. (Multiple-dose vials require air to be inserted equal to the amount of medication that is to be withdrawn. It is not necessary to insert air into a single-dose vial.)

- Insert needle into self-sealing lid, and inject correct amount of air without needle touching medication.

- Invert vial and withdraw correct dose.

- Remove needle from vial.

- Expel excess medication and air bubbles to obtain correct dose.

Δ   **Mixing Injectable Medications From two Vials**

- Draw air into a syringe equal to the amount of solution to be drawn from the second vial. Then, inject air into this vial, not allowing the needle to touch the solution. Withdraw the needle.

- Draw air into the syringe equal to the amount of solution to be drawn from the first vial. Inject air into the first vial, invert vial, and withdraw the desired amount of solution. Remove the needle from the vial.

- Insert needle into second vial, invert vial, and withdraw the desired amount of solution. Remove needle from the vial.

Δ   **Managing and epidural infusion**

- Secure catheter to skin to prevent discomfort.

- Assess and monitor dressing for drainage. Change per facility protocol.

- Use surgical aseptic technique when administering medication and providing other care of catheter.

- Assess/monitor vital signs and pulse oximetry to monitor for respiratory depression. Discontinue infusion if respirations are less than 12/min and notify the primary care provider.

- Assess for pruritis and treat with diphenhydrAMINE (Benadryl).

- Assess for nausea and vomiting and treat with antiemetic.

- Monitor I&O, urinary, and bowel function. Notify the primary care provider if urinary retention and/or constipation occur.

Primary Reference:

Potter, P. A., & Perry, A. G. (2005). *Fundamentals of nursing* (6th ed.). St. Louis, MO: Mosby.

Additional Resources:

Abrams, A. C., & Goldsmith, T. L. (2003). *Clinical drug therapy: Rationales for nursing practice* (7th ed.). Philadelphia: Lippincott Williams & Wilkins.

DeLaune, S, & Ladner, P. (2006). *Fundamentals of nursing* (3rd ed.). Clifton Park: Thomson Delmar.

Lehne, R. A. (2007). *Pharmacology for nursing care* (6th ed.). Philadelphia: W.B. Saunders.

Linton, A. D., & Harris, J. A. (2000). *Pharmacology companion for introductory nursing care of adults* (2nd ed.). Philadelphia: W.B. Saunders.

NANDA International (2004). *NANDA nursing diagnoses: Definitions and classification 2005-2006*. Philadelphia: NANDA.

Chapter 43: Basic Principles of Medication Administration

Application Exercises

1. A nurse is preparing insulin from two different vials. Which of the following actions indicates that she understands correct medication preparation?

   A. The nurse injects fluid from one vial into the other regardless of the medication.

   B. The nurse wipes the needle with alcohol prior to injecting into the vial.

   C. The nurse inserts air into the first vial, but not the second one.

   D. The nurse discards medication if medications are mixed during preparation.

2. An older adult client has had a cerebrovascular accident and is prescribed a metered dose inhaler. Which nursing consideration is a priority when teaching the client how to take the medication?

   A. Dosage and amount of medication

   B. Schedule of administration

   C. Coordination and cognition of the client

   D. The purpose and goal of medication regimen

3. Identify the correct client position for each of the following routes of administration.

   _____ Oral

   _____ Otic

   _____ Vaginal

   _____ Rectal

   A. Lying on the left side with right knee brought up toward the chest (Sims' position)

   B. Sitting, semi-Fowler's, or Fowler's position

   C. Supine with knees bent, feet flat on the bed and close to the hips

   D. Client lying on side with the ear that is receiving the drops facing up

4. Proper administration of eye drops includes which of the following nursing interventions? (Select all that apply.)

   _____ Using medical aseptic technique

   _____ Asking the client to look up at ceiling

   _____ Having the client lie in a side-lying position

   _____ Dropping medication into the center of the client's conjunctival sac

   _____ Instructing the client to close the eye gently

5. Identify the correct equipment needed for each of the following types of injections.

_____ Intradermal

_____ Subcutaneous

_____ Intramuscular

_____ Intravenous

A. Sixteen- to 24-gauge catheters appropriate for most adults, smaller-gauge catheters appropriate for infants and children

B. A tuberculin syringe with a fine-gauge needle (26 to 27)

C. A short, fine-gauge needle (⅜- to ⅝-inch, 25- to 27-gauge)

D. Needle size 18 to 27 (1- to 1 ½-inch, 22- to 25-gauge)

Chapter 43: Basic Principles of Medication Administration

Application Exercises Answer Key

1. A nurse is preparing insulin from two different vials. Which of the following actions indicates that she understands correct medication preparation?

    A. The nurse injects fluid from one vial into the other regardless of the medication.

    B. The nurse wipes the needle with alcohol prior to injecting into the vial.

    C. The nurse inserts air into the first vial, but not the second one.

    D. The nurse discards medication if medications are mixed during preparation.

If the medication from one vial becomes mixed with the medication in the other vial, that vial needs to be discarded because an accurate dose cannot be determined. Medications should not be mixed within vials. The needle is sterile when the needle cover is removed. It should not be wiped with alcohol. If the needle becomes contaminated, begin the preparation over or change the needle. Air needs to be injected into both vials prior to medication withdrawal.

2. An older adult client has had a cerebrovascular accident and is prescribed a metered dose inhaler. Which nursing consideration is a priority when teaching the client how to take the medication?

    A. Dosage and amount of medication

    B. Schedule of administration

    C. Coordination and cognition of the client

    D. The purpose and goal of medication regimen

The client has to have the cognitive and physical capabilities necessary to perform medication self-administration. If the client is able to self-administer the medication, it will then be important to determine the dosage, amount, schedule, purpose, and goal.

3. Identify the correct client position for each of the following routes of administration.

__B__ Oral   A. Lying on the left side with right knee brought up toward the chest (Sims' position)

__D__ Otic   B. Sitting, semi-Fowler's, or Fowler's position

__C__ Vaginal   C. Supine with knees bent, feet flat on the bed and close to the hips

__A__ Rectal   D. Client lying on side with the ear that is receiving the drops facing up

4. Proper administration of eye drops includes which of the following nursing interventions? (Select all that apply.)

_____ Using medical aseptic technique

__X__ **Asking the client to look up at ceiling**

_____ Having the client lie in a side-lying position

__X__ **Dropping medication into the center of the client's conjunctival sac**

__X__ **Instructing the client to close the eye gently**

The client should be asked to look up at the ceiling, the medication should be dropped into the center of the conjunctival sac, and the client should be instructed to close the eye gently. Surgical aseptic technique is used to administer eye drops. The client should be sitting or in a supine position to facilitate proper administration of eye drops.

5. Identify the correct equipment needed for each of the following types of injections.

__B__ Intradermal   A. Sixteen- to 24-gauge catheters appropriate for most adults, smaller-gauge catheters appropriate for infants and children

__C__ Subcutaneous   B. A tuberculin syringe with a fine-gauge needle (26 to 27)

__D__ Intramuscular   C. A short, fine-gauge needle (⅜- to ⅝-inch, 25- to 27-gauge)

__A__ Intravenous   D. Needle size 18 to 27 (1- to 1 ½-inch, 22- to 25-gauge)

Unit 3   Basic Nursing Care
Section: Medication Administration and Error Prevention

Chapter 44:   Safe Medication Administration and Error Prevention
                  Contributor: Denise T. Bynum, MSN, RN,
                       Judith A. Harris, MSN, RNC

 NCLEX® Connections:

Learning Objective: Review and apply knowledge within **"Safe Medication Administration and Error Prevention"** in readiness for performance of the following nursing activities as outlined by the NCLEX® test plans:

Δ   Identify nursing responsibilities of medication administration.

Δ   Assess client data (e.g., vital signs, laboratory values, allergies) before medication preparation and administration.

Δ   Assess/monitor the client for physical and psychosocial factors that impact medication administration.

Δ   Plan/provide care to the client receiving medication therapy.

Δ   Evaluate medication orders for clarity and accuracy.

Δ   Demonstrate appropriate documentation of all medication administration.

Δ   Use the nursing process to reduce the risk of medication errors.

Δ   Follow legal and facility policies in the administration of controlled substances.

Δ   Identify and use various resources to obtain information regarding medication administration.

 Key Points

Δ   Legal Responsibilities

•   The health care providers that are legally permitted to write prescriptions in the United States include physicians, advanced practice nurses, dentists, and physician assistants. These health care providers are responsible for:

◊   Obtaining the client's medical history and physical examination.

◊   Diagnosing.

◊   Prescribing medications.

◊   Monitoring the response to therapy.

◊   Modifying medication orders as necessary.

- Nurses are responsible for:

  ◊ Preparing, administering, and evaluating client responses to medications.

  ◊ Developing and maintaining an up-to-date knowledge base of medications administered, including uses, mechanisms of action, routes of administration, safe dosage range, adverse/toxic responses, precautions, and contraindications.

  ◊ Skill competency.

  ◊ Knowledge of acceptable practice.

  ◊ Determining accuracy of medication orders.

  ◊ Reporting all medication errors.

  ◊ Safeguarding and storing medications.

- The prescribing, dispensing, and administering of medications is controlled by federal, state, and local laws, health care agency policies, and each state's nurse practice act.

Key Procedural Points

Δ Medication Orders

- Each facility/agency will have written policies related to medication orders. Policies include which health care providers can write medication orders, receive medication orders, and transcribe medication orders.

- Types of medication orders include:

  ◊ Routine order/standard order.

    ° A routine/standard order may or may not have a termination date. Without a specified termination date, the order will be in effect until the primary care provider discontinues it, or the client is discharged.

    ° Certain medications (e.g., opioids, antibiotics) must be reordered within a specified amount of time or will automatically be discontinued.

  ◊ Single/one-time order.

    ° A single/one-time order is to be given once at a specified time or as soon as possible. For example, a one-time order instructs the nurse to give furosemide (Lasix) 40 mg PO at 1000.

  ◊ Stat order.

    ° A stat order is only given once, and it is given immediately. For example, a stat order instructs the nurse to give furosemide (Lasix) 40 mg IV right now.

◊ PRN order.

° A PRN order stipulates at what dosage, what frequency, and under what conditions a medication may be given. The nurse uses clinical judgment to determine the client's need for the medication. For example, a PRN order instructs the nurse to give acetaminophen 325 mg PO every 3 hr prn for pain.

◊ Standing orders.

° Standing orders may be written for specific circumstances and/or for specific units. For example, the critical care unit has standing orders to treat a client with asystole.

• Components of a medication order include:

◊ Name of client.

◊ Date and time of order.

◊ Name of medication (may be generic or brand).

◊ Dosage.

◊ Route of administration.

◊ Time and frequency – exact times or number of times per day (dictated by facility/agency policy or specific qualities of the medication).

◊ Signature of prescribing provider.

Assessment

Δ Physiological variables affecting medication response include:

• **Age** – Immature liver function of infants limits the ability to metabolize medications. The aging process can alter liver and kidney function and therefore decrease metabolism and excretion of medications. Decreased circulation can negatively affect medication distribution.

• **Gender/body build** – Differences in hormones, distribution of fat and water, weight, height, and lean body mass can affect medication absorption, metabolism, distribution, and excretion.

• **Chronic disease** – Body organ dysfunction (e.g., peripheral vascular system, liver, kidneys, and genitourinary tracts) influences how medications are absorbed, distributed, metabolized and excreted by the body.

• **Concurrent medication** use – Different medications used together can lead to unexpected and/or unpredictable metabolism, interference with intended therapeutic effect, and an increased risk of adverse medication reactions and interactions.

• **First-pass effect**s – Certain medications, when taken orally, are inactivated on their first pass through the liver and must be given by an alternate route.

- **Nutritional status** – Presence or absence of food in the stomach can alter medication absorption. Decreased nutritional status impairs the client's ability to produce specific medication-metabolizing enzymes, leading to impaired medication metabolism.

- **Pregnancy** – Circulatory changes, hormonal changes, and presence of fetus may influence how medications are absorbed, distributed, metabolized and excreted by the body.

- **Genetic factors** – Inherited traits may have specific influence on metabolism of medications.

Δ Psychosocial variables affecting medication response include:

- Health illness beliefs.

- Previous experiences with medications.

- Knowledge base.

- Cultural beliefs.

- Developmental stage.

- Social support/financial status.

- Potential for medication dependence and misuse.

Δ Obtain all necessary objective data before administering medication (e.g., apical heart rate before giving digitalis preparations).

Nursing Interventions

Δ **Safe Medication Administration**

- **Six Rights**

  ◊ **Right client** – Verify the client's identification each time a medication is given. Check identification band, name, and/or photograph with the medication record.

  ◊ **Right medication** – Correctly interpret medication order (verify completeness and clarity); read label three times: when container is selected, when removing dose from container, and when container is replaced. Leave unit-dose medication in its package until administration.

  ◊ **Right dose** – Calculate correct medication dose; check drug reference to ensure dose is within usual range. Have a second nurse check if unsure or if per facility/agency policy. Use a cutting device to break a scored tablet.

◊ **Right time** – Give medication on time to maintain consistent therapeutic blood level. It is generally acceptable to give the medication **½ hr before or after the scheduled time**. However, refer to the drug reference or facility/agency policy for exceptions. PRN medications are given no sooner than the interval specified by the primary care provider.

◊ **Right route** – Select the correct preparation for the ordered route (e.g., otic vs ophthalmic topical ointment or drops). Know how to safely and correctly administer medication. Give injections only from preparations designed for parenteral use. If route is not designated, or if a specified route is not recommended, contact the primary care provider for clarification.

◊ **Right documentation** – Immediately record pertinent information, including client's response to the medication.

Δ **Resources for medication information** include:

- Nursing drug handbooks.

- Pharmacology textbooks.

- Professional journals.

- Physicians' Desk Reference (PDR).

- Professional web sites

Medication category/ class	Medications may be organized according to pharmacologic action, therapeutic use, body system, chemical makeup, and safe use during pregnancy.
Mechanism of action	This is how the medication produces the desired therapeutic effect.
Therapeutic effect	This is the primary action for which the medication is administered to a specific client. One medication may have more than one therapeutic effect.
Adverse effects	These are undesired and sometimes dangerous effects of the medication. Adverse effects are usually identified according to body system.
Toxicity	Medications can have specific risks and manifestations of toxicity.
Medication interactions	Medications can interact with each other resulting in desired or undesired effects.
Precautions and contraindications	Some medications require caution when used with specific clients. Contraindications for medications may include a specific disease or condition, age, and allergy.
Preparation, dosage, administration	Know any special considerations for preparation, recommended dosages, and how to administer the medication.
Nursing implications	Know how to monitor therapeutic effects, prevent and treat adverse effects, provide for comfort, and instruct clients in the safe use of medications.

Δ   **Medication Errors**

- Common medication errors include:

    ◊   Wrong medication or IV fluid.

    ◊   Incorrect dose or IV rate.

    ◊   Wrong client, route, or time.

    ◊   Administration of known allergic medication.

    ◊   Omission of dose.

    ◊   Incorrect discontinuation of medication or IV fluid.

- Medication error reduction

Assessment	<ul><li>Obtain information about the client's medical diagnoses and conditions related to medication administration (e.g., ability to swallow, allergies; heart, liver, and/or kidney disorders).</li><li>Obtain necessary preadministration data (e.g., heart rate prior to administration of digoxin).</li><li>Identify physical and psychosocial risk factors.</li><li>Learn essential information about each medication to be given.</li><li>Interpret the medication order accurately. The inappropriate use of abbreviations can lead to errors. For example, $ZnSO_4$, the abbreviation for zinc sulfate, can be mistaken for MSO_4, morphine sulfate. In both situations, the full name of the medication should be written out. Also, not leaving enough space between the medication name and the dose can lead to error. For example, atenolol 10 mg may be interpreted as atenolol 110 mg. Make sure there is adequate space between the medication name and dose to prevent an inaccurate dose. The Institute for Safe Medication Practices (ISMP) has developed a list of abbreviations, symbols, and dose designations, which upon use, may lead to medication error. For a complete list of error-prone terms, go to the ISMP Web site, www.ismp.org.</li><li>Question the primary care provider if the prescription is unclear or seems inappropriate for the client's condition.</li><li>Check the labels for the medication name and concentration. Read labels correctly and carefully. Different medications may come in similar colors, shapes, and packages. Be aware of look-alike and sound-alike medication names (e.g., Keflex and Keflin).</li><li>To monitor therapeutic responses, dosage changes are usually made gradually. Question the primary care provider if abrupt and excessive changes in dosages are made.</li><li>Refuse to give a medication if it is believed to be unsafe. Check the prescription with the primary care provider.</li></ul>

Planning	• Calculate doses accurately and verify with a colleague or pharmacist if necessary. Doses are usually 1 to 2 tablets or one single-dose vial. Question multiple tablets or vials for a single dose. • Measure doses accurately and double-check high-alert medications (e.g., insulin, heparin) with a colleague. • Avoid distractions during medication preparation (e.g., poor lighting, ringing phones). Interruptions may increase the risk of error.
Implementation	• Follow Six Rights consistently. Take the medication administration record (MAR) to the bedside. • Medications should only be administered by the individual who has prepared the medication. Do not delegate medication administration to assistive personnel. • Follow correct procedures for all routes of administration. • Communicate clearly both in writing and speaking. Use verbal orders only for emergencies, and follow facility/agency protocol for telephone orders. • Encourage clients to become part of the safety net, teaching them about medications and the importance of proper identification before medications are administered. • Follow all laws and regulations regarding controlled substances when preparing and administering medications.
Evaluation	• Evaluate client response to a medication, and document and report appropriately. • Recognize side/adverse effects, and document and report appropriately. • Omit or delay doses as indicated by the client's condition, and document and report appropriately. • Omit or delay a dose if the client says the dose seems too large (e.g., insulin) or oral medications are different (e.g., color, shape) from those usually taken. Verify the prescription order with the primary care provider. • Report all errors per facility/agency policy, and implement corrective measures immediately. Document on appropriate forms. Complete information will facilitate the facility/agency review process and promote solutions to system-based causes. Promptly administer treatment to decrease injury to the client.

Δ   Self-administration of Medications

- Self-administration of medication typically takes place in the home and community-based settings. Self-administration may also be used in a facility/agency setting when clients wish to use their home medications and have the ability to do so safely.

- Careful preassessment is necessary to determine the client's suitability for safe self-medication (e.g., mental status, physical ability).

- Give the client instructions for each medication (written and verbal) regarding dosage, expected responses, and side/adverse effects.

- Schedule follow-up visits with the primary care provider to monitor compliance.

Primary Reference:

Potter, P. A., & Perry, A. G. (2005). *Fundamentals of nursing* (6th ed.). St. Louis, MO: Mosby.

Additional Resources:

Abrams, A. C., & Goldsmith, T. L. (2003). *Clinical drug therapy: Rationales for nursing practice* (7th ed.). Philadelphia: Lippincott Williams & Wilkins.

Institute for Safe Medication Practices. (2006). ISMP's List of Error-Prone Abbreviations, Symbols, and Dose Designations. Retrieved October 10, 2006, from *www.ismp.org/Tools/errorproneabbreviations.pdf*

Lehne, R. A. (2007). *Pharmacology for nursing care.* (6th ed.). St. Louis, MO: Saunders.

Linton, A. D., & Harris, J. A. (2000). *Pharmacology companion for introductory nursing care of adults* (2nd ed.). Philadelphia: Saunders.

NANDA International (2004). *NANDA nursing diagnoses: Definitions and classification 2005-2006.* Philadelphia: NANDA.

Chapter 44: Safe Medication Administration and Error Prevention

Application Exercises

1. A nurse prepares an injection of an opioid to give to a client who reports pain. Prior to administering the medication, the nurse is called to another room to assist another client onto a bedpan. This nurse then asks a second nurse to give the injection so that she can help the client needing the bedpan. Which of the following actions is the most appropriate for the second nurse to take?

   A. Offer to assist the client needing the bedpan.

   B. Give the injection prepared by the other nurse.

   C. Prepare another syringe and give the injection.

   D. Tell the client needing the bedpan she will have to wait for her nurse.

2. During morning rounds, a nurse enters a client's room and finds medications sitting on the bedside table. The client states that the medications are from last night and asks the nurse if he can take them now. Which of the following actions should the nurse take?

   A. Let the client take the medications with water and document in chart.

   B. Review the medication administration record (MAR), let the client take the medications with water, and document.

   C. Remove the medications, discard them, report the error, and document according to facility/agency policy.

   D. Report medication error to the pharmacist and charge nurse immediately.

3. For a medication that was ordered at 0900, which of the following are acceptable administration times? (Select all that apply.)

   _____ 0905

   _____ 0825

   _____ 1000

   _____ 0840

   _____ 0935

4. Which of the following nursing actions may prevent medication errors from occurring?

   A. Taking all medications out of the unit-dose wrappers before entering the client's room

   B. Checking with the primary care provider when a single dose requires administration of multiple tablets

   C. Giving the ordered medication and then looking up the usual dosage range

   D. Relying on another nurse to clarify a medication order

5. When implementing medication therapy, the nurse's responsibilities include which of the following? (Select all that apply.)

_____ Observing for medication side effects

_____ Monitoring for therapeutic effects

_____ Ordering the appropriate dose

_____ Changing the dose if side effects occur

_____ Maintaining an up-to-date knowledge base

Chapter 44: Safe Medication Administration and Error Prevention

Application Exercises Answer Key

1. A nurse prepares an injection of an opioid to give to a client who reports pain. Prior to administering the medication, the nurse is called to another room to assist another client onto a bedpan. This nurse then asks a second nurse to give the injection so that she can help the client needing the bedpan. Which of the following actions is the most appropriate for the second nurse to take?

    A. Offer to assist the client needing the bedpan.

    B. Give the injection prepared by the other nurse.

    C. Prepare another syringe and give the injection.

    D. Tell the client needing the bedpan she will have to wait for her nurse.

The second nurse should offer to assist the client needing the bedpan. This will allow the nurse who prepared the opioid injection to administer it to the client. A nurse should only administer medications that he/she prepared. Preparing another syringe will delay the administration of the needed pain medication. Telling the client to wait is not an acceptable option for the client needing the bedpan.

2. During morning rounds, a nurse enters a client's room and finds medications sitting on the bedside table. The client states that the medications are from last night and asks the nurse if he can take them now. Which of the following actions should the nurse take?

    A. Let the client take the medications with water and document in chart.

    B. Review the medication administration record (MAR), let the client take the medications with water, and document.

    C. Remove the medications, discard them, report the error, and document according to facility/agency policy.

    D. Report medication error to the pharmacist and charge nurse immediately.

The medications should be removed and discarded. The mistake should be reported and documented according to facility/agency policy. Letting the client take the medication at this time violates the "right time" principle. Reporting the medication error to the pharmacist does not provide the primary care provider with any information, and it neglects the issue of what to do with the medications and the documentation.

3. For a medication that was ordered at 0900, which of the following are acceptable administration times? (Select all that apply.)

__X__ **0905**

_____ 0825

_____ 1000

__X__ **0840**

_____ 0935

A medication may be given within 30 min of the scheduled time. 0905 and 0840 are within that window of time. 0825, 1000, and 0935 are not.

4. Which of the following nursing actions may prevent medication errors from occurring?

A. Taking all medications out of the unit-dose wrappers before entering the client's room.

B. Checking with the primary care provider when a single dose requires administration of multiple tablets.

C. Giving the ordered medication and then looking up the usual dosage range.

D. Relying on another nurse to clarify a medication order.

If a single dose requires multiple tablets, it is possible that an error has occurred in the transcription of the order. Errors may be prevented by taking unit-dose medication out of the wrapper at the bedside. Looking up usual dosage range prior to giving a medication may uncover an inaccurate dosage. If the order is unclear, the nurse must contact the prescribing provider for clarification.

5. When implementing medication therapy, the nurse's responsibilities include which of the following? (Select all that apply.)

__X__ **Observing for medication side effects**

__X__ **Monitoring for therapeutic effects**

_____ Ordering the appropriate dose

_____ Changing the dose if side effects occur

__X__ **Maintaining an up-to-date knowledge base**

The nurse is responsible for observing for medication side effects, monitoring for therapeutic effects, and maintaining an up-to-date knowledge base. The prescribing provider is responsible for ordering the appropriate dose and changing the dose if side effects occur.

Unit 3
Section:

Basic Nursing Care

Medication Administration and Error Prevention

Chapter 45: Dosage Calculation
Contributor: Alison Hewig, MSN, RN

 NCLEX® Connections:

Learning Objective: Review and apply knowledge within **"Dosage Calculation"** in readiness for performance of the following nursing activities as outlined by the NCLEX® test plans:

Δ Apply/use knowledge of dosage calculations to determine correct medication dosage for clients.

Δ Demonstrate the use of dimensional analysis and other methods to calculate and monitor client medication dosages.

 Key Points

Δ Basic medication dose conversion and calculation skills are essential to the provision of safe nursing care.

Δ Regardless of the dosage calculation method used, knowledge of **standard conversions** (e.g., 1 gr = 60 mg) and recognition of **availability data** (e.g., 300 mg/tablet) are used to **solve a clinical problem** (e.g., quantity of tablets to give for a prescribed dose of Tylenol 5 gr).

Δ **Standard conversion factors**:

- 1 mg = 1,000 mcg

- 1 g = 1,000 mg

- 1 kg = 1,000 g

- 1 oz = 30 mL

- 1 L = 1,000 mL

- 1 tsp = 5 mL

- 1 tbs = 15 mL

- 1 tbs = 3 tsp

- 1 kg = 2.2 lb

- 1 gr = 60 mg

Δ General rounding guidelines are to round to the tenths place. For example, 21.81 = 21.8; 21.86 = 21.9.

Methods Used for Dosage Calculations

Δ Dimensional analysis (or the factor-label method) is a method of dosage calculation that involves **systematically arranging a series of factors into a mathematical equation**.

Δ Let's apply the dimensional analysis method to the following clinical problem:

- A primary care provider has prescribed Lasix 40 mg intravenously every day. Available is 10 mg/mL. How many mL should be administered for this dose?

Step	Description	Example
1	What are you solving for (the **desired**)? Write the goal over 1 as a reminder to keep mL on top of the equation.	What is the **quantity** of mL required for the prescribed dose? $$\dfrac{mL}{1}$$
2	Identify what is **available**.	$10 \, mg / mL$
3	Change this to a ratio (or in factor form) with the desired measure that is being solved for on top.	$$\dfrac{1 \, mL}{10 \, mg}$$
4	Identify the **desired** dose.	$$\dfrac{40 \, mg}{1}$$
5	Set up your equation. Remember that you are solving for mL. Follow the rules of mathematics which say that to cross out a unit on the top, you must do the same to the bottom or vice versa. Therefore, the formula should be set up as:	$$\dfrac{1 \, mL}{10 \, mg} \bullet \dfrac{40 \, mg}{1} = \dfrac{mL}{1}$$
6	Do the math. Remember to multiply all the way across the top and all the way across the bottom, then divide.	$$\dfrac{1 \, mL}{10 \, mg} \bullet \dfrac{40 \, mg}{1} = \dfrac{40 \, mL}{10} = 4 \, mL$$

Δ   Another dosage calculation method involves the use of **specific formulas**:

$$\frac{Desired}{Available} \bullet Quantity \ \text{ or } \ \frac{D}{A} \bullet Q$$

$$\frac{Volume}{Time(min)} \bullet Drop\,Factor\,(gtt/mL) = IV\,Flow\,Rate\,(gtt/min)$$

$$\frac{Volume\,(mL)}{Time\,(min)} \bullet \frac{60\,min}{1\,hr} = IV\,Flow\,Rate\,(mL\,/\,hr)$$

Δ   Let's try applying the $\dfrac{D}{A} \bullet Q$ formula to the same clinical problem.

•   A primary care provider has prescribed Lasix 40 mg intravenously every day. Available is 10 mg/mL. How many mL should be administered for this dose?

Step	Description	Example
1	What are you solving for?	**What is the quantity** of mL required for the dose?
2	Identify the **desired** dose.	$40\,mg$
3	Identify what is **available.**	$10\,mg$
4	Identify the quantity in which it is available.	$1\,mL$
5	Set up your equation. Remember that you are solving for mL.	$\dfrac{40\,mg}{10\,mg} \bullet 1\,mL$
6	Do the math.	$\dfrac{40\,mg}{10\,mg} \bullet 1\,mL = 4\,mL$

Primary Reference:

Potter, P. A., & Perry, A. G. (2005). *Fundamentals of nursing* (6th ed.). St. Louis, MO: Mosby.

Additional Resources:

Curren, A. M. (2005). *Dimensional analysis for meds.* (3rd ed.). Albany, NY: Thomson Delmar Learning.

Lehne, R. A. (2007). *Pharmacology for nursing care.* (6th ed.). St. Louis, MO: Saunders.

Mulholland, J. (2006). *The Nurse, the math, the meds: Drug calculations using dimensional analysis.* (1st ed.). St. Louis, MO: Mosby.

NANDA International (2004). *NANDA nursing diagnoses: Definitions and classification 2005-2006.* Philadelphia: NANDA.

Chapter 45: Dosage Calculation

Application Exercises

1. A client is to receive 300 mg of phenytoin (Dilantin) now and every morning. The pharmacy sends 200 mg tablets. How many **tablets** should be given?

2. A client is to receive furosemide (Lasix) 80 mg intravenously every 6 hr for 24 hr. Available is 10 mg/mL. How many **mL** should be administered for each dose?

3. A client is to be given ampicillin (Ampicin) 250 mg orally every 6 hr. Available is 125 mg/5 mL. How many **mL** should be given for each dose?

4. A client is to receive aspirin 10 gr every 4 hr when necessary. Available are 325 mg tablets. How many **tablets** should be given for each dose?

5. A client is to receive acetaminophen (Tylenol) 320 mg every 3 to 4 hr for fever. Available is 160 mg/5 mL. How many **tsp** should be given each day?

6. A primary care provider prescribes atropine 0.5 mg IV for bradycardia. The vial is labeled atropine 400 mcg/mL. How many **mL** should be given?

7. A child weighs 31 lb. The primary care provider prescribes ampicillin 100 mg/kg/day in four divided doses. Available is ampicillin 250 mg/2 mL. How many **mL** per dose should be given?

8. Phenytoin (Dilantin) 5 mg/kg/day is prescribed in two divided doses for a child weighing 16 lb. It is available at 50 mg/mL. What is the total daily dosage in **mL** for this child?

9. Methylprednisolone (Solu-Medrol) 40 mg/kg/day is ordered every 4 hr for an adult weighing 154 lb. It is available at 40 mg/mL. How many **mL** should be given per dose?

10. A client is to receive 1 L of normal saline over 8 hr. The tubing drop factor is 15 gtt/mL. Calculate how many **gtt/min** should be delivered per manual control.

11. A client is to receive metronidazole (Flagyl) 500 mg in 100 mL normal saline intravenous piggyback administered over 1 hr. The tubing drop factor is 60 gtt/mL. Calculate how many **gtt/min** should be delivered per manual control.

12. A client is to receive Zantac 50 mg in 100 mL normal saline intravenous piggyback administered over 20 min. The tubing drop factor is 10 gtt/mL. Calculate how many **gtt/min** should be delivered per manual control.

13. A nurse is to administer 600 mL of D_5W over 8 hr. The IV pump should be set to deliver how many **mL/hr**?

14. An IV medication is to infuse over 20 min on the IV pump. The medication is mixed in 100 mL of normal saline. The IV pump should be set to deliver how many **mL/hr**?

15. An IV medication is to infuse over 30 min on the IV pump. The medication is mixed in 100 mL of normal saline. The IV pump should be set to deliver how many **mL/hr**?

Chapter 45: Dosage Calculation

Application Exercises Answer Key

1. A client is to receive 300 mg of phenytoin (Dilantin) now and every morning. The pharmacy sends 200 mg tablets. How many **tablets** should be given?

Dimensional Analysis	Formula
$\dfrac{1\,tab}{200\,mg} \bullet \dfrac{300\,mg}{1} = \dfrac{300}{200} = 1.5\,tabs$	Step 1: Choose formula. $$\dfrac{D}{A} \bullet Q$$ Step 2: Use formula. $$\dfrac{300\,mg}{200\,mg} \bullet 1\,tab = 1.5\,tabs$$

2. A client is to receive furosemide (Lasix) 80 mg intravenously every 6 hr for 24 hr. Available is 10 mg/mL. How many **mL** should be administered for each dose?

Dimensional Analysis	Formula
$\dfrac{1\,mL}{10\,mg} \bullet \dfrac{80\,mg}{1} = \dfrac{80}{10} = 8\,mL$	Step 1: Choose formula. $$\dfrac{D}{A} \bullet Q$$ Step 2: Use formula. $$\dfrac{80\,mg}{10\,mg} \bullet 1\,mL = \dfrac{80}{10} = 8\,mL$$

3. A client is to be given ampicillin (Ampicin) 250 mg orally every 6 hr. Available is 125 mg/5 mL. How many **mL** should be given for each dose?

Dimensional Analysis	Formula
$\dfrac{5\,mL}{125\,mg} \bullet \dfrac{250\,mg}{1} = \dfrac{1,250}{125} = 10\,mL$	Step 1: Choose formula. $$\dfrac{D}{A} \bullet Q$$ Step 2: Use formula. $$\dfrac{250\,mg}{125\,mg} \bullet 5\,mL = \dfrac{1,250}{125} = 10\,mL$$

4. A client is to receive aspirin 10 gr every 4 hr when necessary. Available are 325 mg tablets. How many **tablets** should be given for each dose?

$$\frac{1\,tab}{325\,mg} \bullet \frac{60\,mg}{1\,gr} \bullet \frac{10\,gr}{1} = \frac{600}{325} = 1.85 = 2\,tab$$	Step 1: Choose formula. $$\frac{D}{A} \bullet Q$$ Step 2: Convert. $$\frac{60\,mg}{1\,gr} \bullet \frac{10\,gr}{1} = 600\,mg$$ Step 3: Use formula. $$\frac{600\,mg}{325\,mg} \bullet 1\,tab = 1.85 = 2\,tab$$

5. A client is to receive acetaminophen (Tylenol) 320 mg every 3 to 4 hr for fever. Available is 160 mg/5 mL. How many **tsp** should be given each day?

$$\frac{5\,mL}{160\,mg} \bullet \frac{320\,mg}{1} \bullet \frac{1\,tsp}{5\,ml} = 2\,tsp$$	Step 1: Choose formula. $$\frac{D}{A} \bullet Q$$ Step 2: Convert. $$5\,mL = 1\,tsp$$ Step 3: Use formula. $$\frac{320\,mg}{160\,mg} \bullet 1\,tsp = 2\,tsp$$

6. A primary care provider prescribes atropine 0.5 mg IV for bradycardia. The vial is labeled atropine 400 mcg/mL. How many **mL** should be given?

$$\frac{1\,mL}{400\,mcg} \bullet \frac{0.5\,mg}{1} \bullet \frac{1{,}000\,mcg}{1\,mg} = 1.25\,mL$$	Step 1: Choose formula. $$\frac{D}{A} \bullet Q$$ Step 2: Convert. $$\frac{1{,}000\,mcg}{1\,mg} \bullet \frac{0.5\,mg}{1} = 500\,mcg$$ Step 3: Use formula. $$\frac{500\,mcg}{400\,mcg} \bullet 1\,mL = 1.25\,mL$$

7. A child weighs 31 lb. The primary care provider prescribes Ampicillin 100 mg/kg/day in four divided doses. Available is Ampicillin 250 mg/2 mL. How many **mL** per dose should be given?

Step 1: $$\frac{2\,mL}{250\,mg} \bullet \frac{100\,mg}{1\,kg} \bullet \frac{1\,kg}{2.2\,lb} \bullet \frac{31\,lb}{1} = \frac{6,200}{550}$$ $$= 11.3\,mL\,/\,day$$ Step 2: Calculate single dose. $$\frac{11.3\,mL}{4\,doses} \bullet \frac{1\,dose}{1} = 2.8\,mL$$	Step 1: Choose formula. $$\frac{D}{A} \bullet Q$$ Step 2: Convert. $$\frac{1\,kg}{2.2\,lb} \bullet \frac{31\,lb}{1} = 14.1\,kg$$ Step 3: Calculate dose ordered for client based on weight. $$\frac{100\,mg}{1\,kg} \bullet \frac{14.1\,kg}{1} = 1,410\,mg\,/\,day$$ Step 4: Use formula. $$\frac{1,410\,mg}{250\,mg} \bullet 2\,mL = 11.3\,mL\,/\,day$$ Step 5: Calculate single dose. $$\frac{11.3\,mL}{4\,doses} \bullet \frac{1\,dose}{1} = 2.8\,mL$$

8. Phenytoin (Dilantin) 5 mg/kg/day is prescribed in two divided doses for a child weighing 16 lb. It is available at 50 mg/mL. What is the total daily dosage in **mL** for this child?

Step 1:	Step 1: Choose formula.
$$\frac{1\,mL}{50\,mg}\bullet\frac{5\,mg}{1\,kg}\bullet\frac{1\,kg}{2.2\,lb}\bullet\frac{16\,lb}{1}=\frac{80}{110}=0.7mL$$	$$\frac{D}{A}\bullet Q$$
	Step 2: Convert.
	$$\frac{1\,kg}{2.2\,lb}\bullet\frac{16\,lb}{1}=7.3\,kg$$
	Step 3: Calculate dose ordered for client based on weight.
	$$\frac{5\,mg}{1\,kg}\bullet\frac{7.3\,kg}{1}=36.5mg\,/\,day$$
	Step 4: Use formula.
	$$\frac{36.5\,mg}{50\,mg}\bullet 1\,mL=0.7mL\,/\,day$$

9. Methylprednisolone (Solu-Medrol) 40 mg/kg/day is ordered every 4 hr for an adult weighing 154 lb. It is available at 40 mg/mL. How many **mL** should be given per dose?

Step 1: $\dfrac{1\,mL}{40\,mg} \cdot \dfrac{40\,mg}{1\,kg} \cdot \dfrac{1\,kg}{2.2\,lb} \cdot \dfrac{154\,lb}{1} = \dfrac{6{,}160}{88}$ $= 70.0\,\text{mL}\,/\,day$ Step 2: Calculate single dose. $\dfrac{70.0\,mL}{6\,doses} \cdot \dfrac{1\,dose}{1} = 11.7\,mL$	Step 1: Choose formula. $\dfrac{D}{A} \cdot Q$ Step 2: Convert. $\dfrac{1\,kg}{2.2\,lb} \cdot \dfrac{154\,lb}{1} = 70\,kg$ Step 3: Calculate dose ordered for client based on weight. $\dfrac{40\,mg}{1\,kg} \cdot \dfrac{70\,kg}{1} = 2{,}800\,mg\,/\,day$ Step 4: Use formula. $\dfrac{2800\,mg}{40\,mg} \cdot 1\,mL = 70.0\,mL/day$ Step 5: Calculate single dose. $\dfrac{70.0\,mL}{6\,doses} \cdot \dfrac{1\,dose}{1} = 11.7\,mL$

10. A client is to receive 1 L of normal saline over 8 hr. The tubing drop factor is 15 gtt/mL. Calculate how many **gtt/min** should be delivered per manual control.

$\dfrac{15\,gtt}{1\,mL} \cdot \dfrac{1{,}000\,mL}{1\,L} \cdot \dfrac{1\,L}{8\,hr} \cdot \dfrac{1\,hr}{60\,min}$ $= 31.25 = 31\,gtt\,/\,min$	Step 1: Choose formula. $\dfrac{Volume}{Time(min)} \cdot Drop\,Factor\,(gtt\,/\,mL) = IV\,Flow\,Rate\,(gtt\,/\,min)$ Step 2: Use formula. $\dfrac{1{,}000\,mL}{480\,min} \cdot 15\,gtt\,/\,mL = 31.25 = 31\,gtt\,/\,min$

11. A client is to receive metronidazole (Flagyl) 500 mg in 100 mL normal saline intravenous piggyback administered over 1 hr. The tubing drop factor is 60 gtt/mL. Calculate how many **gtt/min** should be delivered per manual control.

$$\frac{60\,gtt}{1\,mL} \bullet \frac{100\,mL}{60\,\min} = 100\,gtt/\min$$	**Step 1: Choose formula.** $$\frac{Volume}{Time(\min)} \bullet Drop\,Factor\,(gtt/mL) = IV\,Flow\,Rate\,(gtt/\min)$$ **Step 2: Use formula.** $$\frac{100\,mL}{60\,\min} \bullet 60\,gtt/mL = 100\,gtt/\min$$

12. A client is to receive Zantac 50 mg in 100 mL normal saline intravenous piggyback administered over 20 min. The tubing drop factor is 10 gtt/mL. Calculate how many **gtt/min** should be delivered per manual control.

$$\frac{10\,gtt}{1\,mL} \bullet \frac{100\,mL}{20\,\min} = 50\,gtt/\min$$	**Step 1: Choose formula.** $$\frac{Volume}{Time(\min)} \bullet Drop\,Factor\,(gtt/mL) = IV\,Flow\,Rate\,(gtt/\min)$$ **Step 2: Use formula.** $$\frac{100\,mL}{20\,\min} \bullet 10\,gtt/mL = 50\,gtt/\min$$

13. A nurse is to administer 600 mL of D_5W over 8 hr. The IV pump should be set to deliver how many **mL/hr**?

$$\frac{600\,mL}{8hr} = 75\,mL/hr$$	**Step 1: Choose formula.** $$\frac{Volume(mL)}{Time(\min)} \bullet \frac{60\,min}{1hr} = IV\,Flow\,Rate(mL/hr)$$ **Step 2: Use formula.** $$\frac{600\,mL}{480\,min} \bullet \frac{60\,min}{1hr} = 75\,mL/hr$$

14. An IV medication is to infuse over 20 min on the IV pump. The medication is mixed in 100 mL of normal saline. The IV pump should be set to deliver how many **mL/hr**?

$$\frac{100\,mL}{20\,min} \bullet \frac{60\,min}{1\,hr} = \frac{6{,}000}{20} = 300mL/hr$$	Step 1: Choose formula. $$\frac{Volume(mL)}{Time(\text{min})} \bullet \frac{60min}{1hr} = IVFlowRate(mL/hr)$$ Step 2: Use formula. $$\frac{100mL}{20min} \bullet \frac{60min}{1hr} = 300mL/hr$$

15. An IV medication is to infuse over 30 min on the IV pump. The medication is mixed in 100 mL of normal saline. The IV pump should be set to deliver how many **mL/hr**?

$$\frac{100\,mL}{30\,min} \bullet \frac{60\,min}{1\,hr} = \frac{6{,}000}{30} = 200mL/hr$$	Step 1: Choose formula. $$\frac{Volume(mL)}{Time(\text{min})} \bullet \frac{60min}{1hr} = IVFlowRate(mL/hr)$$ Step 2: Use formula. $$\frac{100mL}{30min} \bullet \frac{60min}{1hr} = 200mL/hr$$

Unit 3   Basic Nursing Care

Section: Medication Administration and Error Prevention

Chapter 46:   Intravenous Therapy

Contributor: Denise T. Bynum, MSN, RN

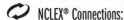 NCLEX® Connections:

Learning Objective: Review and apply knowledge within "**Intravenous Therapy**" in readiness for performance of the following nursing activities as outlined by the NCLEX® test plans:

Δ   Demonstrate appropriate techniques required for maintaining intravenous (IV) therapy.

Δ   Assess/monitor IV therapy site and flow rate.

Δ   Plan and provide care for the client receiving IV therapy.

Δ   Assess/monitor for complications of IV therapy and initiate appropriate actions.

Δ   Evaluate and document the client's condition during IV therapy.

 Key Points

Δ   Advantages and Disadvantages of IV Therapy

Advantages	Disadvantages
• Fast absorption and onset of action • Less discomfort after initial insertion • Maintains constant therapeutic blood levels • Less irritation to subcutaneous and muscle tissue	• Circulatory fluid overload is possible if infusion is large and/or too rapid. • Immediate absorption leaves no time to correct errors. • IV administration can cause irritation to the lining of the vein. • Failure to maintain surgical asepsis can lead to local infection and septicemia.

Δ   **Types of IV Access**

•   Intravenous access can be via a **peripheral** or **central** vein (central line).

•   Central lines can be peripherally inserted or directly inserted into the jugular or subclavian vein.

Δ   **Guidelines for Safe IV Medication Administration**

- Certain medications, such as potassium chloride, can cause serious adverse reactions and should be infused on an IV pump for accurate dosage control and never given IV push.

- Add medication to a new IV fluid container, not to an IV container that is already hanging.

- Never administer IV medication through tubing that is infusing blood, blood products, or parenteral nutritional solutions.

- **Verify compatibility** of medications before infusing a medication through tubing that is infusing another medication.

Δ   **Needlestick Prevention**

- Be familiar with IV insertion equipment.

- Avoid using needles when needleless systems are available.

- Use **protective safety devices** when available.

- **NEVER recap** a needle.

- Dispose of needles immediately in designated puncture-resistant receptacles.

- Do not break, bend, or recap needles.

Key Procedural Points

Δ   **Methods of IV Medication Infusions**

- **IV medication infusions** are mixed in **large volumes of fluid** (500 to 1,000 mL) and given as **continuous IV infusion**. Potassium chloride may be administered this way.

    ◊   The medication can be found in premixed solution bags or can be added to the IV bag by the pharmacy or the nurse.

- **Intermittent IV administration** – Some medications, such as antibiotics, are given intermittently in a small amount of solution (**25 to 250 mL**) through a continuous IV system, or with saline or heparin lock systems.

    ◊   The medications infuse for short periods of time and are given on a scheduled basis.

    ◊   If given with a continuous IV infusion, the medication is "piggybacked" in through secondary tubing. If infused through a saline/heparin lock system, the access is flushed before and after with solution per facility/agency protocol.

- **Bolus IV administration**

    ◊   The medications are typically in **small amounts** of solution that can be injected over a short time (1 to 2 min) in emergent and nonemergent situations.

◊ Some medications are given directly into the peripheral IV or access port to achieve an immediate medication level in the bloodstream, such as pain medication.

◊ Make sure medications are prepared according to recommended concentration and administered according to the safe recommended rate.

◊ Use extreme caution and observe for signs and symptoms of complications (e.g., redness, burning, or increasing pain).

Δ **Special Considerations**

• Older adult clients, clients taking anticoagulants, or clients with fragile veins:

◊ Avoid tourniquets.

◊ Use blood pressure cuff instead.

◊ Do not slap extremity to visualize veins.

• Edema in extremities:

◊ Apply digital pressure over proposed vein to displace edema.

◊ Apply pressure with alcohol pad.

◊ Cannulation must be quick.

• Obese clients may require the use of anatomical landmarks to find veins.

Nursing Interventions

Δ Equipment

• Examine the solution to be infused for clarity, leaks, and expiration date.

• Select correct size catheter:

◊ 16-gauge for trauma clients, rapid fluid volume.

◊ 18-gauge for surgical clients, rapid blood administration.

◊ 22- to 24-gauge for children, older adults, medical clients, and stable postoperative clients.

• Obtain correct tubing, and prime tubing as indicated.

• Obtain infusion pump, if indicated.

• Obtain insertion supplies by following agency/facility protocol.

Δ Initiating Peripheral IV Therapy

• Check the primary care provider's order (e.g., solution, rate).

• Assess the client for allergies to products used in initiating and maintaining IV therapy (e.g., latex, tape, iodine).

• Follow the **Six Rights of medication administration** (including compatibilities of all IV solutions).

- Obtain supplies.

- Wash hands.

- Identify the client and explain procedure.

- Place the client in a comfortable position.

- Apply gloves before insertion.

- **Assess extremities and veins**. If hair removal needed, clip with scissors or shave with electric shaver.

- Using clean tourniquet, apply **4 to 6 inches above** proposed insertion site to compress only venous blood flow.

- Select vein.

  ◊ Choose distal veins first on the nondominant hand.

  ◊ Avoid:

    ° Varicosed veins that are permanently dilated and tortuous.

    ° Veins in inner wrist with bifurcations, in flexion areas, near valves (appear as bumps), in lower extremities, and antecubital fossa.

    ° Veins that are sclerosed or hard.

    ° Veins in an extremity with impaired sensitivity (e.g., scar tissue, CVA), lymph nodes removed, recent infiltration, or arteriovenous fistula/ graft.

  ◊ Choose site that is not painful or bruised and will not interfere with activity.

  ◊ Choose a vein that is resilient with a soft, bouncy feeling upon palpation.

  ◊ Additional methods to enhance venous access include:

    ° Gravity, fist clenching, friction with alcohol, and heat.

    ° Percussion by tapping gently.

    ° Multiple tourniquets and transillumination.

  ◊ **Cleanse area at the site** using friction in a circular motion from middle to outward with alcohol, iodine preparation, or chlorhexidine. Allow to air dry for 1 to 2 min.

  ◊ Remove cover from catheter, grasp plastic hub, and examine device for smooth edges.

  ◊ **Anchor vein** below site of insertion.

  ◊ Pull skin taut and maintain.

  ◊ Warn the client of sharp, quick stick.

◊   Insert the catheter with bevel up at an angle of **15 to 20°** using steady smooth motion (or as recommended by catheter manufacturer). Lower the hub of the catheter close to the skin to prepare for threading into the vein.

◊   Advance the catheter through skin and into the vein. **Flashback of blood** should be seen.

◊   Upon completion of advancing the catheter, **withdraw** the needle.

◊   **Release the tourniquet** before attaching the tubing to maintain sterility.

◊   **Apply dressing** per facility/agency protocol. The dressing is usually left in place until the catheter is removed, unless it becomes damp, loose, or soiled.

◊   Avoid encircling the entire extremity with tape, and taping under the sterile dressing.

◊   On the side of the dressing, document catheter size, date/time of insertion, and the initials of the nurse that inserted the catheter.

◊   Regulate IV infusion rate according to the primary care provider's order.

◊   Dispose of used equipment properly.

◊   Document in chart:

      °   Date and time of insertion.

      °   Insertion site and appearance.

      °   Catheter size.

      °   Type of dressing.

      °   IV fluid and rate (if applicable).

      °   Number, locations, and conditions of site-attempted cannulations.

      °   Client response.

◊   Sample documentation: 1/1/2006, 1635, #22 gauge IV catheter inserted into left wrist cephalic vein (1 attempt) with sterile occlusive dressing applied. IV D_5LR infusing at 100 mL/hr per infusion pump without redness or edema at the site. Tolerated without complications. J. Doe, RN

Δ   Maintaining patency of IV access

-    **Do not stop** a continuous infusion or allow blood to back up into the catheter for any length of time. Clots can form at the tip of the needle or catheter and can be lodged against the vein wall, blocking the flow of fluid.

-    Instruct the client not to manipulate flow rate device, change settings on IV pump, and avoid lying on tubing.

-    Make sure the IV dressing is not too tight.

- **Flush intermittent** IV catheters with heparin or NS after every medication administration or every **8 to 12** hr when not in use.

- Monitor site and infusion rate at least **every hour.**

Δ Discontinuing IV therapy

- Check order/prepare equipment.

- Wash hands.

- Apply gloves.

- Remove tape and dressing, stabilizing IV.

- Clamp IV tubing.

- Apply sterile gauze pad over site without putting pressure on vein. Do not use alcohol.

- Using other hand, withdraw catheter by pulling straight back from the site.

- Elevate and apply pressure for 2 min.

- Assess site.

- Apply tape over gauze.

- Use pressure dressing, if needed.

- Assess catheter for intactness.

- Document.

Complications and Nursing Implications

Δ **Preventing IV Infections**

- **Use standard precautions.**

- Change IV sites according to facility/agency policy (usually 72 hr).

- Remove catheters as soon as they are no longer clinically indicated.

- **Change catheter** if any break in surgical aseptic technique is suspected, such as emergency insertions.

- Use sterile needle/catheter for **each insertion attempt**.

- Avoid writing on IV bags with pens or markers, because ink could contaminate the solution.

- Change tubing immediately if contamination is known or suspected.

- Fluids should not hang more than **24 hr** unless it is a closed system (e.g., pressure bags for hemodynamic monitoring).

- **Wipe all ports** with alcohol or an antiseptic swab before connecting IV lines or inserting a syringe to prevent the introduction of micro-organisms into the system.

- **Never disconnect tubing** for convenience or to position the client.

- Do not allow ports to remain exposed to air.

- Wash hands before and after handling the IV system.

Complication	Signs	Prevention	Treatment
Infiltration	• **Pain, burning** • **Pallor** • **Local swelling at the site** • **Cool skin** • Damp dressing • **Slowed infusion**	• Careful selection of site and catheter • Securing the catheter	• Stopping the infusion and removing the catheter • Elevating the extremity • Encouraging active range of motion • Applying warm compresses three to four times/day • Restarting proximal to the site or other extremity
Phlebitis/ thrombophlebitis	• **Edema** • **Throbbing, burning, or pain at the site** • **Warmth** • **Erythema** • May be a **red line** up the arm with a **palpable band** at the vein site • **Slowed infusion**	• Rotation of sites • Avoiding the lower extremities • Proper handwashing and surgical aseptic technique	• Promptly discontinuing the infusion • Notifying the primary care provider • Elevation • Warm/moist compresses • Restarting with new tubing and fluid • TED hose and/or anticoagulants • Culturing the site and cannula if drainage is present
Hematoma	• Accumulation of clotted blood in the tissue, causing **ecchymosis** (bruising)	• Minimizing tourniquet time • Removing before starting IV fluid • Holding pressure after removal	• Pressure dressing • Avoiding alcohol • After bleeding stops, using warm compresses and elevation

Complication	Signs	Prevention	Treatment
Catheter embolus	• If no migration, may be asymptomatic • With migration, **severe pain at the site** (may be same as pulmonary embolus)	• Never reinsert the stylet into the catheter • Avoid the joints	• Placing the tourniquet high on the extremity to limit venous flow • Preparing for removal under x-ray or surgery • Saving the catheter after removal to determine the cause
Cellulitis	• **Tenderness, pain** • **Warmth** • **Edema** • **Induration** • **Red streaking** • **Fever, chills, malaise**	Same as phlebitis	• Same as phlebitis • Antibiotics • Analgesics • Antipyretics
Septicemia	• Sudden or gradual **rise in temperature**, chills and shaking, **increased HR and RR**, headache, nausea, vomiting, diarrhea, and **confusion** • Bacteria cultured from the blood	• Diligent adherence to maintaining surgical aseptic technique	• Monitoring the client's vital signs and assessing for signs and symptoms of infection • Notifying the primary care provider of changes in status • Blood cultures • Administering antibiotics as ordered
Fluid overload	• Distended neck veins • Increased BP • Tachycardia • Shortness of breath, tachycardia • Crackles in the lungs • Edema	• Using an infusion pump • Monitoring I&O	• Raising the head of the bed • Assessing vital signs • Notifying the primary care provider of changes in status • Possible readjustment of rate

Complication	Signs	Prevention	Treatment
Air embolus	• If occurrence in the pulmonary arteries, signs and symptoms of a pulmonary embolism (e.g., chest pain, shortness of breath) • Rarely occurs with peripheral lines	• Priming/flushing all tubing to prevent air from entering the system • Changing the IV solution containers before empty	• Usually requires immediate intervention • Putting the client in the Trendelenburg position on the left side and instructing him to perform the Valsalva maneuver • Notifying the primary care provider • Performing frequent assessments • Ventilatory support and IV therapy per orders

Primary Reference:

Potter, P. A., & Perry, A. G. (2005). *Fundamentals of nursing* (6th ed.). St. Louis, MO: Mosby.

Additional Resources:

NANDA International (2004). *NANDA nursing diagnoses: Definitions and classification 2005-2006*. Philadelphia: NANDA.

Potter, P. & Perry, A. (2003). *Basic nursing: Essentials for practice*. St. Louis, MO: Mosby.

Chapter 46: Intravenous Therapy

Application Exercises

1. When assessing the IV site for phlebitis, the nurse should look for which of the following signs and symptoms? (Select all that apply.)

_____ Red line on affected extremity

_____ Increased rate of infusion

_____ Local swelling at site

_____ Cool, pale skin

_____ Pain at site

2. Which of the following techniques will minimize the risk of catheter embolism?

A. Use good handwashing technique before and after IV insertion.

B. Rotate the IV sites at least every 72 hr.

C. Administer anticoagulants.

D. Once in the vein, never put the stylet back through the catheter.

3. Which of the following actions is the highest priority if the nurse suspects an air embolism?

A. Remove the IV catheter immediately.

B. Observe for fever and site redness.

C. Place the client in Trendelenburg position on the left side.

D. Assess neck veins and respiratory rate.

4. The nurse checks for patency of an IV saline lock by

A. assessing the site for redness.

B. flushing the IV with NS and assessing the site.

C. asking the client if the site is painful.

D. checking the date of insertion.

Chapter 46: Intravenous Therapy

Application Exercises Answer Key

1. When assessing the IV site for phlebitis, the nurse should look for which of the following signs and symptoms? (Select all that apply.)

__X__ Red line on affected extremity

_____ Increased rate of infusion

_____ Local swelling at site

_____ Cool, pale skin

__X__ Pain at site

Pain at the site and a red line over the vein of the affected extremity are signs and symptoms of phlebitis. The rate of the infusion slows down with phlebitis. The skin is warm and red. Edema might be present, but local swelling at the site is more indicative of infiltration.

2. Which of the following techniques will minimize the risk of catheter embolism?

A. Use good handwashing technique before and after IV insertion.

B. Rotate the IV sites at least every 72 hr.

C. Administer anticoagulants.

D. Once in the vein, never put the stylet back through the catheter.

Reinsertion of the stylet can damage the catheter, causing a small portion to break off and enter the venous system. Good handwashing will prevent infection. Rotating IV sites will prevent phlebitis and thrombosis. A catheter embolism is not related to blood clotting.

3. Which of the following actions is the highest priority if the nurse suspects an air embolism?

    A. Remove the IV catheter immediately.

    B. Observe for fever and site redness.

    C. Place the client in Trendelenburg position on the left side.

    D. Assess neck veins and respiratory rate.

This position and technique prevent the air from entering the bloodstream. Removing the IV catheter immediately; assessing for fever, redness at the site, distended neck veins, and increased respiratory rate are not effective techniques for managing signs and symptoms of air embolism.

4. The nurse checks for patency of an IV saline lock by

    A. assessing the site for redness.

    B. flushing the IV with NS and assessing the site.

    C. asking the client if the site is painful.

    D. checking the date of insertion.

Free flow of solution through the IV indicates patency. Absence of redness and reports of pain are not positive indicators of IV patency. How long an IV has been in will not determine if it is still patent.

Unit 3   Basic Nursing Care
Section: Safety

Chapter 47:   Client Safety
Contributor: Teri W. Scott, MSN, FNP-c, RN

 NCLEX® Connections

Learning Objective: Review and apply knowledge within **"Client Safety"** in readiness for performance of the following nursing activities as outlined by the NCLEX® test plans:

Δ   Use all equipment in a safe manner.

Δ   Remove and report unsafe equipment.

Δ   Assess/monitor client for potential fall risks.

Δ   Plan and implement care to limit the risk of illness or injury while ensuring optimal function of clients in all settings.

Δ   Teach the client to use assistive devices correctly.

Δ   Orient the client to his environment.

Δ   Apply/monitor the use of the least restrictive restraints according to federal/state/laws and facility policies for clients who are a danger to themselves or others.

Δ   Know the fire safety procedures of the health care agency.

 Key Points

Δ   Falls account for up to 90% of all reported hospital accidents.

Δ   Equipment should be used only by the nurse after a safety inspection and instruction.

Δ   Use restraints only as a last resort. The nurse should consult with the primary care provider and obtain a written order stating why the restraint is necessary and for how long.

Δ   All health care workers must be aware of:

    •   Safety procedures.

    •   Response to dangerous situations.

    •   Security plans.

- How to identify incidents.

- Implementation of plans.

- Documentation of the incidents and responses per health care agency policy.

Δ It is the primary care provider's responsibility to assess, report, and document client allergies and to provide client care that avoids exposure to allergens.

Key Procedural Points

Δ **Falls**

- **Older adult clients** may be at an increased risk for falls due to decreased strength, impaired mobility and balance, and endurance limitations combined with decreased sensory perception.

- Other clients at increased risk include those with decreased **visual acuity,** generalized **weakness**, **urinary frequency, gait and balance problems** (e.g., cerebral palsy, injury, MS) and **cognitive dysfunction**. Side effects of medications (e.g., orthostatic hypotension, drowsiness) can also increase the client's risk for falls.

Δ **Seizures**

- Seizures may include sudden onset and violent clonic-tonic movements that can result in injury (e.g., head injury, aspiration, falls).

- Prevent injury by implementing seizure precautions.

Δ **Restraints**

- Have knowledge of and follow federal/state/laws and facility policies that govern the use of restraints.

- Use **restraints** only as a last resort, in consultation with the primary care provider, and with an order stating why the restraint is necessary and for how long.

- **Physical restraints** are any physical, manual, or mechanical method or device attached to a body to restrict movement.

- **Chemical restraints** are medications used to control behavior and are especially dangerous in older adults because the increased sedation, drowsiness, and/or otherwise impaired cognition may increase the risk of falling. Chemical restraints should be used as a last resort.

- Use of restraints without an order is considered false imprisonment and is therefore illegal.

- If a nurse uses restraints in an emergent situation, such as when the client is a danger to self or others, a face-to-face assessment is to be done within 1 hr by the primary care provider.

NANDA Nursing Diagnoses

Δ   Risk for falls

Δ   Risk for injury

Δ   Deficient knowledge

Nursing Interventions

Δ   **Prevention of Falls**

- Complete a **fall-risk assessment** upon admission and at regular intervals on the client for individualization of the care plan to limit the risk of falls.

- Document all identified risks in the health care record, and report risks to the family and primary care providers in order to alert them to the specific needs of this client.

- Provide the client with **nonskid footwear**.

- Keep the **floor free from clutter** with a clear path to the bathroom (e.g., no scatter rugs, cords, furniture).

- Provide **adequate lighting** (a night light for necessary trips to the bathroom).

- **Orient the client to the setting** (e.g., grab bars, call light) to ensure he knows how to use all assistive devices and can locate necessary items.

- Keep **assistive devices** nearby after validation of safe use by the client and family (e.g., glasses, walkers, transfer devices).

- Complete home safety surveys to identify and rectify problems in the home that can contribute to the fall risk.

- Educate the client and family/caregivers on identified risks and the plan of care.

- Report and document all incidents per the health care agency's policy. This provides valuable information that may be helpful in preventing similar incidents.

- Staff should **answer call lights promptly** to prevent the client at risk from trying to ambulate independently.

- Assign clients at risk for falls to **a room close to the nurses' station** to shorten the response time to call lights and ensure more frequent assessments of the client.

- Keep the **bed rails up and the bed in the low position** (when not working with the client) for sedated, unconscious, or high-risk clients.

- **Lock wheels** on beds, wheelchairs, and gurneys to prevent the device from rolling during transfers or stops.

- Use **chair or bed sensors** for clients at risk to alert staff of independent ambulation.

Δ **Restraints**

- Prior to use, the nurse should review the manufacturer's instructions for correct application.

- **Remove or replace restraints frequently** to ensure good circulation to the area and allow for full range of motion to the limb that has been restricted.

- **Pad bony prominences and do neurosensory checks** (to include loosening or removing the restraint and testing temperature, mobility, and capillary refill) every 2 hr to identify any neurological or circulatory deficits.

- Always **tie the restraint to the bed frame** (loose knots that are easily removed) where it will not tighten when the bed is raised or lowered.

- Leave the **restraint loose enough for range of motion** and with enough room to fit two fingers between the device and the client to prevent injury.

- Always **explain the need** for the restraint to the client and family so as to help them understand that these actions are for the safety of the client.

- Regularly **assess the need for continued use** of the restraints to allow for discontinuation of the restraint or limiting the restraint at the earliest possible time while ensuring the client's safety.

- Never leave the client unattended without the restraint.

- Restraints should:

  ◊ Never interfere with treatment.

  ◊ Restrict movement as little as is necessary to ensure safety.

  ◊ Fit properly.

  ◊ Be easily changed to decrease the chance of injury and to provide for the greatest level of dignity.

- **Documentation** for the use of restraints is very specific and must include:

  ◊ The behavior that makes the restraint necessary.

  ◊ Nursing interventions used prior to the placement of restraints.

  ◊ Client's level of consciousness.

  ◊ Type of restraint used and location.

  ◊ Education/explanations to the client and family.

  ◊ Exact time of application and removal.

  ◊ Client's behavior while restrained.

◊ Type and frequency of care (e.g., range of motion, neurosensory checks, removal, integumentary checks).

◊ Attempts to use alternate restraints with client's response.

◊ Client's response when the restraint is removed.

Δ **Seizure Precautions**

- To develop a plan of care, **assess the client** with a history of seizures for:

  ◊ Frequency.

  ◊ Type and date of last seizure.

  ◊ Medications.

  ◊ Triggers or trends of the seizures.

- Ensure **rescue equipment** is at the bedside to include oxygen, an oral airway, and suction equipment. A saline lock may be put in for intravenous access if the client is at high risk for experiencing a generalized seizure.

- Inspect **the client's environment** for items that may cause injury in the event of a seizure, and remove items that are not necessary for current treatment.

- Assist the client at risk for a seizure in **ambulation and transfer** to reduce the risk of injury.

- Advise all caregivers and family **not to put anything in the client's mouth** (except in status epilepticus, where an airway is needed) in the event of a seizure.

- Advise all caregivers and family not to restrain the client in the event of a seizure, ensure the client's safety by **lowering him to the floor** or bed, **protect his head**, remove nearby furniture, **provide privacy**, put the client on his side if possible, and **loosen clothing** to prevent injury and promote dignity of the client.

- After a seizure, explain what happened to the client, provide comfort and understanding and a quiet environment for the client to recover.

- Document the seizure in the client's record with any precipitating behaviors and a description of the event (e.g., movements, any injuries, length of seizure, aura, postictal state), and report it to the primary care provider.

Δ **Equipment Safety**

- Use equipment only after a safety inspection and instruction in its use.

- Equipment is to be regularly inspected by the engineering or maintenance department and by the user prior to use.

- Faulty equipment (e.g., frayed cords, disrepair) can start a fire or cause a shock and should be removed and reported immediately per the health care agency's policy.

- Electrical equipment must be grounded (three-pronged plug and grounded outlet) to decrease the risk for electrical shock.

- Use outlet covers in environments with individuals at risk for sticking items into them.

- Unplug equipment using the plug, not the cord, to prevent bending the plug prongs and increasing the risk for electrical shock.

- Disconnect all electrical equipment prior to cleaning.

- JCAHO (2004) requires all pumps (general and PCA) to have free-flow protection to prevent an overdose of fluids or medications.

- Do not overcrowd outlets, and use extension cords only when absolutely necessary. If extension cords must be used in an open area, tape the cords to the floor.

- Use all equipment only as it is intended to prevent injury.

Δ **Fire Safety**

- All staff must be instructed in the fire response procedures, which include:

  ◊ Knowing the location of exits, fire extinguishers, and oxygen turn-offs.

  ◊ Knowing the evacuation plan.

- **The fire response** in the health care setting always follows this sequence (**RACE**):

  ◊ Protect and evacuate clients in immediate danger (**R**escue).

  ◊ Report the fire (**A**larm).

  ◊ Contain the fire (**C**ontain).

  ◊ Extinguish the fire (**E**xtinguish).

- The **correct fire extinguisher** must be used to promptly and safely extinguish a fire.

  ◊ Class A is for paper, wood, upholstery, rags, or other types of trash.

  ◊ Class B is for flammable liquids and gases.

  ◊ Class C is for electrical fires.

Δ **Teaching plan for home fire safety** – The primary care provider should educate the client and family on home fire safety, which includes:

- Reviewing "**Stop, Drop, and Roll**" with clients of all ages.

- Correcting the **use and storage of oxygen** if used in the home:

  ◊ No open flame.

  ◊ Storing the container as instructed by the manufacturer.

- Keeping **emergency numbers near the phone** for prompt use in the event of an emergency of any type.

- Making sure stairs are well lit and have nonslip tread.

- Having a **family exit and meeting plan** that is practiced and reviewed regularly.

- Having **fire extinguishers and operable smoke and carbon monoxide detectors**.

- In the event of a fire, if possible, closing windows and doors, covering the mouth and nose with a damp cloth when going through a smoky area, and keeping the head as close to the floor as possible to avoid the heaviest smoke.

Primary Reference:

Potter, P. A., & Perry, A. G. (2005). *Fundamentals of nursing* (6th ed.). St. Louis, MO: Mosby.

Additional Resources:

NANDA International (2004). *NANDA nursing diagnoses: Definitions and classification 2005-2006*. Philadelphia: NANDA.

Chapter 47: Client Safety

Application Exercises

1. A client is admitted to the emergency department after a head injury. He is combative and cursing. He has tried to hit and bite the staff. The nurse determines that restraints are necessary for the protection of the client and staff. Identify the appropriate nursing actions by documenting the actions as they would appear in the client's record.

2. A nurse enters a client's room and discovers flames in the trash can. Identify the sequence of actions in response to a fire in a client care area.

3. During his admission assessment, a client has a generalized tonic-clonic seizure. Identify the actions to be taken by the nurse doing the assessment and up to four priority nursing interventions to be included in the plan of care.

4. An older adult client was just admitted to the unit after falling at a nursing home. This client is oriented to person, place, and time and can follow directions. Identify a primary nursing diagnosis for this client and develop a plan of care.

5. Identify the order of priority for completion of each of the following interventions for a newly admitted client with a history of falls.

   _____ Survey the client's belongings.

   _____ Complete a fall-risk assessment.

   _____ Complete a physical assessment.

   _____ Make arrangements for a home safety survey.

   _____ Educate the family and client on the fall risks.

6. When doing an admission, the nurse surveys the personal belongings of an older adult client. The client's belongings include glasses, a hearing aid, cane, and a variety of medications. Identify a priority nursing diagnosis for this client based on that information.

   A. Disturbed sensory perception

   B. Impaired physical mobility

   C. Hopelessness

   D. Risk for falls

Chapter 47: Client Safety

Application Exercises Answer Key

1. A client is admitted to the emergency department after a head injury. He is combative and cursing. He has tried to hit and bite the staff. The nurse determines that restraints are necessary for the protection of the client and staff. Identify the appropriate nursing actions by documenting the actions as they would appear in the client's record.

Upper extremity restraint (right and left wrist) applied at 1715 after the client repeatedly tried to hit and bite the staff. Client was not responsive to repeated requests to stop these behaviors. Client is alert but inappropriately responds to questions. Primary care provider notified at 1725 of the need for restraints and reported he would be in to assess the client within the hour. Restraints applied per hospital protocol (loosely, with 2 fingerbreadths between the client and the device and to the frame of the bed). Client and family are aware of the need for the restraints relative to the client and staff safety. Client continues to try to strike out at the staff with both arms; therefore, unable to release the restraints. Initial circulatory and neurosensory checks show both upper extremities within normal limits and limited ROM relative to the restraints. Restraint care plan and flow chart initiated and added to client chart.

2. A nurse enters a client's room and discovers flames in the trash can. Identify the sequence of actions in response to a fire in a client care area.

The fire response in the health care setting always follows this sequence (RACE):

> **Protect and evacuate clients in immediate danger (Rescue).**
>
> **Report the fire (Alarm).**
>
> **Contain the fire (Contain).**
>
> **Extinguish the fire (Extinguish).**

3. During his admission assessment, a client has a generalized tonic-clonic seizure. Identify the actions to be taken by the nurse doing the assessment and up to four priority nursing interventions to be included in the plan of care.

The nurse should not restrain the client or try to put anything in his mouth. She should ensure the client's safety by lowering him to the floor or bed, protecting his head, removing nearby furniture, providing privacy, putting the client on his side if possible, and loosening clothing.

Assess the client's seizure history for frequency, type and date of last seizure, medications, and triggers or trends of the seizures.

Ensure rescue equipment is at the bedside and includes oral airway, oral suction equipment, padding for the side rails and headboard, and clean gloves.

Inspect the client's environment for items that may cause injury in the event of a seizure, and remove items that are not necessary for current treatment.

Advise all caregivers and family of the importance of following these guidelines in the event of a seizure:

Δ   Do not put anything in the client's mouth in the event of a seizure and explain why (this is likely to cause injury to the caregiver or can break and obstruct the client's airway).

Δ   Do not restrain the client in the event of a seizure.

Δ   Ensure the client's safety by lowering him to the floor or bed, protecting his head, removing nearby furniture, providing privacy, putting the client on his side (if possible), and loosening clothing to prevent injury.

Δ   Promote dignity of the client.

4. An older adult client was just admitted to the unit after falling at a nursing home. This client is oriented to person, place, and time and can follow directions. Identify a primary nursing diagnosis for this client and develop a plan of care.

Risk for injury related to recurrent falls

Client outcomes

Δ   The client will have no injuries from falls during this hospitalization.

Δ   The family/caregivers will understand the specific risks for falls for this client by the time of discharge.

Δ   A home safety inspection will be completed prior to discharge.

Interventions

Δ   Complete a fall-risk assessment on admission and every other day, or in the event of a change in the client's condition, per hospital protocol.

Δ   Assign the client to a room near the nurses' station.

Δ   Be certain the client is oriented to the location of the call light and that it is nearby at all times.

Δ   Orient the client to the use of assistive devices and the location of the bathroom.

Δ   Use a bed alarm.

Δ   Discuss the fall risk with the client and family.

Δ   Advise all staff to keep the floor clear from the bed to the bathroom at all times.

Δ   Advise all staff and educate the client and family on the importance of having the two bed rails up at the head and the bed in low position with the brakes on.

Δ   Answer call lights promptly.

5. Identify the order of priority for completion of each of the following interventions for a newly admitted client with a history of falls.

   3   Survey the client's belongings.

   1   Complete a fall-risk assessment.

   2   Complete a physical assessment.

   5   Make arrangements for a home safety survey.

   4   Educate the family and client on the fall risks.

1. **The client's fall-risk assessment is used to find a safe room and guide how the client will be oriented to his room and the facility/agency.**

2. **In addition to the report information from the emergency department, the physical assessment will help to identify further risks or injuries, as well as provide baseline physical data.**

3. **Surveying the client's belongings may provide further clues to fall risks (e.g., glasses, medications, hearing aids, canes, walkers).**

4. **It is important for family members and any visitors to be aware of the client's risk for falls. Providing instruction to the family will allow them to provide safety to the client.**

5. **The home safety survey is very important and should be completed prior to discharge. However, this survey does not take precedence over any of the other items that may impact safety during the hospital stay.**

6. When doing an admission, the nurse surveys the personal belongings of an older adult client. The client's belongings include glasses, a hearing aid, cane, and a variety of medications. Identify a priority nursing diagnosis for this client based on that information.

    A. Disturbed sensory perception

    B. Impaired physical mobility

    C. Hopelessness

    D. Risk for falls

The decreased visual acuity relative to the glasses, use of a cane, advanced age, and probable impaired cognition from the medications are all risks for falls. Risk for falls would be the priority diagnosis. There is no indication that he has disturbed sensory perception, as he is using corrective devices. The use of a cane does not confirm that impaired mobility may be an issue, but his use of a cane places him at risk for falls. There is no assessment data to validate a nursing diagnosis of hopelessness.

Unit 3   Basic Nursing Care
Section: Safety

Chapter 48:   Ergonomic Principles and Client Positioning
Contributor: Teri W. Scott, MSN, FNP-c, RN

NCLEX® Connections:

> **Learning Objective**: Review and apply knowledge within **"Ergonomic Principles and Client Positioning"** in readiness for performance of the following nursing activities as outlined by the NCLEX® test plans:
>
> Δ   Demonstrate an understanding of the basic elements of good body mechanics to protect both the client and the provider from injury.
>
> Δ   Teach/reinforce the client, family, and caregivers on the necessity of frequent position changes and how to change positions safely and without injury.
>
> Δ   Teach/reinforce the client, family, and caregivers on body positions/movements that reduce risk for repetitive stress injuries.
>
> Δ   Safely position clients with limited mobility while maintaining correct body alignment.
>
> Δ   Implement care using proper body mechanics when lifting, positioning, transporting, or assisting a client.

 Key Points

Δ   Ergonomics are the factors or qualities in an object's design and/or use that contribute to comfort, safety, efficiency, and ease of use.

Δ   Prior to attempting to position or move a client, the nurse should do a **mobility assessment**.

Δ   Begin this assessment with the easiest movements (e.g., range of motion) and progress as long as the client tolerates it (e.g., balance, gait, exercise).

Key Procedural Points

Δ   **Assessing Body Alignment**

•   Correct **body alignment** assists in balance. When the body's center of gravity is stable, there is no strain on the muscles. Without correct body alignment, the client has less control over her balance and is at increased risk for falls. To enhance balance, widen the base of support and ensure the center of gravity is within the base of that support.

◊ **Lying** – best done in a lateral position with no support except for a pillow under the head. The vertebra should be straight without causing discomfort for the client.

◊ **Sitting and standing** – the head is erect, vertebral column is straight and in an S-shape from a lateral view. Shoulder and hips are parallel.

Δ **Bed and Client Positions**

Fowler's position	• The client lies supine with the head of the bed elevated **45 to 90°**, and the knees may be slightly elevated (about **15°**). • This allows for better chest expansion and ventilation and for better dependent drainage after abdominal surgeries.
Semi-Fowler's position	• The client lies supine with head elevated **30 to 40°**, and the knees may be elevated (about 15°). • This position promotes lung expansion and decreases stress on the abdominal muscles.
Supine or dorsal recumbent position	• The client lies on his back with his head and shoulders elevated on a pillow.
Prone position	• The client lies flat on the abdomen with the head to one side. • This position promotes drainage from the mouth for clients with throat or oral surgery, but inhibits chest expansion.
Lateral or side-lying position	• The client **lies on his side** with most of the weight on the dependent hip and shoulder. The arms should be flexed in front of the body. A pillow behind the back and hips may be required to support the client and maintain the position. • This is a good sleeping position, but the client must be turned regularly to prevent development of pressure ulcers on the dependent areas.
Sims' or semi-prone position	• The client is on his side halfway **between lateral and prone positions** (Weight is on the anterior ileum, humerus, and clavicle.). The lower arm is behind the client while the upper arm is in front with the upper leg flexed. • This is a comfortable sleeping position for many clients, and it promotes oral drainage.
Trendelenburg position	• The entire bed is tilted with the **head of the bed lower than the foot of the bed.** • This position is used during postural drainage, and it facilitates venous return.
Reverse Trendelenburg	• The entire bed is tilted with the **foot of the bed lower than the head of the bed.** This position promotes gastric emptying and prevents esophageal reflux.

Δ   Transfers and Use of Assistive Devices

- Assess the client's ability to help with transfers (e.g., balance, muscle strength, endurance).

- Determine the need for additional personnel or assistive devices (e.g., transfer belt, hydraulic lift, sliding board).

- Assess and monitor the client's proper use of mobility aids (e.g., canes, walkers, crutches).

- Include assistance or mobility aids needed for safe transfers and ambulation in plan of care.

NANDA Nursing Diagnoses

Δ   Risk for injury

Δ   Risk for impaired skin integrity

Δ   Impaired physical mobility

Δ   Risk for activity intolerance

Nursing Interventions

Δ   **The Immobile Client**

- The nurse will do a routine and very thorough skin assessment to identify potential areas of breakdown (over bony prominences).

- Position changes should occur every 1 to 2 hr, or per facility/agency protocol or provider's orders, to decrease the risk of pressure ulcers relative to decreased circulation to areas in contact with the bed/chair.

- Assess the client's respiratory status to determine if there is an accumulation of secretions in the lungs (decreased breath sounds in dependent areas of the lungs).

- Have the client turn, cough, and deep breathe, or do incentive spirometry every 2 hr, to reduce stasis of secretions in the lungs and fully expand the lungs, which decreases the risk for pneumonia or respiratory complications.

- Assess the client's circulatory status (pulses, capillary refill, skin temperature) regularly to determine any decrease in circulation increasing the risk for thrombosis (specifically in the lower extremities).

- Encourage leg exercise, ambulation (if able), fluids, and position changes to promote circulation and prevent stasis, which increases the risk for thrombosis.

- Reduce the risk of orthostatic hypotension by ambulating the client as soon as possible to increase venous return. Assist with transfers and ambulation to prevent falls.

- Support treatments, ordered by the primary care provider, to decrease venous return and risk of thrombosis.

  ◊ **Medications** – platelet inhibitors or anticoagulants

  ◊ **Intermittent pneumatic compression** cuffs (**IPC**s), or sequential compression devices (**SCD**s) to increase venous return through external pressure

  ◊ **Therapeutic elastic stockings**, which exert external pressure on muscles promoting venous return

Δ **Ergonomic Principles**

- The **center of gravity** is the center of a mass. In the body, the center of gravity is the pelvis. When an individual moves, the center of gravity also shifts. The closer the line of gravity is to the center of the base of support, the more stable the individual is. To lower the center of gravity, bend the hips and knees. **Avoid twisting the spine or bending at the waist** (flexion) to minimize the risk for injury.

- When **lifting**, use the major muscle groups to prevent back strain, and tighten the abdominal muscles to increase support to the back muscles. Distribute the weight between the large muscles of the arms and legs to decrease the strain on any one muscle group and avoid strain to smaller muscles. When lifting from the floor, flex the hips, knees, and back. Get the object to thigh level keeping the knees bent and straightening the back. Hold the object as close as possible, bringing the load to the center of gravity to increase stability and decrease strain. Use assistive devices whenever possible, and find assistance whenever it is needed.

- When **pushing or pulling** a load, widen the base of support. If pushing, move the front foot forward, and if pulling, move the rear leg back to promote stability. Face the direction of movement if moving a client. It is easier and safer to pull toward than to push away from the center of gravity. Use body weight when pushing or pulling to decrease the strain on muscles, which makes the movement easier. Sliding, rolling, and pushing require less energy than lifting and have less risk for injury.

Δ   **Guidelines to Prevent Injury**

- Plan ahead for activities that require lifting, transfer, or ambulation of a client and ask others to be ready to assist at the time planned.

- Rest between these heavy activities to decrease muscle fatigue.

- Maintain good posture and exercise regularly to increase the strength of arm, leg, back, and abdominal muscles so these activities require less energy.

- Get help from others, use assistive devices, and offer to help others in lifting clients to reduce the load for any one individual.

- Use smooth movements when lifting and moving clients to prevent injury through sudden or jerky muscle movements.

- When standing for long periods of time, flex the hip and knee through use of a foot rest. When sitting for long periods of time, keep the knees slightly higher than the hips.

- The client who is debilitated does not move easily and has difficulty changing positions frequently. It is the responsibility of the caregiver to reposition the client regularly while maintaining good body alignment for the client, and using good body mechanics for the provider's safety.

- Avoid repetitive movements of the hands, wrists, and shoulders. Take a break every 15 to 20 min to flex and stretch joints and muscles.

- Maintain good posture (head and neck in straight line with pelvis) to avoid neck flexion and hunched shoulders which can cause impingement of nerves in the neck.

Primary Reference:

Potter, P. A., & Perry, A. G. (2005). *Fundamentals of nursing* (6th ed.). St. Louis, MO: Mosby.

Additional Resources:

NANDA International (2004). *NANDA nursing diagnoses: Definitions and classification 2005-2006*. Philadelphia: NANDA.

Chapter 48: Ergonomic Principles and Client Positioning

Application Exercises

1. A nurse on the rehabilitation unit is assigned to care for a client who is hemiplegic and preparing to be dismissed to the care of his family. The plan of care includes teaching the family how to prevent injury to themselves and the client through safe positioning. What teaching points should be included in the instructions given to the family?

2. A client is being admitted to the surgical unit postoperatively with strict orders for no ambulation for 4 days. What assessments should be done to evaluate the risk for complications?

3. A postoperative client should be in a semi-Fowler's position. The nurse determines the position is incorrect because

    A. the client is in pain.

    B. the head of the bed is at 50°.

    C. the client's knees and legs are flat.

    D. there is a pillow behind the client's head.

4. Place the following steps in a mobility assessment in the correct sequence.

    _____ Exercise tolerance

    _____ Moving from supine to sitting on the side of the bed

    _____ Gait

    _____ Range of motion

5. Which of the following positions promotes drainage from the mouth for clients with throat or oral surgery, but inhibits chest expansion?

    A. Fowler's position

    B. Semi-Fowler's position

    C. Prone position

    D. Reverse Trendelenburg

Chapter 48: Ergonomic Principles and Client Positioning

Application Exercises Answer Key

1. A nurse on the rehabilitation unit is assigned to care for a client who is hemiplegic and preparing to be dismissed to the care of his family. The plan of care includes teaching the family how to prevent injury to themselves and the client through safe positioning. What teaching points should be included in the instructions given to the family?

> Maintain good posture.

> The wider the base of support, the more stability.

> Exercise regularly to strengthen leg, arm, and abdominal muscles to be the primary muscle groups used in lifting.

> Strong abdominal muscles support the smaller back muscles.

> Carry load as close to the body as possible.

> Pushing, rolling, or sliding a load requires less energy.

> Stop and rest between lifting tasks to give the muscles time to recover.

> When pushing, move the front foot forward for more stability.

> When pulling, move the back foot back to increase stability.

2. A client is being admitted to the surgical unit postoperatively with strict orders for no ambulation for 4 days. What assessments should be done to evaluate the risk for complications?

> Assessment of the skin to identify potential areas of breakdown (over bony prominences) every 1 to 2 hr, or per facility/agency protocol or provider's orders, to decrease the risk of pressure ulcers relative to decreased circulation to areas in contact with the bed/chair

> Assessment of the client's respiratory status to determine if there is an accumulation of secretions in the lungs (decreased breath sounds in dependent areas of the lungs)

> Assessment of the client's circulatory status (pulses, capillary refill, skin temperature) regularly to determine any decrease in circulation, which increases the risk for thrombosis (specifically in the lower extremities)

3. A postoperative client should be in a semi-Fowler's position. The nurse determines the position is incorrect because

    A. the client is in pain.

    B. the head of the bed is at 50°.

    C. the client's knees and legs are flat.

    D. there is a pillow behind the client's head.

While the client is in the semi-Fowler's position, the bed is raised approximately 30 to 40°. The client is currently in the Fowler's position. The client's pain is probably not related to bed position. The legs may be slightly elevated in the semi-Fowler's position, but they do not have to be. A pillow behind the client's head will not alter the bed position.

4. Place the following steps in a mobility assessment in the correct sequence.

    __4__   Exercise tolerance

    __2__   Moving from supine to sitting on the side of the bed

    __3__   Gait

    __1__   Range of motion

5. Which of the following positions promotes drainage from the mouth for clients with throat or oral surgery but inhibits chest expansion?

    A. Fowler's position

    B. Semi-Fowler's position

    C. Prone position

    D. Reverse Trendelenburg

The prone position promotes drainage from the mouth for clients with throat or oral surgery, but it inhibits chest expansion. Fowler's and semi-Fowler's positions promote chest expansion. Reverse Trendelenburg promotes gastric emptying and prevents esophageal reflux.

Unit 3   **Basic Nursing Care**
Section: Infection Control

Chapter 49:   Medical and Surgical Asepsis

Contributor: Terri Astorino, EdD, MSN, RN

 NCLEX® Connections:

> **Learning Objective**: Review and apply knowledge within **"Medical and Surgical Asepsis"** in readiness for performance of the following nursing activities as outlined by the NCLEX® test plans:
>
> Δ   Identify circumstances requiring the use of medical and surgical asepsis.
>
> Δ   Employ medical and surgical aseptic practices correctly to prevent or reduce the risk of infection.

 Key Points

Δ   **Asepsis** – the absence of illness-producing micro-organisms. Asepsis is maintained through the use of **aseptic technique** with hand hygiene being the primary behavior associated with maintenance of asepsis/aseptic technique.

   • **Medical asepsis** – the use of precise practices to reduce the number, growth, and spread of micro-organisms from an object or area. It is also known as "clean technique." Uses include oral medication administration, nasogastric tube management, and providing personal hygiene.

   • **Surgical asepsis** – the use of precise practices to eliminate all micro-organisms from an object or area. Also known as "sterile technique." Uses include parenteral medication administration, insertion of urinary catheters, and surgical procedures.

Key Procedural Points

Δ   **Practices that Promote Medical Asepsis**

- The number one measure to reduce the growth and transmission of infectious agents is through good handwashing. The Centers for Disease Control and Prevention (CDC) states that "handwashing is the single most effective means of preventing the spread of micro-organisms."

- The **three essential components** of good **handwashing** include:

    ◊   **Soap** or a chemical that contains an antimicrobial agent.

    ◊   **Water**.

    ◊   **Friction**.

- All healthcare personnel must wash their hands before and after every client contact, after removing gloves, after contact with body fluids, when hands are visibly soiled, and after using the restroom.

- The CDC recommends a 10- to 15-sec handwashing time to remove transient flora from the hands and up to 2 min when hands are more soiled or in contact with high-risk areas. After washing, hands should be dried with a clean paper towel before turning off the faucet.

- Additional examples of practices that reduce the growth and spread of micro-organisms are changing linens daily, cleaning floors and the client's bedside stand, and separating clean from contaminated materials into different areas.

- The use of masks, gloves, gowns, and protective eyewear helps control the contact and spread of micro-organisms to both the primary care provider and the client.

- Do not place items on the floor in the client environment (even soiled laundry). The floor is considered "grossly" contaminated.

- Educate all clients on the importance of covering their mouth and nose when coughing or sneezing, using and disposing of tissues, and good handwashing to prevent spraying or spreading of droplet infections.

- Do not shake linens to avoid "raising" dust in the client environment, which can be irritating to those in the environment.

- Clean the least soiled areas first to prevent moving more contaminants into the cleaner areas.

- Use plastic bags for moist soiled items (Follow facility/agency protocol on bag selection.) to prevent further contamination of items or individuals handling the soiled items. Put all soiled items directly into the appropriate receptacle to avoid handling soiled items more than once.

- Pour any liquids used in care directly into the drain, and avoid splattering that can spread droplets.

- Primary care providers should:
  - ◊ Follow facility/agency protocols for isolation and protection.
  - ◊ Wash their hair frequently and keep it short or pulled back to prevent contamination of the care area or the client.
  - ◊ Not wear artificial nails while providing care and should keep the nails short and clean. The area around and under the nails can harbor micro-organisms.
  - ◊ Use hand lotion to prevent drying, chapping, and lesions on the hands that present a risk for infection to the provider.
  - ◊ Not wear rings with grooves or stones that are difficult to clean.

Δ **Practices that maintain a sterile field**

- Prolonged exposure to airborne micro-organisms can cause sterile items to become nonsterile.
  - ◊ Avoid coughing, sneezing, or talking directly over a sterile field.
  - ◊ Air movement should be controlled by special ventilation.
- Only sterile items may be in a sterile field.
  - ◊ The outer wrappings and 1-inch edges of packaging that contain sterile items are not sterile.
  - ◊ Only touch sterile materials with sterile gloves.
  - ◊ Sterile materials may touch other sterile surfaces or materials; however, contact with nonsterile materials at any time renders a sterile area contaminated, no matter how short the contact.
- Microbes can move by gravity from a nonsterile item to a sterile item.
  - ◊ Do not reach across or above a sterile field.
  - ◊ Items to be added to a sterile field must be held a minimum of 6 inches above the field.
- Any sterile, nonwaterproof wrapper that comes in contact with moisture becomes nonsterile by a wicking action that allows microbes to travel rapidly from a nonsterile surface to the sterile surface.
  - ◊ Keep all surfaces dry.
  - ◊ Discard any sterile packages that become wet.

Nursing Interventions

Δ Equipment

- Select a clean area in the client's environment (e.g., a bedside stand) to set up the sterile field.
- Check that all sterile packages (additional dressings, sterile bowl, sterile gloves, solution) are dry and within expiration date.
- Make sure there is a waste receptacle.

Δ   Procedure

- Wash hands.

- Open plastic covering of package per manufacturer's directions, slipping the package onto the center of the workspace with the top flap of wrapper opening away from body.

- Reach around the package to open the top flap of the package, grasp the outside flap between the thumb and the index finger, and unfold the top flap away from body.

- Next open the side flaps, using the right hand for the right flap and the left hand for the left flap.

- The last flap should be grasped and turned down toward body.

- Additional sterile packages

    ◊ Open next to the sterile field by holding the bottom edge with one hand and pulling back on the top flap with the other hand. Place the packages that are to be used last furthest from the sterile field, and open these first.

    ◊ Add them directly to the sterile field. Lift the package from the dry surface, holding it 15 cm (6 inches) above the sterile field, pulling the two surfaces apart, and dropping it onto the sterile field.

- Pour sterile solutions by:

    ◊ Removing the bottle cap.

    ◊ Placing the bottle cap face up on the surface.

    ◊ Holding the bottle with the label in the palm of the hand so that the solution does not run down the label.

    ◊ First pouring a small amount (1 to 2 mL) of the solution into an available receptacle.

    ◊ Pouring the solution onto the dressing or site without touching the bottle to the site.

- Once the sterile field is set up, it is necessary to don sterile gloves.

- Sterile gloving includes opening the wrapper and handling only the outside of the wrapper. Don gloves by using the following steps.

    ◊ With the cuff side pointing toward the body, use the left hand and pick up the right-hand glove by grasping the folded bottom edge of the cuff and lifting it up and away from the wrapper.

    ◊ While picking up the edge of the cuff, pull the right glove on the hand.

    ◊ With the sterile right-gloved hand, place the fingers of the right hand inside the cuff of the left glove, lifting it off the wrapper, and put the left hand into it.

◊ When both hands are gloved, adjustments of the fingers in the gloves may be made if necessary.

◊ During that time, only the sterile gloved hand can touch the other sterile gloved hand.

◊ At the close of the sterile procedure, or if the gloves tear, the gloves must be removed. Take off the gloves by grasping the outer part of one glove at the wrist, pulling the glove down over the fingers and into the hand that is still gloved. Then, place the ungloved hand inside the soiled glove and pull the glove off so that it is inside out, and only the clean inside part is exposed. Discard into an appropriate receptacle.

Primary Reference:

Potter, P. A., & Perry, A. G. (2005). *Fundamentals of nursing* (6th ed.). St. Louis, MO: Mosby.

Additional Resources:

Harkreader, H., & Hogan, M. A, (2004). *Fundamentals of nursing: Caring and clinical judgment*. Philadelphia: Elseveir.

NANDA International (2004). *NANDA nursing diagnoses: Definitions and classification 2005-2006*. Philadelphia: NANDA.

Chapter 49: Medical and Surgical Asepsis

Application Exercises

1. When entering a client's room to change a surgical dressing, a nurse notes that the client is coughing and sneezing. When preparing the sterile field, it is important that the nurse

   A. keep the sterile field on the far side of the client's room away from the bedside.

   B. instruct the client to refrain from coughing and sneezing during the dressing change.

   C. place a mask on the client to limit the spread of micro-organisms into the surgical wound.

   D. keep a box of tissues close to the client for the client's use during the dressing change.

2. A nurse is teaching a group of personal care assistants that the most effective way to decrease the spread of infection is by

   A. wearing gloves with all clients.

   B. placing clients with infection in isolation.

   C. wearing gowns and masks at all times when in contact with a client's skin.

   D. basic handwashing.

3. While wearing sterile gloves, a nurse can touch any

   A. object on the sterile field.

   B. object on the bedside stand.

   C. part of the client's gown.

   D. sterile object below the waist.

4. Match each of the following practices to the best example.

   _____ Medical asepsis practice   A. A nurse wears gloves when emptying a bedpan each time.

   _____ Standard precautions   B. A nurse drops a sterile dressing on the floor.

   _____ Sterile field maintenance   C. A nurse keeps her sterile hands above her waist.

   _____ Contamination   D. A nurse wipes off the client's bedside table.

5. Which of the following statements are true of surgical asepsis and a sterile field? (Select all that apply.)

_____ The nurse should turn her back on the sterile field if she needs to cough.

_____ The 1-inch edge around a sterile field is also considered sterile.

_____ A sterile item can touch another sterile item without contaminating it.

_____ Sterile items must remain above the waist.

_____ Surgical asepsis is also called "sterile technique."

6. Describe the proper procedure for pouring a sterile solution.

Chapter 49: Medical and Surgical Asepsis

Application Exercises Answer Key

1. When entering a client's room to change a surgical dressing, a nurse notes that the client is coughing and sneezing. When preparing the sterile field, it is important that the nurse

   A. keep the sterile field on the far side of the client's room away from the bedside.

   B. instruct the client to refrain from coughing and sneezing during the dressing change.

   C. place a mask on the client to limit the spread of micro-organisms into the surgical wound.

   D. keep a box of tissues close to the client for the client's use during the dressing change.

   Placing a mask on the client prevents contamination of the surgical wound during the dressing change. It would be difficult for the nurse to maintain the sterile field if it is on the far side of the room away from the bedside. The client may be unable to refrain from coughing and sneezing during the dressing change. Keeping tissues close by for the client to use still allows for contamination of the surgical wound.

2. A nurse is teaching a group of personal care assistants that the most effective way to decrease the spread of infection is by

   A. wearing gloves with all clients.

   B. placing clients with infection in isolation.

   C. wearing gowns and masks at all times when in contact with a client's skin.

   D. basic handwashing.

   Frequent handwashing is the best way to prevent the spread of infection. Wearing gloves is appropriate when in contact with any client's blood, body fluids, or nonintact skin, but handwashing is still important after removing the gloves. Placing clients with infections in isolation is important for certain types of infections, but it neglects the important aspect of handwashing. Wearing gowns and masks is not necessary if the client's skin is intact.

3. While wearing sterile gloves, a nurse can touch any

    A. object on the sterile field.

    B. object on the bedside stand.

    C. part of the client's gown.

    D. sterile object below the waist.

To maintain a sterile field, the nurse can only touch other sterile items when wearing sterile gloves without causing contamination. Touching an object on the bedside stand, the client's gown, and any sterile object below the waist will break the sterile field.

4. Match each of the following practices to the best example.

  D Medical asepsis practice   A. A nurse wears gloves when emptying a bedpan each time.

  A Standard precautions   B. A nurse drops a sterile dressing on the floor.

  C Sterile field maintenance   C. A nurse keeps her sterile hands above her waist.

  B Contamination   D. A nurse wipes off the client's bedside table.

5. Which of the following statements are true of surgical asepsis and a sterile field? (Select all that apply.)

    _____ The nurse should turn her back on the sterile field if she needs to cough.

    _____ The 1-inch edge around a sterile field is also considered sterile.

    __X__ A sterile item can touch another sterile item without contaminating it.

    __X__ Sterile items must remain above the waist.

    __X__ Surgical asepsis is also called "sterile technique."

A sterile item can touch another sterile item without contaminating it. To maintain the sterility of an item, it must stay above the waist, and surgical asepsis is also called "sterile technique." If the nurse turns her back on the sterile field, the sterile field is considered contaminated. The nurse should step away but continue to face the sterile field. The 1-inch edge around a sterile field is not considered sterile.

6. Describe the proper procedure for pouring a sterile solution.

Remove the bottle cap and place the bottle cap face up on the surface.

Hold the bottle with the label in the palm of the hand so that the solution does not run down the label.

Pour a small amount of the solution into an available receptacle.

Pour the solution onto the dressing or site without touching the bottle to the site.

Unit 3   Basic Nursing Care

Section: Infection Control

Chapter 50:   Infection Control

Contributor: Teri W. Scott, MSN, FNP-c, RN

 NCLEX® Connections:

Learning Objective: Review and apply knowledge within **"Infection Control"** in readiness for performance of the following nursing activities as outlined by the NCLEX® test plans:

Δ   Assess/monitor the client for signs and symptoms of infection, and report findings to the primary care provider for prompt treatment.

Δ   Identify the mode of transmission for various infectious agents.

Δ   Plan and/or provide safe care by employing standard precautions with all clients.

Δ   Prevent the spread of infection by employing the two-tier isolation guidelines.

Δ   Communicate the presence of communicable diseases to the appropriate authorities.

Δ   Use aseptic technique, education, proper nutrition, and good handwashing to protect the biological safety of the client, families, and health care providers.

Δ   Evaluate and document care given to prevent the spread of infection.

Δ   Teach/reinforce to the client and family appropriate infectious control measures such as frequent handwashing.

 Key Points

Δ   An infection occurs when the presence of a pathogen leads to a chain of events. All components of the chain must be present and intact for the infection to occur. The nurse uses infection control practices (e.g., medical asepsis, surgical asepsis, standard precautions) to break the chain and thus stop the spread of infection.

Δ   Components of the chain include:

• An infectious agent (e.g., bacteria, virus, fungi, protozoa).

• A reservoir where the infectious agent grows (e.g., wound drainage, food, oxygen tubing).

• An exit portal of the infectious agent (e.g., skin, respiratory, gastrointestinal tracts).

- A means of transmission (e.g., droplet, person-to-person contact, touching contaminated items).

- An entry portal to a susceptible host (same as exit).

- A host that must be susceptible to the infectious agent.

Key Procedural Points

Δ   **Risks of infection** – The nurse should assess each client for the risks of infection specific to the client, the disease or injury, and the environment. The most common risks include:

- Inadequate handwashing (client and caregivers).

- Individuals that have compromised health or defenses against infection, which include:

  ◊   Those who are immunocompromised.

  ◊   Those who have had surgery.

  ◊   Those with indwelling devices.

  ◊   A break in the skin (the body's best protection against infection).

  ◊   Those with poor oxygenation.

  ◊   Those with impaired circulation.

  ◊   Those who have chronic or acute disease.

- Use of poor medical or surgical asepsis by caregivers.

- The client with poor personal hygiene, poor nutrition, and those that are stressed.

- The client who lives in a very crowded environment.

- The older adult client.

- Individuals that make poor lifestyle choices that put them at risk, which include:

  ◊   Clients that use IV drugs and share needles.

  ◊   Clients who engage in unprotected sex.

- Clients who have recently been exposed to:

  ◊   Poor sanitation.

  ◊   The presence of mosquito-borne or parasitic diseases.

  ◊   Diseases endemic to the area visited, but not in the client's home country.

Δ   Types of Infections

- **Nosocomial infections**

    ◊   This is an infection that is acquired while the client is in the health care system. A nosocomial infection can come from an exogenous source (from outside the client) or endogenous (altered normal flora).

    ◊   The best way to prevent nosocomial infections is through **frequent handwashing**.

    ◊   The most common site of a nosocomial infection is the urinary tract. The most common causative agents in nosocomial infections are *Escherichia coli* and *Staphylococcus aureus*.

Assessment

Δ   **Signs and Symptoms of Infection**

- The signs and symptoms, identifiable in the nursing assessment, of generalized or **systemic infection** include:

    ◊   Fever.

    ◊   Increased pulse and respiratory rate (in response to the high fever).

    ◊   Malaise.

    ◊   Anorexia, nausea, and/or vomiting.

    ◊   Enlarged lymph nodes (repository for "waste").

- The signs and symptoms of a **localized infection** include:

    ◊   Redness (from dilation of arterioles bringing blood to the area).

    ◊   Edema.

    ◊   Pain or tenderness.

    ◊   Presence of exudates (dead phagocytes and tissue cells that leak from the vessels).

    ◊   Warmth of the area on palpation.

    ◊   Loss of use of the affected part.

- In addition to the items found on physical assessment, **laboratory results** indicating infection include:

    ◊   Leukocytosis (WBCs > 11,000/µL).

    ◊   Increases in the specific types of WBCs on differential (left shift = an increase in neutrophils).

    ◊   Elevated erythrocyte sedimentation rate (ESR).

    ◊   Presence of micro-organism on culture of the specific fluid/area.

NANDA Nursing Diagnoses

Δ   Impaired tissue integrity

Δ   Risk for infection

Δ   Risk for social isolation

Δ   Risk for impaired tissue integrity

Nursing Interventions

Δ   General Guidelines

- Use of **frequent and effective handwashing** by all health care providers and support staff between visits to the client is the most important intervention to prevent infection.

- Educate the client on the **required and recommended immunizations** and where immunizations can be obtained. The target groups include children, older adults, those with chronic disease, and those that are immunocompromised and their families/contacts.

- Educate the client and ask for a return demonstration on **good oral hygiene**. Good oral hygiene decreases the protein in the oral cavity, which thereby decreases the growth of micro-organisms (Protein attracts micro-organisms.) that can migrate through breaks in the oral mucosa.

- Encourage the client to consume an **adequate amount of fluids**. Adequate fluid intake prevents the stasis of urine by "flushing" the urinary tract and decreasing the growth of micro-organisms. Adequate hydration will also keep the skin from breaking down. Intact skin prevents micro-organisms from entering the body.

- In immobile clients, ensure that **pulmonary hygiene** (turning, coughing, and deep breathing or incentive spirometry) is done every 2 hr, or as ordered by the primary care provider. Good pulmonary hygiene decreases the growth of micro-organisms and development of pneumonia by prevention of stasis of pulmonary excretions, stimulation of ciliary movement and clearance, and expansion of the lungs.

- Use of **aseptic technique** and proper **personal protective equipment** in the provision of care to all clients prevents unnecessary exposure to micro-organisms.

Δ   Isolation Guidelines

- Isolation guidelines include a group of actions that include hand hygiene and the use of barrier precautions, which are intended to reduce the transmission of infectious organisms.

- The precautions apply to every client, regardless of the diagnosis, and must be implemented whenever contact with a potentially infectious material is anticipated.

- Personal protective equipment is changed after contact with each client, or between procedures with the same client if in contact with large amounts of blood and body fluids.

- **Standard Precautions (Tier One)**

  ◊ This tier of standard precautions applies to **all body fluids** (except sweat), nonintact skin, or mucous membranes.

  ◊ Hands are washed after contact with the client, body fluids, contaminated equipment/articles, and after removal of gloves.

  ◊ Gloves are worn when touching all body fluids, nonintact skin, mucous membranes, and contaminated equipment/articles.

  ◊ Gloves are removed and hand hygiene is completed between all clients.

  ◊ Masks, eye protection, or face shields are required when care may cause splashing or spraying of body fluids.

  ◊ Gowns are worn if the caregiver's clothes may be soiled during care. Hand hygiene is required after removal of the gown. A sturdy moisture-resistant bag should be used for soiled items, and the bag should be tied securely in a knot at the top.

  ◊ All equipment used in client care is to be properly cleaned; one-time use items are to be disposed of according to facility/agency policy.

  ◊ Contaminated laundry should be bagged and handled to prevent leaking or contamination of clothing or skin.

  ◊ Safety devices on all equipment/supplies must be enabled after use; all sharps must be disposed of in a puncture-resistant container.

  ◊ A private room is not necessary, unless the client's hygiene necessitates it.

- **Transmission Precautions (Tier Two)**

  ◊ **Airborne precautions** are to protect against droplet infections **smaller than 5 μm** (e.g., measles, varicella, pulmonary or laryngeal tuberculosis). Airborne precautions require a:

    ° Private room.

    ° Mask/respiratory protection device for caregivers and visitors.

    ° Negative pressure airflow exchange in the room of at least six exchanges per hour.

◊ **Droplet precautions** protect against droplets **larger than 5 µm** (e.g., streptococcal pharyngitis or pneumonia, scarlet fever, rubella, pertussis, mumps, mycoplasma pneumonia, meningococcal pneumonia/sepsis or pneumonic plague). Droplet precautions require a:

° Private room or a room with other clients with the same infectious disease.

° Mask for providers and visitors.

◊ **Contact precautions** protect the visitors and caregivers against **direct client/environmental contact infections** (e.g., respiratory syncytial virus, shigella, enteric diseases caused by micro-organisms, wound infections, herpes simplex, scabies, varicella zoster, and multidrug-resistant organisms). Contact precautions require:

° A private room or a room with other clients with the same infection.

° Gloves and gowns worn by the caregivers and visitors.

° Disposal of infectious dressing material into a single, nonporous bag without touching the outside of the bag.

Δ **Cleaning Contaminated Equipment Guidelines**

• Always wear gloves.

• Rinse first in cold water (hot water coagulates proteins, making them adhere).

• Wash the article in hot water with soap.

• Use a brush or abrasive to clean corners or hard-to-reach areas.

• Rinse well in warm or hot water.

• Dry the article – it is considered clean at this point.

• Clean the equipment used in cleaning and the sink (still considered dirty unless a disinfectant is used).

• Remove gloves and wash hands.

Δ **Reporting of Communicable Diseases**

• A complete list of reportable diseases and the reporting system are available through the Centers for Disease Control and Prevention Web site, *www.cdc. gov*. There are more than 60 communicable diseases that must **be reported to the public health departments** to allow for officials to:

◊ Ensure appropriate medical treatment of diseases (tuberculosis).

◊ Monitor for common-source out breaks (e.g., foodborne – hepatitis A).

◊ Plan and evaluate control and prevention plans (e.g., immunizations for preventable diseases).

◊ Identify outbreaks and epidemics.

◊ Determine public health priorities based on trends.

Primary Reference:

Potter, P. A., & Perry, A. G. (2005). *Fundamentals of nursing* (6th ed.). St. Louis, MO: Mosby.

Additional Resources:

Centers for Disease Control and Prevention. (2006). *Reported diseases*, Retrieved February, 2006 from *www.cdc.gov/epo/dphsi/casedef/introduction.htm*

NANDA International (2004). *NANDA nursing diagnoses: Definitions and classification 2005-2006*. Philadelphia: NANDA.

Chapter 50: Infection Control

Application Exercises

1. Match the component of the chain of infection with the example of each component.

_____ Infectious agent   A. Client

_____ Reservoir   B. Bacteria, virus, fungi, protozoa

_____ Means of transmission   C. Wound drainage, food, oxygen tubing

_____ Exit and entry portal   D. Person-to-person contact

_____ Host   E. Skin, respiratory, and gastrointestinal tracts

2. Which of the following are reasons health care professionals are required to report communicable/infectious diseases? (Select all that apply.)

_____ Planning and evaluating of control and prevention plans

_____ Determining public health priorities

_____ Ensuring proper medical treatment

_____ Identifying endemic disease

_____ Monitoring for common-source outbreaks

3. A client is experiencing gastric pain with vomiting and diarrhea. A nurse is setting up the room. Which of the following is required until an enteric micro-organism is ruled out? (Select all that apply.)

_____ Gloves

_____ Gown

_____ Mask

_____ Handwashing

_____ Private room

4. Place an (S) next to the signs and symptoms that indicate a systemic infection and an (L) in front of the signs and symptoms that indicate a local infection.

	Fever
	Edema
	Pain or tenderness
	Malaise
	Warmth of the area on palpation
	Increased pulse and respiratory rate

Chapter 50: Infection Control

Application Exercises Answer Key

1. Match the component of the chain of infection with the example of each component.

  B   Infectious agent   A. Client

  C   Reservoir   B. Bacteria, virus, fungi, protozoa

  D   Means of transmission   C. Wound drainage, food, oxygen tubing

  E   Exit and entry portal   D. Person-to-person contact

  A   Host   E. Skin, respiratory, and gastrointestinal tracts

2. Which of the following are reasons health care professionals are required to report communicable/infectious diseases? (Select all that apply.)

   X   **Planning and evaluating of control and prevention plans**

   X   **Determining public health priorities**

   X   **Ensuring proper medical treatment**

   _____   Identifying endemic disease

   X   **Monitoring for common-source outbreaks**

Reporting of communicable/infectious diseases assists with planning and evaluating of control and prevention plans, determining public health policies, ensuring proper medical treatment is available, and monitoring for common-source outbreaks. Endemic disease is already prevalent within a population, so reporting is not necessary.

3. A client is experiencing gastric pain with vomiting and diarrhea. A nurse is setting up the room. Which of the following is required until an enteric micro-organism is ruled out? (Select all that apply.)

   X   **Gloves**

   X   **Gown**

   _____   Mask

   X   **Handwashing**

   X   **Private room**

Gloves, gown, handwashing, and a private room will help prevent the spread of infection from micro-organisms from the gastrointestinal tract. A mask is necessary to prevent the spread of infection from airborne exposures.

4. Place an (S) next to the signs and symptoms that indicate a systemic infection and an (L) in front of the signs and symptoms that indicate a local infection.

S	Fever
L	Edema
L	Pain or tenderness
S	Malaise
L	Warmth of the area on palpation
S	Increased pulse and respiratory rate

Unit 3   Basic Nursing Care
Section: Comfort and Basic Needs

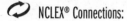

Chapter 51:   Hygiene Care
                Contributor: Wendy Buenzli, MN, RN

 NCLEX® Connections:

Learning Objective: Review and apply knowledge within **"Hygiene Care"** in readiness for performance of the following nursing activities as outlined by the NCLEX® test plans:

Δ   Assess/monitor the client's hygiene and grooming practices.

Δ   Assist the client with hygiene needs and privacy needs that he is unable to perform.

Δ   Plan and provide care to promote optimal level of independence.

Δ   Instruct the client and family about resources available to assist the client with activities of daily living.

Δ   Evaluate and document the client's ability to perform hygiene and grooming practices independently as the client approaches discharge.

Key Points

Δ   Bathing

•   The purpose of bathing is to **cleanse** the body, relax it, and enhance healing.

•   Perform skin assessment and wound care at this time.

•   Clients with diseases and disabilities that have exhausted them or limited their mobility should be bathed.

◊   Complete baths are given when the client is able to tolerate it, and the client's hygiene needs warrant it (usually reserved for debilitated clients).

◊   Partial baths are useful when the client needs to only have odorous or uncomfortable areas cleansed or can perform part of the bath himself. The client should be assessed to see how much of the bath he can complete himself.

Δ   Proper oral hygiene helps to **decrease infections** in clients living in nursing homes, especially the transmission of pneumonia.

Δ   **Foot care** is given to prevent skin breakdown, pain, and infection. Foot care is extremely important for clients with diabetes and must be done by a trained professional.

Δ   **Perineal care** maintains skin integrity, relieves discomfort, and prevents transmission of infection (catheter care).

Key Procedural Points

Δ   **Cultural and Social Practices**

- Each client will require different hygiene preferences and practices. This includes bathing routines, oral care, grooming preferences, body image issues, health beliefs, and physical condition. Culture also plays an important role, because specific cultures may adhere to their own hygiene practices. Be sure to be respectful and observant of each client's specific cultural needs.

- Socioeconomic status may play a role in the client's hygiene status. If the client is homeless, discharge instructions and follow up care may need to be altered.

- **Respect the client's dignity**. Many clients are dealing with a loss of control when allowing another person to provide for their hygiene needs. Reassuring the client and allowing her to have as much control as possible may help.

Δ   **Safety**

- Before starting any care, understand how to complete each task to avoid injuring the client. This includes knowing the equipment and what the proper techniques are for each hygiene item.

- Never leave the client in a position where injury could occur during routine hygiene care (e.g., Avoid leaving a client who is at risk for aspiration alone with oral hygiene supplies).

Δ   **Special Considerations for Older Adult Clients**

- The older adult's skin is **drier and thinner** and may not tolerate as much bathing as a younger adult.

- The older adult has a higher incidence of **infection** and **periodontal disease** because of the weakening of the periodontal membrane.

- Dentures and partials must be fitted correctly, or they can cause digestive issues, pain, and discomfort. **Dentures are a client's personal property. Never leave them on a meal tray or in a place where they could be damaged.**

- **Dry mouth** is common in the older adult due to decreased saliva production and medications used by this population (e.g., antihypertensives, diuretics, anti-inflammatory agents, and antidepressants).

- **Poor nutritional status** is often due to dental problems, socioeconomic status, and a decrease in the ability to prepare healthy foods.

Assessment

Δ   Assess the client's skin for color, hydration, texture, and the presence of any lesions.

Δ   Note the condition of the client's gums and teeth.

Δ   Assess the client's skin surfaces including the feet, nails, shape and size of foot, any lesions, and areas of dryness or inflammation. Abnormal assessment findings may indicate the presence of neuropathies and/or vascular insufficiency.

Δ   **Hygiene preferences** should be identified to understand how the client conducts hygiene at home and where the nurse will need to provide education and extra care.

Δ   Assess the client for **safety issues** (e.g., positioning, ability to ambulate) and ability to participate in self-care.

NANDA Nursing Diagnoses

Δ   Risk for injury

Δ   Risk for infection

Δ   Bathing/self-care deficit

Δ   Dressing/grooming deficit

Nursing Interventions

Δ   Steps in performing a bed bath include:

- Collecting equipment, providing for privacy, and explaining the procedure to the client.

- Placing a bath blanket over the client and removing the client's gown.

- Obtaining bath water.

- Washing the client's face first. Allow the client to perform this task if able.

- Performing the bath systematically by starting with the client's upper body and continuing on to her lower extremities. Change water as indicated using fresh water to perform perineum care.

- Applying lotion, powder, and a clean gown.

- Documenting skin assessment, type of bath, and client response.

- Changing an occupied bed.

  ◊ Roll the old bottom linens up in the bottom sheet or mattress pad under the client who is turned on his side, facing the opposite direction.

  ◊ Apply clean bottom linens to the bed, and smooth to the middle of the bed with the remainder of the linen fan folded underneath the client.

  ◊ The client should roll over the linens and face the opposite direction while the nurse removes the old linens and applies the new linens.

  ◊ Apply upper sheet and blanket.

  ◊ Remove the pillow case by inserting the hand into the opening, grabbing the pillow, and turning the pillowcase inside out.

  ◊ Apply the clean pillow case by grasping the center of the closed end, turning the case inside out, fitting the pillow into the corner of the case, and pulling the case until it is right side out over the pillow.

Δ Oral Hygiene

- Clients who have fragile oral mucosa require gentle brushing and flossing.

- Perform denture care for the client who is unable to do it himself.

  ◊ Remove the dentures with a gloved hand, pulling down and out at the front of the upper denture, and lifting up and out at the front of the lower denture.

  ◊ Place dentures in a denture cup or emesis basin.

  ◊ Brush them with a soft brush and denture cleaner.

  ◊ Rinse them in water.

  ◊ Store the dentures, or assist the client with reinserting the dentures.

Δ Foot Care

- It is important to prevent any infection or pain that may interfere with the client's gait. This care is extremely important for clients with diabetes and must be done by a trained professional.

- Instruct the client at risk for injury to:

  ◊ Inspect feet daily, paying special attention to between the toes.

  ◊ Use lukewarm water and dry the feet thoroughly.

  ◊ Apply moisturizer to the feet but avoid applying it between the toes.

  ◊ Avoid over-the-counter products that contain alcohol or other strong chemicals.

  ◊ Wear clean cotton socks daily.

◊   Check shoes for any objects that may cause injury.

◊   Cut nails straight across and use emery board to file edges.

◊   Avoid self-treating corns or calluses.

◊   Buy and wear comfortable shoes that do not cut off circulation.

◊   Avoid using heat applications.

◊   Contact her primary care provider if any signs of infection or inflammation appear.

Δ   Perineal care – maintains skin integrity, relieves discomfort, and prevents transmission of infection (catheter care). Principles of perineal care include:

- Providing privacy.

- Maintaining a professional demeanor.

- Removing fecal material away from the skin if present.

- Cleansing the client from front to back.

- Drying thoroughly.

- Retracting the foreskin in male clients to wash the tip of the penis. Then, replace the foreskin.

Δ   Nail Care

- Assess the client's nails for size, shape, and condition of nail beds.

- Assess for cracking, clubbing, or any fungus that may be present.

- Use caution and have proper training when cutting nails. The nails of a diabetic client should only be trimmed by a primary care provider or specialist.

Δ   Shaving

- Safety is important. Clients prone to bleeding or receiving anticoagulants should use an electric razor.

- With a razor blade, the nurse applies soap or shaving cream to warm, moist skin.

- The razor is moved over the skin in the direction of hair growth using short strokes.

- Communication with the client about personal shaving preferences is important.

Primary Reference:

Potter, P. A., & Perry, A. G. (2005). *Fundamentals of nursing* (6th ed.). St. Louis, MO: Mosby.

Additional Resources:

DeLaune, S, & Ladner, P. (2006). *Fundamentals of nursing* (3rd ed.). Clifton Park: Thomson Delmar.

NANDA International (2004). *NANDA nursing diagnoses: Definitions and classification 2005-2006*. Philadelphia: NANDA.

Chapter 51: Hygiene Care

Application Exercises

1. A client is transferred from a long-term care facility to an acute care setting. An indwelling Foley catheter was inserted just prior to her transfer. Which of the following tasks will help prevent the development of a nosocomial infection?

    A. Assessing the client's ability to void independently

    B. Placing an absorbent pad under the client to protect the bed in case of incontinence

    C. Frequently cleaning the client's perineal area and properly caring for her catheter

    D. Properly hydrating the client and giving her a diet high in fiber to prevent constipation

2. Which of the following are appropriate teaching measures related to care of the feet for a client with diabetes mellitus? (Select all that apply.)

    _____ Inspect feet daily.

    _____ Use moisturizing lotions on feet.

    _____ Wash with warm water and let air dry.

    _____ Use over-the-counter products to treat abrasions.

    _____ Check shoes for any foreign objects.

3. A client is in balanced suspension traction following a motor vehicle crash. He is unable to perform his own personal hygiene and must have it performed by the nurse. Which of the following factors will have the most influence on his comfort level?

    A. The client's position

    B. The attitude of the nurse

    C. The gender of the nurse

    D. The amount of pain medicine he has received

4. A client experiences dyspnea and reports feeling tired after completing her morning care. Which of the following should the nurse include in the client's plan of care for the next day?

    A. Plan for several rest periods during morning care.

    B. Do not offer any morning care.

    C. Perform all of the client's care as quickly as possible.

    D. Ask a family member to come in and give the client a bath.

Chapter 51: Hygiene Care

Application Exercises Answer Key

1. A client is transferred from a long-term care facility to an acute care setting. An indwelling Foley catheter was inserted just prior to her transfer. Which of the following tasks will help prevent the development of a nosocomial infection?

    A. Assessing the client's ability to void independently

    B. Placing an absorbent pad under the client to protect the bed in case of incontinence

    C. Frequently cleaning the client's perineal area and properly caring for her catheter

    D. Properly hydrating the client and giving her a diet high in fiber to prevent constipation

Most nosocomial infections develop in the urinary tract, and regular cleaning of the perineal area along with catheter care reduces the number of micro-organisms. Assessing the client's ability to void independently is not a priority on admission for a client who is ill enough to be admitted to an acute care setting. The client has not been assessed yet for incontinence or constipation.

2. Which of the following are appropriate teaching measures related to care of the feet for a client with diabetes mellitus? (Select all that apply.)

    __X__ **Inspect feet daily.**

    __X__ **Use moisturizing lotions on feet.**

    _____ Wash with warm water and let air dry.

    _____ Use over-the-counter products to treat abrasions.

    __X__ **Check shoes for any foreign objects.**

A client with diabetes is at increased risk for infection and should inspect feet daily. The client should also use moisturizing lotions to help keep the skin smooth and supple. Feet should be washed with warm water and dried thoroughly. Over-the-counter products often contain harmful chemicals that can cause skin impairment. Shoes should be checked for foreign objects because decreased sensation may prevent the client from feeling an object that can cause an injury.

3. A client is in balanced suspension traction following a motor vehicle crash. He is unable to perform his own personal hygiene and must have it performed by the nurse. Which of the following factors will have the most influence on his comfort level?

    A. The client's position

    B. The attitude of the nurse

    C. The gender of the nurse

    D. The amount of pain medicine he has received

The nurse understands that performing perineal care on a client could cause embarrassment. The best way to increase the client's comfort level is to behave in a professional manner.

4. A client experiences dyspnea and reports feeling tired after completing her morning care. Which of the following should the nurse include in the client's plan of care for the next day?

    A. Plan for several rest periods during morning care.

    B. Do not offer any morning care.

    C. Perform all of the client's care as quickly as possible.

    D. Ask a family member to come in and give the client a bath.

Planning for several rest periods during morning care will help prevent fatigue and continue to foster independence. Fatigue and dyspnea are not reasons to eliminate morning care. Performing all of the client's care or having a family member do it will prevent the client from maintaining independence.

Unit 3
Section:

Basic Nursing Care
Comfort and Basic Needs

Chapter 52:   **Application of Heat and Cold**
Contributor: Wendy Buenzli MN, RN

 NCLEX® Connections:

Learning Objective: Review and apply knowledge within **"Application of Heat and Cold"** in readiness for performance of the following nursing activities as outlined by the NCLEX® test plans:

Δ   Assess/monitor the need for heat and/or cold applications.

Δ   Use heat applications in a safe manner to relieve pain.

Δ   Use cold applications in a safe manner to decrease inflammation.

Δ   Evaluate and document the effectiveness of heat and/or cold applications.

 Key Points

Δ   Therapeutic effects of heat and cold applications include:

Heat	Cold
• Increases blood flow • Increases tissue metabolism • Relaxes muscles • Is helpful in easing joint stiffness and pain	• Decreases inflammation • Prevents swelling • Reduces bleeding • Reduces fever • Diminishes muscle spasms • Decreases pain by decreasing the velocity of nerve conduction

Key Procedural Points

Δ   **Clients at Risk for Injury from Heat/Cold Applications**

• Use extreme caution with the very young, fair-skinned, and older adults, as they have fragile skin.

• Clients who are immobile may not be able to move away from the application if it becomes uncomfortable, and they are at risk for skin injuries.

• Clients who have impaired sensory perceptions may not feel pain or burning.

- Avoid extremely long applications of either heat or cold, as they will result in an opposite reaction from the desired response.

- Heat

  ◊ Boney prominences are more sensitive to heat applications and need to be monitored carefully.

  ◊ Avoid the use of heat applications over metal devices (e.g., pacemakers and artificial joints) to prevent deep tissue burns.

  ◊ Do not apply heat to the abdomen of a pregnant woman to prevent harm to the fetus.

  ◊ Placing a heat application under an immobile client may increase the risk of burns.

  ◊ Cold application is inappropriate for clients with cold intolerance, vascular insufficiency, and conditions aggravated by cold, such as Raynaud's phenomenon.

Δ Make sure the primary care provider has written a specific order for the application, which includes:

- Location.

- Duration and frequency.

- Specific type (e.g., moist or dry).

- Temperature to use.

NANDA Nursing Diagnosis

Δ Acute/chronic pain

Δ Risk for injury

Δ Risk for impaired skin integrity

Nursing Interventions

Δ Equipment

- Heat application supplies may include:

  ◊ Moist

    ° Hot compresses – towel, bath thermometer, hot water, plastic covering, hot pack, or aquathermia pad (with distilled water), and tape.

    ° Hot soaks – water, bath thermometer, basin, and waterproof pads.

    ° Sitz baths – sitz bath (disposable or built-in), bath thermometer, bath blanket, and towels.

◊ Dry

  ° Hot pack (disposable or reusable) or an aquathermia pad with distilled water, and a pillowcase.

  ° Warming blanket.

- Cold application supplies may include:

  ◊ Moist

    ° Large basin of ice.

    ° Cold water.

    ° Cold pack to be used in place of ice.

  ◊ Dry

    ° Ice bag, ice collar, ice glove, or a cold pack.

    ° Cooling blanket.

Δ Apply the application to the area correctly.

Δ Make sure the client's call light is in reach, and instruct the client to report any discomfort.

Δ Assess the site every 5 to 10 min to check for:

- Redness or pallor.

- Pain or burning.

- Numbness.

- Shivering (with cold applications only).

- Blisters.

- Decreased sensation.

- Cyanosis (with cold applications only).

Δ Discontinue the application if any of the above occur, or remove the application at the set time (usually 15 to 20 min).

Δ Document:

- Location, type, and length of the application.

- Condition of the skin prior to and after the application.

- The client's ability to tolerate the application.

Primary Reference:

Potter, P. A., & Perry, A. G. (2005). *Fundamentals of nursing* (6th ed.). St. Louis, MO: Mosby.

Additional Resources:

DeLaune, S, & Ladner, P. (2006). *Fundamentals of nursing* (3rd ed.). Clifton Park: Thomson Delmar.

NANDA International (2004). *NANDA nursing diagnoses: Definitions and classification 2005-2006*. Philadelphia: NANDA.

Chapter 52: Application of Heat and Cold

Application Exercises

1. Which of the following clients would benefit from the application of cold? (Select all that apply.)

   _____ A 45-year-old client with a sprained ankle
   _____ A 27-year-old client with Raynaud's phenomenon
   _____ A 62-year-old client who just had knee-replacement surgery
   _____ A 35-year-old client with a toothache
   _____ A 10-year-old client with a nosebleed

2. A nurse is conducting morning rounds and notices an immobile client lying on an aquathermia pad. Which of the following nursing interventions is the most important for the nurse to include in the morning assessment?

   A. Pain assessment to determine the client's level of pain
   B. Evaluation of the heating pad to check for a malfunction
   C. A thorough skin assessment to check for skin damage
   D. The client's ability to express if treatment is eliminating pain

3. True or False: Moist cold compresses are left in place for at least 45 min.

4. True or False: Cyanosis is a complication of cold applications.

5. True or False: Heat applications increase muscle tension.

Chapter 52: Application of Heat and Cold

Application Exercises Answer Key

1. Which of the following clients would benefit from the application of cold? (Select all that apply.)

   X   A 45-year-old client with a sprained ankle

   _____   A 27-year-old client with Raynaud's phenomenon

   X   A 62-year-old client who just had knee-replacement surgery

   X   A 35-year-old client with a toothache

   X   A 10-year-old client with a nosebleed

A client with a sprained ankle, a client who just had knee-replacement surgery, and a client with a toothache may benefit from the application of cold to reduce pain and decrease inflammation. A client with a nosebleed may benefit from cold application to reduce/stop bleeding. Cold could trigger Raynaud's phenomenon.

2. A nurse is conducting morning rounds and notices an immobile client lying on an aquathermia pad. Which of the following nursing interventions is the most important for the nurse to include in the morning assessment?

   A. Pain assessment to determine the client's level of pain

   B. Evaluation of the heating pad to check for a malfunction

   C. A thorough skin assessment to check for skin damage

   D. The client's ability to express if treatment is eliminating pain

An immobile client cannot get away from the heat under her and may suffer damage to the skin. Options A, B, and D are valid assessments, but the safety of the client and prevention of injury takes priority.

3. True or False: Moist cold compresses are left in place for at least 45 min.

False: Heat and cold applications are kept in place for 15 to 20 min.

4. True or False: Cyanosis is a complication of cold applications.

True: Cold applications cause vasoconstriction, and cyanosis can occur if circulation is not adequate.

5. True or False: Heat applications increase muscle tension.

False: Heat applications cause muscle relaxation.

Unit 3
Section:

Basic Nursing Care
Comfort and Basic Needs

Chapter 53:   Mobility and Immobility
Contributor: Catherine B. Talley, MSN, RN, PAHM

 NCLEX® Connections:

Learning Objective: Review and apply knowledge within **"Mobility and Immobility"** in readiness for performance of the following nursing activities as outlined by the NCLEX® test plans:

Δ   Assess/monitor the client's strength, gait, and overall mobility with or without assistive devices.

Δ   Assess/monitor the client's physiologic responses to prolonged immobility (e.g., atelectasis, thrombus formation).

Δ   Use and discontinue immobilizers correctly.

Δ   Plan/provide interventions to decrease the risk of complications caused by immobility.

Δ   Plan/provide interventions to maintain or increase the client's strength and mobility.

Δ   Evaluate the effectiveness of interventions to decrease immobility risks and increase mobility.

 Key Points

Δ   Mobility is the ability to be free and independent in purposeful movement. Mobility refers to adapting and having self-awareness of the environment. The musculoskeletal and nervous systems are essential to mobility.

Δ   Immobility is not being able to move on one's own volition. There is an increased risk of complications the greater the amount of immobility and the longer the immobilization.

Δ   Immobility may be:

• Temporary, such as following surgery for a total knee replacement.

• Permanent, such as paraplegia.

- Sudden onset, such as a fractured arm and leg following a motor vehicle crash.

- Slow onset, such as multiple sclerosis.

Δ The principles of body mechanics are based on alignment, balance, gravity, and friction.

Δ Movement is dependent on an intact skeletal system, skeletal muscles, and nervous system.

Δ Assessment of the client focuses on mobility, range of motion, gait, exercise status, activity tolerance, and body alignment in respect to standing, sitting, and lying.

Δ Nursing interventions are designed to maintain mobility and prevent or minimize the complications of immobility.

Key Procedural Points

Δ Factors affecting mobility include:

- Alteration in muscles.

- Injury to the musculoskeletal system.

- Abnormal posture.

- Impaired central nervous system.

- Client's health status and age.

Δ Changes that occur in body systems include:

Body System	Changes
Integumentary	• **Increased pressure** on skin, which is aggravated by metabolic changes • **Decreased circulation** to tissue causing ischemia, which can lead to pressure ulcers
Respiratory	• **Decreased respiratory** movement resulting in decreased oxygenation and carbon dioxide exchange • **Stasis of secretions** and decreased and weakened respiratory muscles resulting in atelectasis and hypostatic pneumonia • Decreased cough response
Cardiovascular	• **Orthostatic hypotension** • Less fluid volume in the circulatory system • Stasis of blood in the legs • Less autonomic response • **Decreased cardiac output** leading to poor cardiac effectiveness, which results in increased workload on the heart • Increased oxygenation requirement • **Increased risk of thrombus** development

Body System	Changes
Metabolic	<ul><li>Altered endocrine system</li><li>**Decreased basal metabolic rate**</li><li>Change in protein, carbohydrate, and fat metabolism</li><li>Decreased appetite with altered nutritional intake</li><li>Negative nitrogen balance</li><li>**Decreased protein** resulting in loss of muscle</li><li>Loss of weight</li><li>Alteration of calcium, fluid, and electrolytes</li><li>**Resorption of calcium** from bones</li><li>Decreased urinary elimination of calcium resulting in **hypercalcemia**</li></ul>
Elimination	<ul><li>Genitourinary<ul><li>◊ Change in calcium metabolism with hypercalcemia resulting in renal calculi</li><li>◊ Decreased fluid intake, poor perineal care, and indwelling Foley catheters resulting in urinary tract infections</li></ul></li><li>Gastrointestinal<ul><li>◊ Decreased peristalsis</li></ul></li><li>Decreased fluid intake</li><li>Constipation, then fecal impaction, then diarrhea</li></ul>
Musculoskeletal	<ul><li>Decreased muscle endurance, muscle strength, and muscle mass</li><li>Decreased balance</li><li>Atrophy of muscles</li><li>Decreased stability</li><li>Altered calcium metabolism</li><li>Osteoporosis</li><li>Contractures</li><li>Foot drop</li><li>Altered joint mobility</li></ul>
Psychosocial	<ul><li>Changes in emotional status – depression, alteration in self-concept, and anxiety</li><li>Behavioral changes – withdrawal, altered sleep/wake pattern, hostility, inappropriate laughter, and passivity</li><li>Altered sensory perception</li><li>Ineffective coping</li></ul>

Body System	Changes
Developmental	• Infants, toddlers, and preschoolers ◊ **Slower progression** in gross motor skill, intellectual, and musculoskeletal development ◊ Body aligned with line of gravity, resulting in unbalanced posture • Adolescents ◊ Growth spurt that is imbalanced and possibly altered with immobility ◊ **Delayed development of independence** ◊ Social isolation • Adults ◊ Alterations in every **physical system** ◊ Alterations in family and social systems ◊ Alterations in job identity • Older adults ◊ **Alteration in balance** resulting in a major risk for falls and injuries ◊ Steady loss of bone mass resulting in weakened bones ◊ Decreased coordination ◊ Walking more slowly ◊ Taking tiny steps ◊ **Alteration in functional status** ◊ Increased dependence on staff, family, and significant others

NANDA Nursing Diagnoses

Δ   Activity intolerance

Δ   Risk for constipation

Δ   Ineffective airway clearance

Δ   Risk for disuse syndrome

Δ   Bathing/hygiene self-care deficit

Δ   Disturbed sleep pattern

Δ   Social isolation

Δ   Impaired tissue integrity

Assessment and Nursing Interventions

Assessment	Nursing interventions
Integumentary – Maintain intact skin.	
• Observe skin for breakdown, warmth, and change in color. Look for pallor or redness in fair-skinned clients and purple or blue in dark-skinned clients. • Observe bony prominences. • Check skin turgor. • Use a pressure ulcer scale such as Norton or Braden. • Assess at least every 2 hr. • Observe for urinary or bowel incontinence.	• Identify clients at risk for pressure ulcer development. • Position the client using correct devices such as pillows, foot boots, trochanter rolls, and wedge pillows. • **Turn the client every 1 to 2 hr,** and use devices for support or per protocol. • Teach the client who can move independently to turn at least every 15 min. • Provide the client sitting in a chair with a device to decrease pressure. • Limit sitting in a chair to less than 2 hr. Instruct client to shift weight every 15 min. • Use therapeutic beds or mattresses if the client is in a bed for an extended time. • Monitor nutritional intake. • Provide skin and perineal care.
Respiratory – Maintain patent airway, achieve optimal lung expansion and gas exchange, and mobilize airway secretions.	

• Complete the following every 2 hr:
  ◊ Observe the client's chest wall movement for symmetry.
  ◊ Auscultate breath sounds.
  ◊ Observe for productive cough, and note the color, amount, and consistency of secretions.
	• Reposition the client every 1 to 2 hr.
	• **Teach the client to turn, cough, and deep breathe (TCDB) every 1 to 2 hr while awake.**
	• Teach the client to yawn every hour while awake.
	• Teach the client to use an incentive spirometer while awake.
	• Remove abdominal binders every 2 hr, and ensure correct placement on the client.
	• Use chest physiotherapy (CPT).
	• Auscultate lungs for effectiveness of chest physiotherapy or respiratory therapy.
	• Teach the client to consume a minimum of 2,000 mL of fluid, unless the client is on restricted intake.
	• Monitor the client's ability to expectorate secretions.
	• Monitor secretions for color, amount, and consistency.
	• Use suction if the client is unable to expectorate secretions.

Assessment	Nursing interventions
Cardiovascular – Maintain cardiovascular function, increase activity tolerance, and prevent thrombus formation.	
• Take orthostatic blood pressure and pulse (lying to sitting to standing), and assess for vertigo. • Palpate the apical and peripheral pulses. • Auscultate the heart at apex for S_3 (an early symptom of heart failure). The older adult client may not adapt well to immobility. • Palpate for edema in sacrum, legs, and feet. • Palpate skin for warmth in peripheral areas to include nose, ear lobes, hands, and feet. • Assess for deep vein thrombosis (DVT) by observing calves for redness and palpating for warmth and tenderness. • Measure circumference of both calves and thighs and compare in size (calf – 10 cm below middle of patella).	• **Increase activity** as soon as possible (dangle feet on side of bed or transfer to chair). • Perform isometric exercises to increase tolerance for activity. • Change position as often as possible. • Teach the client to avoid the Valsalva maneuver. • Increase activity. • Give a stool softener to prevent straining. • Teach **range of motion (ROM)** such as ankle pumps or knee flexion. • Teach the client to avoid placing pillows under the knees or lower extremities, crossing the legs, wearing tight clothes around the waist or on the legs, sitting for long periods of time, and massaging the legs. • Use elastic stockings. • Use sequential compression devices (SCD) or intermittent pneumatic compression (IPC). • Increase fluid intake. • Give low-dose heparin (5,000 units every 8 to 12 hr). • Contact the primary care provider immediately if assessment data indicates venous thrombosis.
Metabolic – Decrease injuries to skin, and maintain metabolism within normal functioning.	
• Record anthropometric measurements of height, weight, and skin fold. • Assess I&O. • Assess food intake. • Review urinary and bowel elimination status. • Auscultate bowel sounds. • Check skin turgor. • Review laboratory values for electrolytes, serum, total protein, and BUN levels.	• Provide a high-calorie and high-protein diet with additional vitamins B and C. • Monitor and evaluate oral intake. If the client is unable to take oral intake, enteral or parenteral nutritional therapy may be indicated.

Assessment	Nursing interventions
Elimination – Maintain or achieve normal urinary and bowel elimination patterns.	
• Observe every shift. • Assess I&O. • Assess bladder distention. • Observe urine for color, amount, clarity, and frequency. • Auscultate bowel sounds. • Observe feces for color, amount, frequency, and consistency.	• Maintain hydration (at least 2,000 mL unless on fluid restriction.) • Teach the client to consume a diet that includes fruits, vegetables, and high fiber. • Give a stool softener. Use laxatives (e.g., cathartics, enemas) as a last resort. • Provide perineal care. • Teach bladder and bowel training if needed. • Insert straight or Foley catheter if the bladder is distended. • Promote urination by pouring warm water over the perineal area if the client has difficulty urinating.
Musculoskeletal – Maintain or regain body alignment and stability, decrease skin and musculoskeletal system changes, achieve full or optimal ROM, and prevent contractures.	
• Range of motion capability • Muscle tone and mass • Contractures • Gait • Nutritional intake for calcium • Use of assistive devices to assist in ADLs	• Assist/instruct the client to change position in bed every 2 hr (minimum) and perform weight shifts in his wheelchair every 15 min. • Provide active and/or passive range of motion (ROM) two or three times a day. • Teach the client to perform ROM while bathing, eating, grooming, and dressing. • Monitor nutritional intake of calcium. • Develop an individualized program for each client. The older adult client may require a program specific to the aging process. • Request the primary care provider to order physical therapy for the client with decreased mobility. • Advise the client to follow program developed by Physical Therapy. • Use a continuous passive motion (CPM) device. **Cane instructions** • Maintain two points of support on the ground at all times. • Keep the cane on the stronger side of the body. • Support body weight on both legs, move cane forward 6 to 10 inches, then move the weaker leg forward toward the cane. • Next, advance the stronger leg. **Crutch instructions** • Do not alter crutches after proper fit has been determined. • Follow crutch gait prescribed by physical therapy. • Support body weight at hand grips with elbows flexed at 30°. • Position crutches on unaffected side when sitting or rising from a chair.

Assessment	Nursing interventions
Psychosocial – Maintain normal sleep/wake pattern, achieve socialization, and achieve independent completion of self-care.	
• Emotional status • Mental status • Behavior and decision-making skills • Mobility status • Unusual alteration in sleep/wake pattern • Coping skills especially to loss • Activities of daily living (ADLs) • Family support and relationships • Social activities	• Assist in using normal coping skills or in developing new coping skills. • Maintain orientation to time (e.g., clock and calendar with date), person (e.g., call by name and introduce self) and place (e.g., talk about treatments and therapy and length of stay). • Develop a schedule of therapies and place on calendar in room. • Arrange for the client to be in a semiprivate room with an alert roommate. • Involve the client in daily care. • Provide daily stimuli such as books, television, newspapers, and radio. • Maintain body image by having the client perform or have assistance with hygiene and grooming to include either shaving or wearing makeup. • Have nurses and other staff interact on an informal social basis. • Recommend to the primary care provider a referral for consultation (psychological, spiritual, or social worker), if the client is not coping well.

Assessment	Nursing interventions
Developmental – Continue normal development and achieve physical and mental stimulation.	
• Infancy through school age ◊ Gross motor skill, intellectual, and musculoskeletal development ◊ Body alignment and posture ◊ Developmental tasks specific to age • Adolescents ◊ Growth development specific to age ◊ Level of independence ◊ Social activities • Adults ◊ All physical systems ◊ Family relationships ◊ Social status ◊ Meaning of career/job • Older adults ◊ Balance ◊ Coordination ◊ Gait ◊ Functional status ◊ Level of independence ◊ Social isolation	• Infancy through school age ◊ Initiate events that stimulate the physical and psychosocial systems. Increase mobility, and involve play therapist in age-appropriate activities. ◊ Use measures to prevent falls. ◊ Develop strategies for maintaining or enhancing the developmental process. ◊ Teach the family that their perception of immobility can affect the child's progress and ability to cope. ◊ Encourage the parents to stay with the child. ◊ Incorporate the involvement of the child, if it is age appropriate, in his treatments. ◊ Place the child in a room with others that are age appropriate. • Adolescents ◊ Initiate care that facilitates independence. ◊ Involve adolescents in decision making of ADLs. ◊ Provide stimulus to promote socialization (e.g., involve interaction with peers and use of adolescent activity room). • Adults ◊ Provide care that promotes activity in all physical systems. ◊ Discuss with the family the importance of interaction with the client. ◊ Discuss the client's social involvement. ◊ Discuss the meaning of the client's career/job. • Older adults ◊ Plan care with the client and family to increase independence with activities of daily living and decision-making skills. ◊ Teach the staff to facilitate the client's independence in all activities. ◊ Maintain stimuli such as a clock, newspaper, calendar, and/or weather status. ◊ Encourage the family to visit to maintain socialization. ◊ Plan for staff to spend some time talking and listening to the client.

Primary Reference:

Potter, P. A., & Perry, A. G. (2005). *Fundamentals of nursing* (6th ed.). St. Louis, MO: Mosby.

Additional Resources:

Rush, K. L., & Ouellet, L. L. (1993). Mobility: A concept analysis. *Journal of Advanced Nursing, 18*, 486-492.

NANDA International (2004). *NANDA nursing diagnoses: Definitions and classification 2005-2006*. Philadelphia: NANDA.

Chapter 53: Mobility and Immobility

Application Exercises

1. A client has been sitting in a chair for 2 hr. What is the client most at risk for developing?

    A. Stasis of secretions

    B. Muscle atrophy

    C. Pressure ulcer

    D. Fecal impaction

2. Which of the following nursing interventions should be implemented to maintain a patent airway in a client on bedrest?

    A. Perform isometric exercises.

    B. Suction every 8 hr.

    C. Give low-dose heparin.

    D. Teach to use an incentive spirometer while awake.

3. Which of the following findings should be reported to the primary care provider for a client on bedrest?

    A. Palpable pedal pulses

    B. Weight gain of .45 kg (1 lb) since admission 7 days ago

    C. Orthostatic hypotension

    D. Crackles heard in bases of lungs bilaterally that clear with coughing

4. Which of the following nursing interventions will reduce the risk of thrombus development? (Select all that apply.)

    _____ Teach the client not to use the Valsalva maneuver.

    _____ Apply elastic stockings.

    _____ Review laboratory values for total protein level.

    _____ Place pillows under the client's knees and lower extremities.

    _____ Assist the client to change position often.

Chapter 53: Mobility and Immobility

Application Exercises Answer Key

1. A client has been sitting in a chair for 2 hr. What is the client most at risk for developing?

    A. Stasis of secretions

    B. Muscle atrophy

    C. Pressure ulcer

    D. Fecal impaction

Unrelieved pressure over a bony prominence for too long increases the risk for skin breakdown. Sitting up in a chair will help prevent stasis of secretions. Muscle atrophy and fecal impaction would be complications for a client on prolonged bed rest.

2. Which of the following nursing interventions should be implemented to maintain a patent airway in a client on bedrest?

    A. Perform isometric exercises.

    B. Suction every 8 hr.

    C. Give low-dose heparin.

    D. Teach to use an incentive spirometer while awake.

Use of an incentive spirometer will assist in keeping the airways open and preventing atelectasis. Performing isometric exercises strengthens skeletal muscles. Suctioning should not be done routinely. Low-dose heparin helps prevent thrombus formation.

3. Which of the following findings should be reported to the primary care provider for a client on bedrest?

    A. Palpable pedal pulses

    B. Weight gain of .45 kg (1 lb) since admission 7 days ago

    C. Orthostatic hypotension

    D. Crackles heard in bases of lungs bilaterally that clear with coughing

Orthostatic hypotension indicates a change in cardiovascular status. This should be reported to the primary care provider. Pedal pulses should be palpable. Weight gain of .45 kg 1 lb in a week is not significant. Crackles that clear with coughing are not an abnormal finding.

4. Which of the following nursing interventions will reduce the risk of thrombus development? (Select all that apply.)

_____ Teach the client not to use the Valsalva maneuver.

__X__ Apply elastic stockings.

_____ Review laboratory values for total protein level.

_____ Place pillows under the client's knees and lower extremities.

__X__ Assist the client to change position often.

Elastic stockings promote venous return and prevent thrombus formation. Frequent position changes will prevent venous stasis. Performance of the Valsalva maneuver increases the workload of the heart, but it does not impact peripheral circulation. Review of total protein level would be important to monitor to assess the client's ability to heal and prevent skin breakdown. Placing pillows under the knees and lower extremities further impairs circulation of the lower extremities and should be avoided.

Unit 3   **Basic Nursing Care**
Section: Comfort and Basic Needs

Chapter 54:   **Rest and Sleep**

            Contributor: Wendy Buenzli MN, RN

 NCLEX® Connections

> **Learning Objective**: Review and apply knowledge within **"Rest and Sleep"** in readiness for performance of the following nursing activities as outlined by the NCLEX® test plans:
>
> Δ   Assess/monitor behaviors and treatments that put the client at risk for sleep disturbances (e.g., diet, exercise, illness, medications, substances).
>
> Δ   Compare the client's quality and quantity of sleep to expected developmental requirements.
>
> Δ   Instruct the client on stress management techniques that promote rest and sleep.
>
> Δ   Communicate to the primary care provider any signs and symptoms of sleep disorders.

 Key Points

Δ   **Sleep Cycle**

• The sleep cycle consists of nonrapid eye movement (NREM) sleep and rapid eye movement (REM) sleep. Typically, after a person experiences Stage 1 of NREM sleep, he cycles 4 to 6 times through the other stages of sleep during the course of a night.

Stage	Characteristics
Stage 1 NREM	• Very light sleep • Only a few minutes long • Vitals signs and metabolism beginning to diminish • Can be awakened easily • Feels relaxed and drowsy

Stage	Characteristics
Stage 2 NREM	• Deeper sleep • 10 to 20 min in length • Vitals signs and metabolism continuing to diminish • Can still be awakened easily • Increased relaxation
Stage 3 NREM	• Deep sleep • 15 to 30 min in length • Vital signs continuing to decrease • Difficult to awaken • Relaxation such that the person seldom moves
Stage 4 NREM	• Deepest sleep • 15 to 30 min in length • Vital signs very low as compared to when awake • Very difficult to awaken • Stage at which the body achieves physical rest and restoration • Stage at which enuresis and talking and walking in one's sleep occur
REM	• Occurrence of dreams • 20 min long and starts about 50 to 90 min after falling asleep • Varying vital signs • Very difficult to awaken • Stage at which mental rest and restoration occur

Key Procedural Points

Δ   Normal Developmental Sleep Patterns

Age	Sleep Averages
Birth to 3 months	16 hr a day
Infants (3 months to 1 year)	8 to 10 hr at night with two to three naps during the day
Toddlers	12 hr a day with some of the sleep coming during a daytime nap
Preschoolers	12 hr a night with less napping during the day
School-age	11 to 12 hr a night for younger children with 9 to 10 hr a night for older ones
Adolescents	7.5 hr a night
Young Adults	6 to 8.5 hr a night
Middle Adults	6 to 8.5 hr a night
Older Adults	6 to 8.5 hr per day with daytime naps possibly accounting for some of the hours

Δ   **Common Sleep Disorders**

- **Insomnia** is difficulty falling asleep or the inability to receive restorative sleep. It is more common in women than men. Causes of insomnia include stress, illness, and work-related issues.

- **Sleep apnea** is a disorder caused by the lack of airflow to the nose and mouth for > 10 sec or longer during sleep. Sleep apnea is caused by a single disorder or a mixture of the following:

  ◊   Central – central nervous system dysfunction that fails to trigger breathing during sleep.

  ◊   Obstructive – occurs when the upper airway becomes occluded by relaxed structures in the mouth and throat.

- **Narcolepsy** – a disorder of the sleep and wake mechanism. The person may lose the ability to stay awake. It often happens at inappropriate times and can put the person at risk for injury.

Assessment

Δ   Ask the client about sleep patterns, history, and if any changes have occurred.

Δ   Ask the client about sleep problems, which include:

- Type of problem.

- Symptoms.

- Timing.

- Seriousness.

- Related factors.

- How the lack of sleep has impacted the client.

Δ   Use a linear scale or visual with "best night sleep" on one end and "worst night sleep" on the opposite end. Also, the nurse could ask the client to rate sleep on a 0 to 10 scale.

Δ   Assess for common factors that interfere with sleep, which include:

- Illness – may require more sleep or disrupt sleep, such as nocturia.

- Current life events (e.g., traveling more, change in work hours).

- Emotional stress or mental illness (e.g., anxiety, fear).

- Diet (e.g., caffeine consumption, heavy meals before bed).

- Exercise – promotes sleep if done at least 2 hr before bedtime; otherwise, it can disrupt sleep.

- Sleep environment that is too light, the wrong temperature, or too noisy (e.g., children, pets, loud noise, snoring partner).

- Medications – may induce sleep but interfere with the restorative sleep cycles.

NANDA Nursing Diagnoses

Δ Sleep deprivation

Δ Fatigue

Δ Disturbed sleep pattern

Nursing Interventions

Δ Assist the client in establishing and following a bedtime routine.

Δ Attempt to minimize the number of times the client is awakened during the night while hospitalized.

Δ Offer to assist the client with personal hygiene needs and/or a back rub prior to sleep to increase comfort.

Δ Instruct the client to:

- Exercise regularly at least 2 hr before bedtime.

- Arrange the sleep environment to what is comfortable.

- Limit alcohol, caffeine, and nicotine in the late afternoon and evening.

- Limit fluids 2 to 4 hr before bedtime.

- Engage in muscle relaxation if anxious or stressed.

Δ Instruct the client with narcolepsy to:

- Participate in regular exercise.

- Eat small meals that are high in protein.

- Avoid activities that increase sleepiness (e.g., sitting too long, warm environments, alcohol).

- Avoid activities that would cause injury should the client fall asleep (e.g., driving, heights).

- Take naps when narcoleptic events are likely to occur.

- Take stimulants as prescribed by a primary care provider.

Δ Apply continuous positive airway pressure (CPAP) devices as ordered by a primary care provider for clients with sleep apnea.

Δ As a last resort, provide a pharmacological agent as prescribed.

Δ Evaluate the effectiveness of interventions.

Primary Reference:

Potter, P. A., & Perry, A. G. (2005). *Fundamentals of nursing* (6th ed.). St. Louis, MO: Mosby.

Additional Resources:

NANDA International (2004). *NANDA nursing diagnoses: Definitions and classification 2005-2006*. Philadelphia: NANDA.

Chapter 54: Rest and Sleep

Application Exercises

1. A client presents to the clinic reporting fatigue and an inability to sleep at night. Which of the following assessment findings supports the client's statement?

      A. The client is attentive with good posture.

      B. The client's eyes are puffy and red, and he is irritable.

      C. The client is patient, understanding, and has a quiet demeanor.

      D. The client's speech is coordinated and clear.

2. Which of the following recommendations should be given to a client to promote sleep and rest? (Select all that apply.)

      _____ Avoid all caffeinated beverages.

      _____ Participate in regular exercise each morning.

      _____ Take an afternoon nap.

      _____ Practice relaxation exercises before bedtime.

      _____ Limit fluid intake after dinner.

3. A client is diagnosed with obstructive sleep apnea. Which of the following nursing diagnoses should be the highest priority?

      A. Ineffective breathing pattern

      B. Altered tissue perfusion

      C. Disturbed sleep pattern

      D. Fatigue

4. Since admission to the hospital, a client has bathed in the morning following facility/agency routine; however, at home, she always takes a warm bath just before bed. Now she is having difficulty sleeping. Which of the following interventions is most beneficial to the client at this time?

      A. Rub her back for 15 min before bed.

      B. Offer her warm milk and crackers at 2100.

      C. Allow her to take a bath in the evening.

      D. Ask her primary care provider for a sleeping medication.

Chapter 54: Rest and Sleep

Application Exercises Answer Key

1. A client presents to the clinic reporting fatigue and an inability to sleep at night. Which of the following assessment findings supports the client's statement?

      A. The client is attentive with good posture.

      B. The client's eyes are puffy and red, and he is irritable.

      C. The client is patient, understanding, and has a quiet demeanor.

      D. The client's speech is coordinated and clear.

Puffy, red eyes and irritability are indications of lack of sleep. Attentiveness with good posture; a patient, understanding, and quiet demeanor; and coordinated, clear speech are all normal findings.

2. Which of the following recommendations should be given to a client to promote sleep and rest? (Select all that apply.)

      _____ Avoid all caffeinated beverages.

      __X__ **Participate in regular exercise each morning**.

      _____ Take an afternoon nap.

      __X__ **Practice relaxation exercises before bedtime.**

      __X__ **Limit fluid intake after dinner**.

Establishing a regular exercise routine helps promote sleep and should be completed at least 2 hr prior to sleep. Relaxation exercises can decrease stress and tension and thereby promote rest. Limiting fluid intake after dinner will help prevent nocturia. It is not necessary to avoid all caffeinated beverages but to limit consumption of these after dinner. An afternoon nap disrupts nighttime sleep. Fluid should be limited 2 to 4 hr before bedtime to prevent nocturia.

3. A client is diagnosed with obstructive sleep apnea. Which of the following nursing diagnoses should be the highest priority?

    A. Ineffective breathing pattern

    B. Altered tissue perfusion

    C. Disturbed sleep pattern

    D. Fatigue

Ineffective breathing pattern is the highest priority. Ineffective breathing pattern can lead to altered tissue perfusion, disturbed sleep pattern, and fatigue.

4. Since admission to the hospital, a client has bathed in the morning following facility/agency routine; however, at home, she always takes a warm bath just before bed. Now she is having difficulty sleeping. Which of the following interventions is most beneficial to the client at this time?

    A. Rub her back for 15 min before bed.

    B. Offer her warm milk and crackers at 2100.

    C. Allow her to take a bath in the evening.

    D. Ask her primary care provider for a sleeping medication.

Allowing a client to follow her normal bedtime routine is helpful in promoting sleep. Rubbing her back and offering warm milk and crackers are not a stated part of this client's routine. It would be most beneficial to allow her to follow her stated routine. Requesting a sleeping medication may be the next step to offer if the nonpharmacologic intervention is not working.

Unit 3   Basic Nursing Care
Section: Comfort and Basic Needs

Chapter 55:   Pain Management
                 Contributors: Sally Swenson, MA, RN
                               Lora McGuire RN, MS

 NCLEX® Connections:

Learning Objective: Review and apply knowledge within **"Pain Management"** in readiness for performance of the following nursing activities as outlined by the NCLEX® test plans:

Δ   Discuss pain transmission, perception, and interpretation.

Δ   Assess/monitor the client for symptoms of impaired comfort using standardized pain rating scales.

Δ   Assess/monitor the client for physiologic and behavioral responses to impaired comfort.

Δ   Provide effective pain relief, and serve as client advocate through the use of pharmacologic and nonpharmacologic interventions.

Δ   Assess/monitor and document effectiveness of pain treatment.

Δ   Evaluate/monitor the client's reaction to pain relief measures, and modify the plan of care as needed.

Δ   Provide/reinforce client teaching regarding management of the client's health problem – acute/chronic pain.

Δ   Recognize how culture influences the client's perception of and reaction to pain.

 Key Points

Δ   Clients have a right to adequate assessment and management of pain. Nurses are accountable for the assessment of pain. The nurse's role is that of an advocate and educator for proper pain management.

Δ   Undertreatment of pain is a serious healthcare problem in the United States. Consequences of undertreatment of pain include physiological and psychological components.

•   Acute/chronic pain can cause anxiety/fear and depression.

- Poorly managed acute pain may lead to chronic pain syndrome.

Δ Assessment challenges may occur with clients who are cognitively impaired and ventilator dependent.

Δ Proper pain management includes the use of pharmacological and nonpharmacological pain management therapies. Invasive therapies such as nerve ablation may be appropriate for intractable cancer-related pain.

Δ Physiology of pain

- **Transduction** is the conversion of painful stimuli to an electrical impulse.

- **Transmission** occurs as the electrical impulse travels along the nerve fibers and is regulated by neurotransmitters.

↑ pain transmission	↓ pain transmission
• Substance P • Prostaglandins • Bradykinin • Histamine	• Serotonin • Endorphins

- **Perception** or awareness of pain occurs in the brain and is influenced by thought and emotional processes.

- **Modulation** occurs in the spinal cord, causing muscles to reflexively contract, moving the body away from painful stimuli.

Δ **Pain Categories**

Acute Pain	Chronic Pain
• Acute pain is protective, temporary, usually self-limiting, and resolves with tissue healing. • Physiological responses (SNS) are fight-or-flight responses (e.g., tachycardia, hypertension, anxiety, diaphoresis, muscle tension). • Behavioral responses may be seen as grimacing, moaning, flinching, and guarding. • Interventions include treatment of the underlying problem.	• Chronic pain is not protective; it is ongoing or reoccurs frequently, lasting > 6 months and persisting beyond tissue healing. • Physiological responses – there is usually no alteration in vital signs, but the client may experience depression, fatigue, and decreased level of functioning. • Psychosocial implications may lead to disability. • Chronic pain may not have a known cause, and it may not respond to interventions. • Management is aimed at symptomatic relief. • Pain rating is not useful. • Chronic pain can be malignant or nonmalignant.

Nociceptive Pain	Neuropathic Pain

• Nociceptive pain is typical processing of stimuli that has damaged normal tissues. It arises from injured body tissues.
• It is usually throbbing, aching, and localized.
• This pain typically responds to opioids and nonopioid medications.
• Types of nociceptive pain include:
  ◊ **Somatic** – coming from bone, muscle, skin, or connective tissues.
  ◊ **Visceral** – coming from internal organs such as the stomach or intestines. It is usually poorly localized. It can cause referred pain in other body locations not associated with the stimulus.
  ◊ **Cutaneous** – originates in the skin or subcutaneous tissue.
	• This pain is atypical processing of stimuli by the peripheral or central nervous system.
	• It is associated with damaged nerve fibers and includes phantom limb pain, pain below the level of a spinal cord injury, and diabetic neuropathy.
	• Neuropathic pain is usually intense, shooting, burning, or described as "pins and needles."
	• This pain typically responds to adjuvant medications (e.g., antidepressants, antispasmodic agents, skeletal muscle relaxants).

Key Procedural Points

Δ **Risk factors** for undertreatment of pain include:

• Cultural and societal attitudes.

• Lack of knowledge.

• Fear of addiction.

• Exaggerated fear of respiratory depression.

Δ **Populations at risk** for undertreatment of pain include:

• Infants.

• Children.

• Older adults.

• Clients with substance abuse problems.

Δ **Causes of acute and chronic pain** include:

• Trauma.

• Surgery.

• Cancer (e.g., tumor invasion, nerve compression, bone metastases).

• Arthritis.

• Fibromyalgia.

• Neuropathy.

• Treatment procedure (e.g., injection, intubation, radiation).

Δ   The pain experience can be impacted by:

- **Age.**
    - ◊   Infants cannot verbalize or understand their pain.
    - ◊   The older adult client may have multiple pathologies that cause pain and limit function.
- **Fatigue**, which can increase sensitivity to pain.
- **Genetic sensitivity**, which can increase or decrease the amount of pain tolerated.
- **Cognitive function.**
    - ◊   Clients who are cognitively impaired may not be able to report pain or report pain accurately.
- **Prior experiences**, which can increase or decrease sensitivity depending on whether or not adequate relief was obtained.
- **Anxiety and fear**, which can increase sensitivity to pain.
- **Support systems** that are present and can decrease sensitivity to pain.
- **Culture**, which may influence how a client expresses pain or the meaning given to pain.

Assessment

Δ   Pain is whatever the person experiencing it says it is, and existing whenever the person says it does. The **client's report of pain** is the most reliable diagnostic measure of pain. **Self-report** using standardized pain scales are useful in clients over the age of 7.

Δ   Pain assessment should be done and recorded frequently, and may be considered the fifth vital sign.

Δ   **Subjective data** can be obtained using a symptom analysis.

Location is described using anatomical terminology and landmarks.	Ask "Where is your pain?", "Does it radiate anywhere else?" Ask the client to point to the location.
Quality refers to how the pain feels. Feelings of pain include: sharp, dull, aching, burning, stabbing, pounding, throbbing, shooting, gnawing, tender, heavy, tight, tiring, exhausting, sickening, terrifying, torturing, nagging, annoying, intense, and unbearable.	Ask "What does the pain feel like?" Give more than two choices (e.g., "Is the pain throbbing, burning, or stabbing?").

Intensity, strength, and severity are "measures" of the pain. **Visual analog scales** (e.g., description scale, number rating scale) can be used to: • Measure pain. • Monitor pain. • Evaluate effectiveness of interventions.	Ask the following questions: • "How much pain do you have now?" • "What is the worst/best the pain has been?"
Timing – onset, duration, frequency	Ask the following questions: • "When did it start?" • "How long does it last?" • "How often does it occur?" • "Is it constant or intermittent?"
Setting	Ask the following questions: • "Where are you when the symptoms occur?" • "What are you doing when the symptoms occur?"
Associated symptoms may include fatigue, depression, nausea, and anxiety, and they should be noted.	Ask "What other symptoms do you experience when you are feeling pain?"
Aggravating/relieving factors	Ask the following questions: • "What makes the pain better?" • "What makes the pain worse?" • "Are you currently taking any prescription or over-the-counter medications?"

Δ   Objective Data

- **Behaviors** complement self-report and assist in pain assessment of nonverbal clients.

    ◊   Facial expressions (e.g., grimacing, wrinkled forehead), body movements (e.g., restlessness, pacing, guarding)

    ◊   Moaning, crying

    ◊   Decreased attention span

Δ   **Physiologic measures** of blood pressure, pulse, and respiratory rate will be temporarily increased by acute pain. Initially, increased vital signs will return to normal despite the persistence of pain. Therefore, physiologic indicators may not be an accurate measure of pain over time.

NANDA Nursing Diagnoses

Δ Acute/chronic pain

Δ Disturbed sleep pattern

Δ Fatigue

Δ Impaired physical mobility

Δ Powerlessness

Δ Self-care deficit

Nursing Interventions

Δ Nurses have a priority responsibility for the continuous assessment of the client's pain level and to provide effective interventions. The effectiveness of interventions should be assessed 30 to 60 min after the implementation.

Δ Nonpharmacological Pain Management

- Cutaneous (skin) stimulation – transcutaneous electrical nerve stimulation (TENS), heat, cold, therapeutic touch, and massage

  ◊ Interruption of pain pathways

  ◊ Cold for inflammation

  ◊ Heat to increase blood flow and to reduce stiffness

- Distraction

  ◊ May include ambulation, deep breathing, visitors, television, and music

- Imagery

  ◊ Focusing on a pleasant thought to divert focus

  ◊ Requires an ability to concentrate

- Acupuncture – vibration or electrical stimulation via tiny needles inserted into the skin and subcutaneous tissues at specific points

- Reduction of pain stimuli in the environment

- Elevation of edematous extremities to promote venous return and decrease swelling

Δ Pharmacological Interventions

- **Analgesics** are the mainstay for relieving pain. The three classes of analgesics are: **nonopioids, opioids, and adjuvants**.

- **Nonopioid** analgesics are appropriate for the treatment of **mild to moderate pain.**

◊ The nurse should be aware of the hepatotoxic effects of acetaminophen. **No more than 4 g/day should be given to a client with a healthy liver**.

◊ Monitor for salicylism (tinnitus, vertigo, and decreased hearing acuity).

◊ **Prevent gastric upset** by administering the medication with food or antacids.

◊ Monitor for bleeding with long-term NSAID use.

- **Opioid** analgesics (e.g., morphine sulfate, codeine) are appropriate for the treatment of moderate to severe pain (e.g., postoperative pain, myocardial infarction pain, cancer pain).

    ◊ Manage acute severe pain with short-term (24 to 48 hr) around-the-clock administration of opioids rather than following a PRN schedule.

    ◊ The parenteral route is preferred for immediate, short-term relief of acute pain. The oral route is the preferred route for chronic, nonfluctuating pain.

    ◊ Consistent dosing and timing of administration of opioids will provide consistent pain control.

    ◊ Monitor and intervene for **adverse effects** of opioid use.

        ° Constipation – Use a preventative approach (e.g., monitoring of bowel movements, fluids, fiber intake, exercise, stool softeners, stimulant laxatives, and enemas).

        ° Orthostatic hypotension – Advise the client to sit or lie down if symptoms of lightheadedness or dizziness occur. Instruct the client to avoid sudden changes in position by slowly moving from a lying to a sitting or standing position. Provide assistance with ambulation as needed.

        ° Urinary retention – Monitor the client's I&O, assess for distention, administer bethanechol (Urecholine), and catheterize as needed.

        ° Nausea/vomiting – Administer antiemetics, advise the client to lie still and/or move slowly, and eliminate odors.

        ° Sedation – Monitor the client's level of consciousness and take safety precautions. Sedation usually precedes respiratory depression.

        ° Respiratory depression – Monitor the client's respiratory rate prior to and following administration of opioids (especially in opioid-naïve clients). Initial treatment of respiratory depression and sedation is generally a reduction in opioid dose. If necessary, slowly administer diluted naloxone (Narcan) to reverse opioid effects.

- **Adjuvant analgesics** enhance effects of nonopioids, help alleviate other symptoms that aggravate pain (e.g., depression, seizures, inflammation), and are useful for treatment of neuropathic pain.

◊ Medications include:

- ° Anticonvulsants: carbamazepine (Tegretol).

- ° Antianxiety agents: diazepam (Valium).

- ° Tricyclic antidepressants: amitriptyline (Elavil).

- ° Antihistamine: hydroxyzine (Vistaril).

- ° Glucocorticoids: dexamethasone (Decadron).

Δ **Patient controlled analgesia (PCA)** is a medication delivery system that allows the client to self-administer safe doses of opioid narcotics.

- Constant plasma levels are maintained by small, frequent doses.

- The client experiences less lag time between identified need and delivery of medication, which increases sense of control and may decrease the amount of medication needed.

- Morphine sulfate and hydromorphone are commonly used opioids.

- Make sure the client understands that he is the only person who should push the PCA button to prevent inadvertent overdosing.

Δ Follow a clinical approach (ABCDE) to pain assessment and management.

- **A – Ask** about pain regularly, **ASSESS** pain systematically.

- **B – BELIEVE** the client and family.

- **C – CHOOSE** appropriate pain control options.

- **D – DELIVER** interventions in a timely fashion.

- **E – EMPOWER** the client and family.

Δ Other strategies for effective pain management include:

- Taking a proactive approach by giving analgesics before pain becomes too severe. Less medication is needed to prevent pain than to treat pain.

- Instructing the client to report developing or recurrent pain and not waiting until pain is severe (for PRN orders of pain medication).

- Educating the client regarding misconceptions about pain.

- Assisting the client to reduce fear and anxiety.

- Creating a treatment plan that includes both nonpharmacological and pharmacological pain relief measures.

Complications and Nursing Implications

Δ   **Undertreatment of pain** is a serious complication and may lead to increased anxiety with acute pain and depression with chronic pain. Assess/monitor the client for pain frequently, and intervene as appropriate.

Δ   **Sedation, respiratory depression, and coma** can occur as a result of overdosing. Sedation always precedes respiratory depression.

- Identify high-risk clients (e.g., the older adult client, the opioid-naïve client).

- Carefully titrate doses while closely monitoring respiratory status.

- Stop the opioid and give the antagonist naloxone (Narcan) if the client's respirations are less than 8/min, shallow, and the client is difficult to arouse.

- Identify the cause of sedation.

- Use a sedation scale in addition to a pain rating scale to assess a client's pain, especially when administering opioids.

Primary Reference:

Potter, P. A., & Perry, A. G. (2005). *Fundamentals of nursing* (6th ed.). St. Louis, MO: Mosby.

Additional Resources:

American Pain Society. (2003). *Principles of analgesic use in the treatment of acute pain and cancer pain* (5th ed.). Glenview, IL: American Pain Society.

Bickley, L. S. (2003). *Bates' guide to physical examination and history taking.* New York: Lippincott Williams & Wilkins.

Ignatavicius, D. D., & Workman, M. L. (2006). *Medical-surgical nursing* (5th ed.). St. Louis, MO: Saunders.

McCaffery, M, & Pasero, C. (1999). *Pain: A clinical manual.* St. Louis, MO: Mosby.

NANDA International (2004). *NANDA nursing diagnoses: Definitions and classification 2005-2006.* Philadelphia: NANDA.

St. Marie, B. (Ed.) (2002). *Core curriculum for pain management nursing.* Philadelphia: Saunders.

Chapter 55: Pain Management

Application Exercises

1. A nurse is performing a pain assessment on a client who has come to the emergency department with a report of severe abdominal pain. The nurse asks the client if he has experienced nausea and vomiting. The nurse is assessing

    A. presence of associated symptoms.

    B. location of the pain.

    C. pain quality.

    D. aggravating and relieving factors.

2. Frequent pain assessment includes assessing the intensity of the pain. The nurse can best assess the intensity of a client's pain by

    A. asking about what precipitates the pain.

    B. questioning the client about the location of the pain.

    C. offering the client a pain scale to measure his pain.

    D. using open-ended questions to find out about the sensation.

3. Which of the following statements are true regarding pain? (Select all that apply.)

    _____ All cultures have the same attitudes regarding pain.

    _____ Feelings of anger and guilt may be caused by pain.

    _____ It may be difficult to adequately assess pain in a client with cognitive impairment.

    _____ A client who is sleeping could not be experiencing pain.

    _____ It is best to wait until pain is severe before administering analgesics.

4. A nurse taking a history on a client with pain knows that

    A. most clients exaggerate their level of pain.

    B. pain must have an identifiable source to justify the use of opioids.

    C. objective data is essential in assessing pain.

    D. pain is whatever the client says that it is.

5. Match the following types of pain with their descriptors: V = Visceral, S = Somatic, and N = Neuropathic.

     _____   Phantom limb pain

     _____   Poorly localized pain

     _____   Referred pain

     _____   Fracture pain

     _____   Burning ("pins and needles") pain

     _____   Sharp, aching pain

6. A nurse is assessing a client who had surgery 3 hr ago. The client reports incisional pain rating at a 7 on a scale of 0 to 10. His pulse, respirations, and blood pressure are elevated, and his pupils are dilated. Explain these physical findings in relation to his pain.

7. A nurse is assessing a client with pneumonia who also has a history of osteoarthritis of her knees. Although she is reporting pain rated at a 6 on a scale of 0 to 10, her vital signs are within normal limits, and she does not show any muscle tension. Explain these physical findings in relation to her pain.

Chapter 55: Pain Management

Application Exercises Answer Key

1. A nurse is performing a pain assessment on a client who has come to the emergency department with a report of severe abdominal pain. The nurse asks the client if he has experienced nausea and vomiting. The nurse is assessing

    A. presence of associated symptoms.

    B. location of the pain.

    C. pain quality.

    D. aggravating and relieving factors.

Nausea and vomiting are common associated symptoms experienced with pain. The location of the pain is where the pain is felt. Pain quality is assessed by identifying what the pain feels like, such as throbbing and aggravating. Relieving factors are what might make the pain better or worse.

2. Frequent pain assessment includes assessing the intensity of the pain. The nurse can best assess the intensity of a client's pain by

    A. asking about what precipitates the pain.

    B. questioning the client about the location of the pain.

    C. offering the client a pain scale to measure his pain.

    D. using open-ended questions to find out about the sensation.

A pain scale can help the client measure the amount of pain he has and its intensity. Assessment of pain triggers, and identification of the location of the client's pain will provide valuable information important to the selection of pain-control interventions, but neither provides information about the intensity of pain. Asking open-ended questions is important in pain assessment, but it does not provide for consistent quantification of pain intensity.

3. Which of the following statements are true regarding pain? (Select all that apply.)

_____ All cultures have the same attitudes regarding pain.

__X__ **Feelings of anger and guilt may be caused by pain.**

__X__ **It may be difficult to adequately assess pain in a client with cognitive impairment.**

_____ A client who is sleeping could not be experiencing pain.

_____ It is best to wait until pain is severe before administering analgesics.

Clients may experience feelings of anger and guilt with pain. Clients with cognitive impairment may not be able to express what they are feeling. Attitudes about pain may vary among different cultures. A client can still sleep even when experiencing pain; less pain medication will be needed if pain is treated before it becomes severe.

4. A nurse taking a history on a client with pain knows that

A. most clients exaggerate their level of pain.

B. pain must have an identifiable source to justify the use of opioids.

C. objective data is essential in assessing pain.

D. pain is whatever the client says that it is.

Pain is a subjective experience, and the client is the best source of information. A misconception about pain is that clients exaggerate their pain level. The client can experience pain without being able to identify the source. Objective data is not always present when the client is experiencing pain.

5. Match the following types of pain with their descriptors: V = Visceral, S = Somatic, and N = Neuropathic.

__N__ Phantom limb pain

__V__ Poorly localized pain

__V__ Referred pain

__S__ Fracture pain

__N__ Burning ("pins and needles") pain

__S__ Sharp, aching pain

6. A nurse is assessing a client who had surgery 3 hr ago. The client reports incisional pain rating at a 7 on a scale of 0 to 10. His pulse, respirations, and blood pressure are elevated, and his pupils are dilated. Explain these physical findings in relation to his pain.

Pain elicits a physiological response from the sympathetic nervous system. The client can experience tachycardia, hypertension, anxiety, diaphoresis, muscle tension, pallor, and dilated pupils.

7. A nurse is assessing a client with pneumonia who also has a history of osteoarthritis of her knees. Although she is reporting pain rated at a 6 on a scale of 0 to 10, her vital signs are within normal limits, and she does not show any muscle tension. Explain these physical findings in relation to her pain.

As the pain continues, the body is not able to sustain the level of sympathetic response, and the parasympathetic nervous system takes over. The client can still be experiencing pain without showing a physiological response to it.

Unit 3   Basic Nursing Care
Section: Comfort and Basic Needs

Chapter 56:   Nutrition and Oral Hydration
Contributor: Wendy Buenzli, MN, RN

NCLEX® Connections:

Learning Objective: Review and apply knowledge within **"Nutrition and Oral Hydration"** in readiness for performance of the following nursing activities as outlined by the NCLEX® test plans:

Δ   Assess/monitor the client for signs/symptoms of fluid overload or dehydration (e.g., significant difference in I&O, tenting, edema, dry membranes).

Δ   Assess/monitor the client's nutritional state (e.g., diet history, caloric intake, weight).

Δ   Evaluate factors that impact the client's fluid or nutritional status (e.g., disease, food availability, food preferences, medications).

Δ   Plan/provide for nutritional supplementation (e.g., high-calorie or protein drinks, tube feedings).

Δ   Instruct the client and/or family on dietary recommendations (e.g., low-calorie or low-sodium diets).

Δ   Communicate with or make referrals to the dietician as needed.

Δ   Assist the client with feeding as needed.

Key Points

Δ   **Basic Nutrients Required by the Body**

- **Carbohydrates** provide most of the body's energy and fiber.

- **Fats** are also used for energy and provide vitamins. No more than 30% of caloric intake should be from this source.

- **Proteins** are used for body growth and repair.

- **Vitamins** need to be consumed daily and are necessary for metabolism (e.g., vitamins A, B-complex, C, D, E, K, folic acid).

- **Minerals** are needed to complete essential biochemical reactions in the body (e.g., calcium, potassium, sodium, iron).

- **Water** is needed to replace fluids lost through perspiration, elimination, and respiration.

Key Factors

Δ **Religious practices** may guide a client's food preparation or choices.

Δ **Finances** may prevent clients from buying foods that are higher in protein or vitamins and minerals.

Δ **Appetite** can be decreased by illness, medications, pain, depression, or unpleasant environmental stimuli.

Δ **Preferences** may be determined by prior bad experiences with certain foods or with familiarity of foods that the client has tried and liked before.

Δ **Disease/illness** can impact the functional ability of the client to prepare and eat food.

Δ **Medications** can alter taste and appetite, as well as interfere in the absorption of certain nutrients.

Δ **Age** can affect nutritional requirements.

Age	Requirements
Infants (Birth to 1 year)	• Breast (preferred) or formula feed to provide: ◊ 108 kcal/kg of weight the first 6 months. ◊ 98 kcal/kg of weight the second 6 months. • Solid food is introduced at 4 to 6 months of age.
Toddlers (12 months to 3 years) and preschoolers (3 to 5 years)	• Toddlers and preschoolers need fewer calories per kg of weight than infants. • Toddlers and preschoolers need increased protein from sources other than milk.
School-age (5 to 12 years)	• School-age children need to be supervised to consume adequate protein and vitamins C and A. • School-age children tend to eat too many foods high in carbohydrates, fats, and salt.
Adolescents (13 to 19 years)	• Metabolic demands are high and require more energy. • Protein, calcium, iron, iodine, folic acid, and B vitamin needs are high. • One fourth of dietary intake comes from snacks. • Increased water consumption is important for active adolescents.
Young (20 to 40 years) and middle adults (40 to 60 years)	• There is a decreased need for most nutrients (except during pregnancy). • Calcium and iron consumption are important for women.
Older adults (over 60 years)	• Slower metabolic rate requires fewer calories. • Older adults need the same amount of vitamins and minerals as younger adults.

Δ **Eating Disorders**

- Anorexia nervosa

  ◊ Body weight less than 85% of ideal

  ◊ Fear of being fat

  ◊ Feeling fat

  ◊ In female clients, no menses for at least 3 consecutive months

- Bulimia – a cycle of binge eating followed by purging (e.g., vomiting, using diuretics or laxatives, exercise, fasting)

- Obesity

  ◊ Determine body mass index by dividing weight (in kg) by height (in meters^2).

  ◊ Adult with a basal metabolic index (BMI) of 30 or greater is considered obese.

Assessment

Δ Dietary history should include:

- Number of meals per day.

- Fluid intake.

- Food preferences and amounts.

- Food preparation/purchasing practices (includes access to food).

- History of indigestion, heartburn and/or gas.

- Allergies.

- Taste.

- Chewing and swallowing.

- Appetite.

- Elimination patterns.

- Use of any medications.

Δ Clinical Measures

- Height and weight to calculate BMI and ideal body weight (IBW)

- Laboratory values of cholesterol, triglycerides, hemoglobin, electrolytes, and albumin levels if available

Δ I&O

- Attention to accuracy is important.

- I&O should be monitored on any client with fluid or electrolyte alterations.

- Weight should be taken each day at the same time after the client voids, and while he is wearing the same clothes (type of clothes) each day.

- If using bed scales, use the same amount of linen each day, and zero out the scale if possible.

Δ   Clinical assessment of poor nutrition includes:

- Muscle tone flaccidity.

- Mental status changes.

- Loss of appetite.

- Change in bowel pattern.

- Spleen or liver enlargement.

- Dry, brittle hair.

- Loss of subcutaneous fat.

- Dry, scaly skin.

- Inflammation and bleeding of gums.

- Poor dental health.

- Dry, dull eyes.

- Enlarged thyroid.

- Prominent protrusions over bony areas.

NANDA Nursing Diagnoses

Δ   Constipation

Δ   Deficient/excess fluid volume

Δ   Imbalanced nutrition: less/more than body requirements

Δ   Feeding self-care deficit

Nursing Interventions

Δ   Assist the client in advancing diet as disease process allows.

Δ   Provide education to client on diet regimen.

Δ   Provide interventions to promote appetite (e.g., good oral hygiene, favorite foods, decreasing environmental odors).

Δ   Educate the client on medications that may affect nutritional intake.

Δ   Assist the client with feeding to promote optimal independence.

Δ   Assess for and assist with preventing aspiration.

- Position the client in a Fowler's position or in a chair.

- Support the upper back, neck, and head.

- Have the client tuck her chin when swallowing to better enable food to pass down the esophagus.

- Observe for aspiration and/or pocketing of food in the cheeks or other areas of the mouth.

- Maintain the client in a semi-Fowler's position for at least 1 hr after meals.

- Provide oral hygiene after meals/snacks.

Δ   Provide therapeutic diets as directed by the primary care provider/dietician.

- Clear liquid – leave little residue (e.g., clear fruit juices, gelatin, broth)

- Full liquid – clear liquids plus liquid dairy products, all juice, puréed vegetables

- Puréed – clear and full liquids plus puréed meats and fruits, and scrambled eggs

- Mechanical soft – clear and full liquids, plus foods that are diced or ground

- Soft/low-residue – foods that are low in fiber and easy to digest

- High-fiber (e.g., whole grains, raw and dried fruits)

- Low sodium – no added salt or 1 to 2 g of sodium

- Low cholesterol – no more than 300 mg/day of dietary cholesterol

- Diabetic – balanced intake of protein, fats, and carbohydrates with a total caloric intake of about 1,800 calories

- Dysphagia – puréed food and thickened liquids

- Regular – no restrictions

Δ   Administer and monitor enteral feedings via nasogastric, gastrostomy, or jejunostomy tubes.

Δ   Administer and monitor parenteral nutrition to clients who are unable to use their gastrointestinal tract to acquire nutrients.

- Types of nutrients given parenterally include:

  ◊   Lipids.

  ◊   Electrolytes.

  ◊   Minerals.

◊ Vitamins.

◊ Dextrose.

◊ Amino acids.

- Initiating parenteral nutrition

  ◊ If using central venous circulation, the placement is confirmed on x-ray prior to starting the feeding.

  ◊ The solution's contents are compared to the primary care provider's order.

  ◊ The solution is infused using a pump, and the rate is gradually increased until the desired rate is achieved.

- Maintaining/monitoring parenteral nutrition

  ◊ Frequent tubing changes every 24 hr for lipids and 48 hr for other solutions

  ◊ Sterile dressing changes of the central venous circulation access site

  ◊ Monitoring laboratory electrolyte values and blood glucose levels frequently until stable

Δ Maintain fluid balance by:

- Administering IV fluids.

- Restricting oral fluid intake.

  ◊ Remove the water pitcher from the bedside.

  ◊ Communicate with the dietary staff the amount of fluid to be served with each meal tray.

  ◊ Communicate with each shift the amount of fluid the client is allowed besides what is served with each meal.

- Encouraging oral intake of fluids.

  ◊ Provide fresh drinking water.

  ◊ Ask the client about beverage preferences.

Primary Reference:

Potter, P. A., & Perry, A. G. (2005). *Fundamentals of nursing* (6th ed.). St. Louis, MO: Mosby.

Additional Resources:

NANDA International (2004). *NANDA nursing diagnoses: Definitions and classification 2005-2006* Philadelphia: NANDA.

Chapter 56: Nutrition and Oral Hydration

Application Exercises

1. When conducting a nursing assessment on a family with a low income, the nurse discovers that the family is deficient in protein. Which of the following would be the best choice for increasing protein intake for this family?

     A. Red meat and fish

     B. Potatoes and rice

     C. Beans and rice

     D. Peas and beans

2. A client is diagnosed as being high risk for aspiration. Which of the following is an appropriate nursing intervention?

     A. Give the client thin liquids.

     B. Instruct the client to tuck chin when swallowing.

     C. Have the client use a straw.

     D. Encourage the client to lie down and rest after meals.

3. Which nutrient is the body's preferred energy source?

     A. Fat

     B. Protein

     C. Vitamins

     D. Carbohydrates

4. School-age children tend to have a dietary deficiency in which of the following if their diet is not adequately supervised?

     A. Carbohydrates

     B. Fats

     C. Minerals

     D. Vitamins

5. Which of the following is most appropriate for a client on a low-residue diet?

     A. Whole grains

     B. Fruits and vegetables

     C. Dairy products

     D. Nuts and legumes

Chapter 56: Nutrition and Oral Hydration

Application Exercises Answer Key

1. When conducting a nursing assessment on a family with a low income, the nurse discovers that the family is deficient in protein. Which of the following would be the best choice for increasing protein intake for this family?

      A. Red meat and fish

      B. Potatoes and rice

      C. Beans and rice

      D. Peas and beans

Beans and rice are a complete source of protein and are the most affordable. Peas and beans are an affordable choice, but without a grain, they do not provide a complete protein. Red meat and fish can be expensive. Potatoes and rice are not a good source of protein.

2. A client is diagnosed as being high risk for aspiration. Which of the following is an appropriate nursing intervention?

      A. Give the client thin liquids.

      B. Instruct the client to tuck chin when swallowing.

      C. Have the client use a straw.

      D. Encourage the client to lie down and rest after meals.

Tucking the chin when swallowing allows food to pass down the esophagus more easily. Thin liquids and using a straw both increase the client's risk for aspiration. Sitting for an hour after meals helps prevent gastroesophageal reflux and possible aspiration of the contents after a meal.

3. Which nutrient is the body's preferred energy source?

      A. Fat

      B. Protein

      C. Vitamins

      D. Carbohydrates

Most of the body's energy comes from carbohydrates. Fat provides energy but should be less than 30% of total caloric intake. Protein is responsible for growth and repair of body tissues. Vitamins do not provide energy.

4. School-age children tend to have a dietary deficiency in which of the following if their diet is not adequately supervised?

> A. Carbohydrates
>
> B. Fats
>
> C. Minerals
>
> **D. Vitamins**

School-age children need to have their dietary intake supervised to ensure adequate intake of protein and vitamins C and A. They tend to eat too many foods high in carbohydrates, fats, and salt.

5. Which of the following is most appropriate for a client on a low-residue diet?

> A. Whole grains
>
> B. Fruits and vegetables
>
> **C. Dairy products**
>
> D. Nuts and legumes

A soft/low-residue diet consists of foods that are low in fiber and easy to digest. Processed foods are low in fiber and easy to digest. Whole grains, fruits, vegetables, nuts, and legumes all have a lot of fiber.

Unit 3   Basic Nursing Care
Section: Nursing Care of Wounds

Chapter 57:   Wound Healing and Management
                 Contributor: Linda Turchin, MSN, RN

 NCLEX® Connections:

Learning Objective: Review and apply knowledge within **"Wound Healing and Management"** in readiness for performance of the following nursing activities as outlined by the NCLEX® test plans:

Δ   Identify risk factors for impaired skin integrity.

Δ   Assess/monitor the client for factors that may interfere with wound healing.

Δ   Plan/provide care for clients with impaired skin integrity.

Δ   Plan/provide fluids and nutrition to promote wound healing.

Δ   Evaluate client's wound for response to interventions.

Δ   Intervene in emergency wound situations (e.g., dehiscence, evisceration).

Key Points

Δ   **Stages of Wound Healing**

- **Inflammatory** stage is the first 3 days after the initial trauma. Attempts are made at the site to:

   ◊   Control bleeding with clot formation.

   ◊   Deliver oxygen, white blood cells, and nutrition to the area via blood supply.

- **Proliferative** stage lasts the next 3 to 24 days. Effects to the wound include:

   ◊   Replacing lost tissue with connective or granulated tissue.

   ◊   Occurrence of contracting of the wound.

   ◊   Resurfacing of new epithelial cells.

- **Maturation or remodeling** stage involves the strengthening of the collagen scar and the resumption of a more normal appearance. It can take more than 1 year to complete, depending on the extent of the original wound.

Δ   **Healing Processes**

Type of Healing	Characteristics	Wound Type
Primary intention	• Has little or no tissue loss • Edges that are approximated, such as a surgical incision	• Will heal rapidly • Has low risk of infection • Will have no or minimal scarring
Secondary intention	• Has loss of tissue • Wound edges that are widely separated (e.g., pressure ulcers, stab wounds)	• Will have a longer healing time • Increased risk of infection • Scarring
Tertiary intention	• Widely separated • Deep • Spontaneous opening of a previously closed wound • Possible presence of infection	• Will likely have extensive drainage and tissue debris • Will be closed later • Long healing time

Δ   Factors Affecting Wound Healing

- **Increased age** potentates poor healing because of:

    ◊   Loss of skin turgor.

    ◊   Skin fragility.

    ◊   Decreased peripheral circulation and oxygenation.

    ◊   Slower tissue regeneration.

    ◊   Decreased absorption of nutrients.

    ◊   Decreased collagen.

    ◊   Impaired function of the immune system.

- **Overall client wellness** – For example, a compound fracture of the femur in a client with a head injury will present greater healing problems.

- **Immune function** is the body's ability to fight infection by destroying invading pathogens.

- **Medications** may interfere with the body's ability to respond to and/or prevent infection.

- **Nutrition** provides elements required for wound healing and energy requirements.

- **Tissue perfusion** provides the circulation needed to deliver the required elements for tissue repair and infection control.

- **Obesity** – fatty tissue lacks blood supply.

- **Chronic diseases** present additional stress on the body's healing mechanisms (e.g., diabetes mellitus).

- **Chronic stress** creates additional stressors that impede healing.

- **Smoking** impairs oxygenation and clotting.

- **Wound stress**, such as vomiting or coughing, stresses the suture line and disrupts the wound healing process.

Key Procedural Points

Δ **General Principles of Wound Management**

- A wound is a disruption of the skin.

- **Inflammation** is a localized protective response brought on by injury or destruction of tissue.

- Wounds heal by various **processes** and in **stages.**

- Wounds may become **infected** by the invasion of a pathogenic micro-organism.

- Principles of wound care include assessment, cleansing, and protection.

- **Wound care** is a nursing responsibility that has a high impact on wound healing.

Assessment

Δ Appearance

- Note color of **open** wounds. The following colors reflect wound condition:

  ◊ **Red** – healthy regeneration of tissue.

  ◊ **Yellow** – presence of purulent drainage and slough (dead tissue).

  ◊ **Black** – presence of eschar (thick, necrotic material) that hinders healing and must be removed.

- Closed wounds – Skin edges should be well-approximated.

Δ Drainage is a normal result of the healing process and occurs during the inflammatory and proliferative phases of healing.

- Note the amount of drainage from a drain or on a dressing.

- Skin around a drain should be observed for skin irritation and breakdown with each cleansing.

- Character of drainage is distinguished by consistency, color, and odor.

  ◊ **Serous** drainage is the serous portion of the blood. It is watery and clear or slightly yellow in appearance.

  ◊ **Sanguineous** drainage contains serum and red blood cells. It is thick and appears reddish.

◊ **Serosanguineous** drainage contains both serum and blood. It is watery and appears blood-streaked or blood tinged.

◊ **Purulent drainage** is the result of infection. It is composed of white blood cells, tissue debris, and bacteria. It may have a foul odor, is thick and appears colored by the specific type of organism present (e.g., green may indicate a pseudomonas infection).

Δ Wound closure (e.g., staples, sutures, steri-strips)

Δ Pain

NANDA Nursing Diagnoses

Δ Pain

Δ Risk for infection

Δ Impaired skin integrity

Δ Impaired tissue integrity

Δ Disturbed body image

Δ Imbalanced nutrition

Nursing Interventions

Δ Provide **adequate hydration** and meet **protein** and calorie needs.

- Encourage intake of 2,000 to 3,000 mL of water/day, if not contraindicated (heart failure, renal failure).

- Provide client education regarding **high sources of protein** (meat, fish, poultry, eggs, dairy products, beans, nuts, whole grains).

- Note if serum albumin levels are low (< 3.5 g/dL), because a lack of protein puts the client at greater risk for delayed wound healing and infection.

- Provide nutritional support as indicated (vitamin and mineral supplements, nutritional supplements, enteral nutrition, parenteral nutrition).

Δ Perform wound cleansing.

- Cleanse in a direction from least contaminated toward the most contaminated.

- Gentle friction is used when cleansing or applying solutions to the skin to avoid bleeding or further injury to the wound.

- While other mild cleansing agents may be ordered, isotonic solution remains the preferred cleansing agent.

- Never use the same gauze to cleanse across an incision or wound more than once.

- Irrigation using a solution-filled syringe held 1 inch above the wound may be used.

Δ Perform wound dressing using:

- Woven gauze (sponges) – absorbs exudate from the wound.

- Nonadherent – does not adhere to the wound bed.

- Self adhesive, transparent film – temporary second skin that is ideal for small, superficial wounds.

- Hydrocolloid – occlusive dressing that swells in the presence of exudate.

  ◊ Used to maintain a granulating wound bed

  ◊ May be left in place up to 5 days

- Hydrogel (Aquasorb)

  ◊ May be used on infected, deep wounds

  ◊ Provides a moist wound bed

Δ Perform debridement, if prescribed, to remove dead wound tissue that prevents wound healing using a wet-to-dry dressing.

Δ Use the negative pressure of a wound vacuum-assisted closure if ordered.

Δ Remove sutures/staples as ordered.

Δ Administer analgesics as needed.

Δ Administer antimicrobials (topical and/or systemic) as ordered.

Δ Document location and type of wound/incision, status of wound and type of drainage, type of dressing and materials used, client teaching provided, and how the client tolerated the procedure.

Complications and Nursing Implications

Δ **Dehiscence** is a partial or total rupture (separation) of a sutured wound usually with separation of underlying skin layers. **Evisceration** is a dehiscence that involves the protrusion of visceral organs through the surgical incision. It is usually caused by the increased flow of serosanguineous fluid occurring approximately 3 to 11 days postoperatively.

- Signs/symptoms of dehiscence include:

  ◊ Appreciable increase in the flow of serosanguineous fluid on the wound dressings.

  ◊ Immediate history of sudden straining (e.g., coughing, sneezing, and/or vomiting).

  ◊ Client states, "Something just happened to my stomach."

◊ Visualization of visceral organs.

- Risk factors include:

  ◊ Chronic disease.

  ◊ Advanced age.

  ◊ Obesity.

  ◊ Invasive abdominal cancer.

  ◊ Vomiting.

  ◊ Dehydration/malnutrition.

  ◊ Ineffective suturing.

  ◊ Abdominal surgery.

- Evisceration requires immediate emergency treatment.

  ◊ Call for help.

  ◊ Stay with the client.

  ◊ Cover the wound and any protruding organs with sterile towels or dressings that have been soaked in saline solution. **Do not attempt to reinsert organs.**

  ◊ Position the client supine with hips and knees bent.

  ◊ Observe the client for signs of shock.

  ◊ Maintain a calm environment.

Δ **Infection**

- Risk factors

  ◊ Extremes in age (e.g., immature immune system, decreased immune function)

  ◊ Impaired circulation and oxygenation (e.g., COPD, peripheral vascular disease)

  ◊ Wound condition/nature (e.g., gunshot wound vs surgical incision)

  ◊ Impaired/suppressed immune system

  ◊ Malnutrition such as with alcoholism

  ◊ Chronic disease

  ◊ Poor wound care such as breaches in sterile technique

- Signs and symptoms are usually apparent within 2 to 7 days of injury/surgery.

  ◊ Purulent drainage

  ◊ Pain

◊ Redness and edema (in and around the wound)

◊ Fever

◊ Chills

◊ Increased pulse and respiratory rate

◊ Increase in white blood cell count

- Interventions

◊ Prevent infection from occurring by using appropriate aseptic technique when performing dressing changes.

◊ Provide good nutrition to promote the immune response.

◊ Provide for adequate rest to promote healing.

◊ Administer antibiotic therapy per primary care provider orders.

Primary Reference:

Potter, P. A., & Perry, A. G. (2005). *Fundamentals of nursing* (6th ed.). St. Louis, MO: Mosby.

Additional Resources:

Brown, P., & Phelps Maloy, J. (2005). *Quick reference to wound care* (2nd ed.). Boston: Jones and Bartlett Publishers.

Ignatavicius, D. D., & Workman, M. L. (2006). *Medical-surgical nursing* (5th ed.). St. Louis, MO: Saunders.

NANDA International (2004). *NANDA nursing diagnoses: Definitions and classification 2005-2006*. Philadelphia: NANDA.

Chapter 57: Wound Healing and Management

Application Exercises

Scenario: An adolescent client with diabetes is recovering from an appendectomy. This is the third postoperative day. The client has been ordered a regular diet and is tolerating it well. He has ambulated successfully around the unit with the help of his parents and is requesting pain medication every 6 to 8 hr while reporting pain at a 2 on a scale of 0 to 10 after medication is given. His incision is approximated and free of redness with scant serous drainage noted on the dressing.

1. What type of healing process would the nurse expect this wound to be undergoing? Explain.

2. Which of the following risk factors does this client possess? (Select all that apply.)

_____ Extremes in age

_____ Impaired circulation

_____ Impaired/suppressed immune system

_____ Malnutrition

_____ Poor wound care such as breaches in sterile technique

3. What is the single most important nursing intervention to protect this client from developing a postoperative infection?

4. An entry in a client's chart states the wound drainage is "sanguineous." That means it is

A. watery in appearance.

B. green-tinged or yellow.

C. bright red.

D. foul-smelling.

5. Which of the following is an example of a wound or injury healing by secondary intention?

A. An open burn area

B. A bone fracture that is casted

C. Sprained ankle

D. A sutured surgical incision

Scenario: An older adult woman has undergone surgery for a bowel obstruction 6 days ago. Prior to surgery, she experienced nausea and vomiting for 3 days. During the last 24 hr, she has reported nausea, and she has vomited small amounts of clear liquid three times in the last 8 hr. Her vital signs are stable. The client weighs 81.6 kg (180 lb) and is 5 ft 2 in tall and smokes two packs of cigarettes a day. Currently, her incision is well approximated and free of redness, tenderness, or swelling.

6. What assessment findings would indicate development of a wound infection?

7. What risk factors for poor healing does this client exhibit?

8. Later that day, the client becomes confused and pulls off her surgical dressing. The nurse enters the room and finds the client with an extensive dehiscence. Which of the following nursing interventions are appropriate? (Select all that apply.)

_____ Repack the wound.

_____ Call for help.

_____ Assist the client to a chair.

_____ Cover the wound with a sterile dressing moistened with normal saline.

_____ Stay with the client.

9. What placed this client at risk for a wound dehiscence/evisceration?

Chapter 57: Wound Healing and Management

Application Exercises Answer Key

Scenario: An adolescent client with diabetes is recovering from an appendectomy. This is the third postoperative day. The client has been ordered a regular diet and is tolerating it well. He has ambulated successfully around the unit with the help of his parents and is requesting pain medication every 6 to 8 hr while reporting pain at a 2 on a scale of 0 to 10 after medication is given. His incision is approximated and free of redness with scant serous drainage noted on the dressing.

1. What type of healing process would the nurse expect this wound to be undergoing? Explain.

   This wound is healing by primary intentions because it is a surgical incision.

2. Which of the following risk factors does this client possess? (Select all that apply.)

   _____ Extremes in age
   _**X**_ **Impaired circulation**
   _**X**_ **Impaired/suppressed immune system**
   _____ Malnutrition
   _____ Poor wound care such as breaches in sterile technique

   Diabetes places this client at risk for impaired circulation and impaired immune system. The client is not at either extreme of the age spectrum, and there is no indication that he is malnourished or that there have been any breaches in sterile technique during wound care.

3. What is the single most important nursing intervention to protect this client from developing a postoperative infection?

   Proper wound care

4. An entry in a client's chart states the wound drainage is "sanguineous." That means it is

    A. watery in appearance.

    B. green-tinged or yellow.

    C. bright red.

    D. foul-smelling.

Sanguineous drainage is bright red and a result of active bleeding. A watery appearance is characteristic of serous or serosanguineous drainage. Green-tinged or yellow and foul-smelling are characteristics of purulent drainage.

5. Which of the following is an example of a wound or injury healing by secondary intention?

    A. An open burn area

    B. A bone fracture that is casted

    C. Sprained ankle

    D. A sutured surgical incision

A burn has loss of tissue and the skin edges are not together. A fractured bone and sprained ankle are injuries to underlying structures and do not require healing of the skin. A sutured surgical incision heals by primary intention.

Scenario: An older adult woman has undergone surgery for a bowel obstruction 6 days ago. Prior to surgery, she experienced nausea and vomiting for 3 days. During the last 24 hr, she has reported nausea, and she has vomited small amounts of clear liquid three times in the last 8 hr. Her vital signs are stable. The client weighs 81.6 kg (180 lb) and is 5 ft 2 in tall and smokes two packs of cigarettes a day. Currently, her incision is well approximated and free of redness, tenderness, or swelling.

---

6. What assessment findings would indicate development of a wound infection?

Purulent drainage

Pain

Redness and edema (in and around the wound)

Fever

Chills

Increased pulse and respiratory rate

Increased white blood cell count

7. What risk factors for poor healing does this client exhibit?

    Obesity, dehydration, smoker

8. Later that day, the client becomes confused and pulls off her surgical dressing. The nurse enters the room and finds the client with an extensive dehiscence. Which of the following nursing interventions are appropriate? (Select all that apply.)

        _____ Repack the wound.

        _**X**_ **Call for help.**

        _____ Assist the client to a chair.

        _**X**_ **Cover the wound with a sterile dressing moistened with normal saline.**

        _**X**_ **Stay with the client.**

It is appropriate for the nurse to call for help, stay with the client, and cover the wound with a sterile dressing moistened with normal saline. The nurse should not attempt to reinsert the organs and repack the wound. The client should be placed in the supine position with hips and knees bent.

9. What placed this client at risk for a wound dehiscence/evisceration?

    Age

    Obesity

    Abdominal surgery 6 days ago

    Recent vomiting

Unit 3   Basic Nursing Care
Section: Nursing Care of Wounds

Chapter 58:   **Pressure Ulcers**

Contributor: Linda Turchin, MSN, RN

↻ NCLEX-RN® Connections

Learning Objective: Review and apply knowledge within **"Pressure Ulcers"** in readiness for performance of the following nursing activities as outlined by the NCLEX® test plans:

Δ   Assess/monitor the client for skin impairment.

Δ   Identify risk factors for the development of pressure ulcers.

Δ   Plan and provide care to the client with a pressure ulcer that promotes wound healing and restoration and maintenance of skin integrity.

Δ   Plan and provide care to promote adequate nutrition, hydration, and wound healing.

Δ   Plan and provide care to promote mobility and/or position changes.

Δ   Implement measures to prevent complications such as infection, sepsis, and septic shock.

Δ   Evaluate and document the client's response to nursing interventions.

 Key Points

Δ   A pressure ulcer is a specific **tissue injury caused by external forces** that result in unrelieved **pressure that results in ischemia** and damage to the underlying tissue.

Δ   Pressure ulcers range from blanchable tissue redness to full thickness skin loss with damage to underlying muscle and bone. They are categorized as Stage I, II, III, and IV.

Δ   Excellent nursing care is the primary factor in the prevention of pressure ulcers.

Δ   The primary focus of **prevention and treatment** is to **relieve the pressure** and provide for good nutrition and hydration.

Δ　All clients must be **assessed** regularly for skin-integrity status and evaluated regularly for **risk factors** that contribute to the development of impaired skin integrity.

Δ　Pressure ulcers are a significant source of morbidity and mortality among older adults and persons of any age who suffer mobility limitations.

Key Procedural Points

Δ　Risk factors for development of pressure ulcers include:

- Skin changes related to aging.

- Immobility.

- Incontinence or excessive moisture.

- Skin friction and shearing.

- Vascular disorders.

- Obesity.

- Inadequate nutrition and or hydration.

- Anemia.

- Fever.

- Impaired circulation.

- Edema.

- Sensory deficits.

- Impaired cognitive functioning, neurological disorders.

- Chronic diseases (e.g., diabetes mellitus, chronic renal failure, congestive heart disease, chronic lung disease).

- Sedation that impairs spontaneous repositioning.

Assessment

Stage I	Stage II	Stage III	Stage IV
• Epidermal involvement only • Lightly pigmented skin: redness; darker skin tones: red, blue, or purple in tone • Reversible if pressure is relieved	• Partial-thickness skin loss involving epidermis and/or dermis • Lesion presenting as an abrasion, shallow crater, or blister • May appear swollen and may be painful • Takes several weeks to heal when pressure is relieved	• Full-thickness skin loss, including subcutaneous tissue and underlying fascia • Lesion presenting as a deep crater with or without undermining of adjacent tissue, may have foul-smelling, purulent drainage if locally infected • Yellow slough and/or necrotic tissue in wound bed • May require months to heal after pressure is relieved	• Extensive damage to underlying structures including tendons, muscles, and bones • Lesion appearing small on the surface but can have extensive tunneling out of sight beneath superficial tissue • Local infection easily spread, which can cause sepsis • May take months or years to heal after pressure is relieved
Skin intact	Superficial	Shallow to deep	Deep

- **Some ulcers cannot be staged** because they are covered with **eschar** – dark, leathery scab (crust) made of necrotic tissue – and the wound bed cannot be visualized.

NANDA Nursing Diagnoses

Δ   Pain

Δ   Impaired skin integrity

Δ   Impaired tissue integrity

Δ   Ineffective tissue perfusion

Nursing Interventions

Δ   Prevention

- Maintain clean, dry skin and wrinkle-free linens.

◊   Appropriately use pressure-reducing surfaces and pressure-relieving devices.

◊   Inspect skin frequently and document risk using a tool such as the Braden scale.

◊ Clean and dry skin immediately following urinary or stool incontinence.

◊ **Apply moisture barrier** creams to the skin of clients who are incontinent.

◊ Use **tepid** water (not hot), minimal scrubbing, and **pat skin dry**.

• **Reposition** the client in bed **at least every 2 hr** and every 1 hr when sitting in a chair. Document position changes.

◊ Place **pillows strategically between bony surfaces**.

◊ Maintain the **head of the bed at or below a 30°** angle (or flat), unless contraindicated, to relieve pressure on sacrum, buttocks, and heels.

◊ **Prevent the client from sliding down** in bed, as this increases shearing forces that pull tissue layers apart and cause damage.

◊ **Lift rather than pull** a client up in bed or in a chair, because pulling creates friction that can damage the client's outer layer of skin (epidermis).

◊ Raise the client's **heels off of the bed** to prevent pressure on the heels.

◊ Ambulate the client as soon as possible and as often as possible.

◊ Implement active/passive exercises for immobile clients.

◊ **Do not massage** bony prominences.

• Provide **adequate hydration** (2,000 to 3,000 mL/day) and meet **protein** and calorie needs.

◊ Note if serum albumin levels are low (< 3.5 g/dL), because a lack of protein puts the client at greater risk for skin breakdown, slowed healing, and infection.

◊ Provide nutritional support as indicated, such as vitamin and mineral supplements, nutritional supplements, enteral nutrition, and parenteral nutrition.

Δ   Treatment

Stage	Interventions
Stage I	• Relieve pressure. • Encourage frequent turning/repositioning. • Use pressure-relieving devices, such as an air-fluidized bed. • Implement pressure-reduction surfaces (air mattress, foam mattress). • Keep the client dry, clean, well-nourished, and hydrated.
Stage II	• Maintain a moist healing environment (saline or occlusive dressing). • Promote natural healing while preventing formation of scar tissue. • Provide nutritional supplements as needed. • Administer analgesics as needed.
Stage III	• Clean and/or debride: ◊ Wet-to-dry dressing. ◊ Surgical intervention. ◊ Proteolytic enzymes. • Provide nutritional supplements as needed. • Administer analgesics as needed. • Administer antimicrobials (topical and/or systemic).
Stage IV	• Perform nonadherent dressing change every 12 hr. • Treatment may require skin grafts. • Provide nutritional supplements as needed. • Administer analgesics as needed. • Administer antimicrobials (topical and/or systemic).

Complications and Nursing Implications

Δ   **Deterioration** to a Higher Stage Ulceration and/or Infection

- Assess/monitor the ulcer frequently and report increases in the size or depth of the lesion, changes in granulation tissues (e.g., color, texture), and changes in exudates (e.g., color, quantity, odor).

- Follow protocol for ulcer treatment.

Δ   **Systemic Infection**

- Assess/monitor the client for signs of sepsis (e.g., changes in level of consciousness, persistent recurrent fever, tachycardia, tachypnea, hypotension, oliguria, increased white blood cell count).

- Prevent infection from occurring by using appropriate aseptic technique when performing ulcer treatment and dressing changes.

- Provide good nutrition to promote the immune response.

- Provide for adequate rest to promote healing.

- Administer antibiotic therapy per primary care provider orders.

Primary Reference:

Potter, P. A., & Perry, A. G. (2005). *Fundamentals of nursing* (6th ed.). St. Louis, MO: Mosby.

Additional Resources:

Brown, P., & Phelps Maloy, J. (2005). *Quick reference to wound care* (2nd ed.). Boston: Jones and Bartlett Publishers.

Ignatavicius, D. D., & Workman, M. L. (2006). *Medical-surgical nursing* (5th ed.). St. Louis, MO: Saunders.

NANDA International (2004). *NANDA nursing diagnoses: Definitions and classification 2005-2006*. Philadelphia: NANDA.

Chapter 58: Pressure Ulcers

Application Exercises

Scenario: An older adult client with diabetes mellitus and Alzheimer's disease must now use a wheelchair after a cerebral vascular accident 2 years ago that affected her right side. She does not respond to verbal commands or pain on the right side of her body. Her fluid and food intake is good, but she does require help with eating. She is continent for stool but is frequently incontinent for urine.

1. What risk factors does this client have for developing pressure ulcers?

2. What usual risk factor(s) does this client NOT have?

3. What can the nurse do to prevent skin breakdown?

Scenario: A client has developed a red area approximately 1 cm x 1 cm on his elbow. It does not blanch.

4. A client has developed a red area approximately 1 cm x 1 cm on his elbow. It does not blanch. To which stage has the client's skin lesion progressed, and which layer(s) of the skin are most likely damaged?

5. The primary focus of prevention and treatment of pressure ulcers is _____, _____, and _____.

6. Which of the following statements best describes a Stage III pressure ulcer?

    A. The skin is reddened and does not blanch with pressure.

    B. The ulcer is an abrasion or blister.

    C. The bone is exposed at the center of the ulcer.

    D. The ulcer extends past the subcutaneous tissue to the muscle.

Chapter 58: Pressure Ulcers

Application Exercises Answer Key

Scenario: An older adult client with diabetes mellitus and Alzheimer's disease must now use a wheelchair after a cerebral vascular accident 2 years ago that affected her right side. She does not respond to verbal commands or pain on the right side of her body. Her fluid and food intake is good, but she does require help with eating. She is continent for stool but is frequently incontinent for urine.

1. What risk factors does this client have for developing pressure ulcers?

   Wheelchair confinement (immobile)

   Right-side (immobile)

   Lack of pain sensations on the right side (decreased sensations)

   Alzheimer's disease (impaired mental status)

   Incontinence of urine (moisture)

   Older adult client (advanced age)

2. What usual risk factor(s) does this client NOT have?

   Poor nutrition and dehydration

3. What can the nurse do to prevent skin breakdown?

   Encourage repositioning every 15 to 30 min while the client is in a wheelchair.

   Keep the client clean and dry (incontinent).

   Perform a thorough daily assessment (particularly areas of decreased pain sensation and coccyx).

   Provide good, frequent skin care.

   Implement pressure-reducing devices when the client is in her wheelchair.

   Encourage and facilitate good nutrition.

Scenario: A client has developed a red area approximately 1 cm x 1 cm on his elbow. It does not blanch.

4. A client has developed a red area approximately 1 cm x 1 cm on his elbow. It does not blanch. To which stage has the client's skin lesion progressed, and which layer(s) of the skin are most likely damaged?

Stage I pressure ulcer – epidermal damage

5. The primary focus of prevention and treatment of pressure ulcers is _____, _____, and _____.

Relieving pressure, providing good nutrition, providing good hydration

6. Which of the following statements best describes a Stage III pressure ulcer?

   A. The skin is reddened and does not blanch with pressure.
   B. The ulcer is an abrasion or blister.
   C. The bone is exposed at the center of the ulcer.
   D. The ulcer extends past the subcutaneous tissue to the muscle.

A Stage III ulcer may extend past all the layers of skin and subcutaneous tissue to the muscle. Reddened skin that does not blanch is characteristic of Stage I. An abrasion or blister is seen with Stage II. Exposed bone is characteristic of Stage IV.

Unit 4   Supporting Psychosocial, Family, Cultural, and Spiritual Health
Section: Psychosocial Health

Chapter 59:   Stress, Adaptation, Coping, and Compliance
Contributor: Shari Goldberg, MS, ARNP

 NCLEX® Connections

Learning Objective: Review and apply knowledge within **"Stress, Adaptation, Coping, and Compliance"** in readiness for performance of the following nursing activities as outlined by the NCLEX® test plans:

Δ   Assess/monitor the client and family for stressors, coping mechanisms, and emotional reactions to illness.

Δ   Provide/plan strategies the client and family can use to manage stress, decrease anxiety, and increase coping.

Δ   Reduce stressful environmental stimuli (e.g., temperature extremes, noise, environmental contaminates).

Δ   Determine the family/support systems available to assist in client care.

Δ   Identify reasons for noncompliance and/or barriers the client has with implementing treatment plans.

 Key Points

Δ   **Stress** is a term that describes an individual's capacity to meet **stressors** of environmental demands. Stress contributes to illness vulnerability, and symptoms of stress may be addressed through nursing interventions.

Δ   **Adaptation** is a coping behavior that describes how an individual handles demands imposed by the environment.

Δ   **Coping** is a term that describes how an individual deals with problems and/or issues.

Δ   **Compliance** is the ability of the client/family to adhere to a given treatment regimen.

Key Factors

Δ **Stress**

- Stress may be situational (e.g., adjusting to a chronic disease or a stressful job change).

- Stress may be developmental (varying with life stage). An adult stressor may include losing parents.

- Stress may be caused by sociocultural factors to include substance abuse and lack of education.

Δ **Adaptation** – General Adaptation Syndrome (GAS)

- **Alarm reaction** – Body functions are heightened to respond to a stressor (e.g., elevated blood pressure and heart rate, heightened mental alertness, and increased secretion of epinephrine and norepinephrine).

- **Resistance stage** – Body functions normalize while responding to the stressor.

- **Exhaustion stage** – Body functions are no longer able to maintain a response to the stressor.

Δ **Coping**

- Factors influencing an individual's ability to cope include the number, duration, and intensity of the stressors, the experiences that an individual has had in the past, and the current support system.

- Caregiver burden refers to the accumulated stress that family members may experience after caring for a loved one over a period of time. Some responses may include fatigue and difficulty sleeping.

Δ **Compliance**

- Complicated regimens interfere with compliance.

- Side effects of medications diminish compliance.

- Coping mechanisms such as denial can cause noncompliance.

Assessment

Δ Ask the client questions related to:

- Current stress, meaning of stressors, and ability to cope.

- Support systems.

- Compliance with the treatment regimen.

- Sleep patterns.

Δ   Observe the client's appearance and eye contact.

Δ   Measure vital signs.

Δ   Observe for irritability, anxiety, and tension.

NANDA Nursing Diagnoses

Δ   Anxiety

Δ   Caregiver role strain

Δ   Decisional conflict

Δ   Ineffective coping

Δ   Disturbed sleep pattern

Nursing Interventions

Stress	• Encourage health promotion strategies including regular exercise, optimal nutrition, and adequate sleep and rest. • Encourage appropriate relaxation techniques including breathing exercises, massage, imagery, yoga, and meditation. • Listen attentively, and take the time to understand the client's perspective. • Control the environment to reduce the number of external stressors including noise and breaks in continuity of care. • Identify available support systems. • Use effective communication techniques to foster the expression of feelings.
Coping	• Be empathetic in communication, and encourage the client to verbalize feelings. • Identify the strengths and abilities of the client and family. • Discuss the client and family's ability to deal with the current situation. • Encourage the client to describe coping skills that were effectively used in the past. • Identify available community resources, and refer for counseling if needed.
Compliance	• Put instructions in writing. • Allow the client to give input into the treatment regimen. • Simplify treatment regimens as much as possible. • Follow-up with the client to see if there are any questions or problems.

Primary Reference:

Potter, P. A., & Perry, A. G. (2005). *Fundamentals of nursing* (6th ed.). St. Louis, MO: Mosby.

Additional Resources:

Ackley, B. & Ladwig, G. (2005). *Nursing diagnosis handbook* (7th ed.). St. Louis, MO: Mosby.

Berman B., Erb, G., Kozier, B., & Snyder, S. (2004). *Fundamentals of nursing* (7th ed.). Upper Saddle River, NJ: Prentice Hall.

NANDA International (2004). *NANDA nursing diagnoses: Definitions and classification 2005-2006*. Philadelphia: NANDA.

Chapter 59: Stress, Adaptation, Coping, and Compliance

Application Exercises

Scenario: A nurse is caring for a client whose partner passed away 4 months ago in a motor vehicle crash. The client was diagnosed with diabetes at about the same time. He is tearful and states that he has had a difficult time adjusting to all of the recent difficulties in his life. He is unable to concentrate at work and is having a hard time managing his diabetes. His family lives nearby, and he sees them every week or two, but he does not want to burden them.

1. What would be a priority nursing diagnosis for this client?

2. While working with this client, he becomes very short-tempered and states, "How could you possibly understand what I am going through?" What would be an appropriate response?

3. What are two priority interventions for this client?

4. A client is diagnosed with cancer and is scheduled for testing and treatment. The client's partner responds to this by keeping a busy work schedule and asking when the client will return to work. Which of the following nursing diagnoses apply to the partner of this client? (Select all that apply.)

   _____ Coping, ineffective

   _____ Caregiver role strain

   _____ Fear

   _____ Anxiety

   _____ Readiness for enhanced family processes

5. Which of the following types of stress is being experienced by a middle adult client who is stressed by the concerns of caring for young adults still in the home and aging parents?

   A. Developmental

   B. Situational

   C. Social

   D. Cultural

Chapter 59: Stress, Adaptation, Coping, and Compliance

Application Exercises Answer Key

Scenario: A nurse is caring for a client whose partner passed away 4 months ago in a motor vehicle crash. The client was diagnosed with diabetes at about the same time. He is tearful and states that he has had a difficult time adjusting to all of the recent difficulties in his life. He is unable to concentrate at work and is having a hard time managing his diabetes. His family lives nearby, and he sees them every week or two, but he does not want to burden them.

1. What would be a priority nursing diagnosis for this client?

   Ineffective coping related to situational crisis and chronic condition secondary to the partner's sudden death and diagnosis of diabetes, as evidenced by the statement of inability to cope and difficulty adjusting to diabetes

2. While working with this client, he becomes very short-tempered and states, "How could you possibly understand what I am going through?" What would be an appropriate response?

   The nurse should validate that she is not in his situation. The nurse should also create a supportive and nonjudgmental environment so that that the client is able to express his frustrations.

3. What are two priority interventions for this client?

   Explore the client's methods of dealing with life problems in the past.

   Assess his knowledge of diabetes, and develop a teaching plan.

   Identify resources in the community, including family and friends.

4. A client is diagnosed with cancer and is scheduled for testing and treatment. The client's partner responds to this by keeping a busy work schedule and asking when the client will return to work. Which of the following nursing diagnoses apply to the partner of this client? (Select all that apply.)

   X   **Coping, ineffective**

   _____   Caregiver role strain

   X   **Fear**

   X   **Anxiety**

   _____   Readiness for enhanced family processes

The partner of the client is not coping effectively as evidenced by maintaining her current work schedule. Fear and anxiety are also appropriate nursing diagnoses due to the uncertainly of the client's health and what to expect from this diagnosis. The partner is not currently experiencing caregiver role strain but may at a future time. Readiness for enhanced family processes would be demonstrated by her willingness to openly communicate with her partner and modify her work schedule as needed to meet the family's new psychosocial needs.

5. Which of the following types of stress is being experienced by a middle adult client who is stressed by the concerns of caring for young adults still in the home and aging parents?

   A. Developmental

   B. Situational

   C. Social

   D. Cultural

This type of stress is related to the stages of life. Situational stress is an unexpected, sudden stressor like a job loss. Social and cultural stresses may include widespread problems like poverty that affect a community as a whole.

Unit 4

Section:

Chapter 60:

Supporting Psychosocial, Family, Cultural, and Spiritual Health

Psychosocial Health

Self-Concept, Body Image, and Sexuality

Shari Goldberg, MS, ARNP

 NCLEX® Connections:

Learning Objective: Review and apply knowledge within "**Self-Concept, Body Image, and Sexuality**" in readiness for performance of the following community health nursing activities as outlined by the NCLEX® test plans:

Δ Compare the client's response to unanticipated body image changes with the norm.

Δ Provide/plan support strategies for the client with an altered body image to achieve an optimal level of independence.

Δ Assess/monitor the client and family's feelings or thoughts on sexuality.

Δ Advise the client and/or family regarding issues of sexuality.

Δ Allow the client to verbalize issues associated with sexuality.

Δ Respect the sexual identity and lifestyle choices of the client.

Δ Encourage the client's healthy self-concept.

 Key Points

Δ **Self-concept**

- Self-concept is the way an individual views one's self. This involves conscious and unconscious thoughts, attitudes, and perceptions.

- Self-concept is subjective and includes self-identity, body image, role performance, and self-esteem.

- An individual with a positive self-concept tends to feel good about one's self.

- An individual's self-concept may be adversely affected by physical, spiritual, emotional, sexual, familial, or sociocultural stressors.

Δ **Body Image**

- Body image is a component of self-concept and refers to the way an individual perceives his/her appearance, size, body structure and/or function.

- Body image may be altered by normal growth and developmental changes. During adolescence, hormonal changes, including the development of secondary sex characteristics, influence one's body image. In the older population, changes in mobility, thinning and graying of hair, and decreased visual acuity impact body image.

- Body image may also be affected by external influences (e.g., movies, books, magazines).

Δ **Sexuality**

- Sexuality and sexual health are vital components of an individual's health, and like other aspects of health, they need to be part of a nursing assessment.

- A nurse needs to assess his/her own comfort level with issues related to sexuality. A client will sense any discomfort on the part of the nurse.

- Aspects of sexual health include knowledge of sexual behavior, understanding of normal growth and development, and the access to appropriate health care resources for the prevention and treatment of issues related to sexual health.

- Some of the skills that the nurse uses in dealing with client sexuality issues are knowledge of sexual growth and development and an understanding of what health problems and treatments may affect sexuality.

- An individual's sexuality and sexual health are influenced by self-concept, body image, gender identity, and sexual orientation.

Key Factors

Δ Self-concept

- Individuals with a high self-esteem are better equipped to cope successfully with life stressors.

- Stressors that affect self-concept include unrealistic expectations, surgery, chronic illness, and a change in role performance.

Δ Body Image

- Stressors that affect body image may include a loss of body parts secondary to an amputation, mastectomy or hysterectomy, a loss of body function secondary to arthritis, a spinal cord injury, a stroke, or an unattainable body ideal.

Δ Sexuality

- Sexuality is affected by one's developmental stage. For example, during adolescence, primary and secondary sex characteristics develop, menarche occurs, relationships involving sexual activity may develop, and masturbation is common.

- Sexuality is influenced by culture. Premarital sex, homosexuality, and polygamy may be viewed differently according to one's culture.

- An individual's health status is affected by one's sexuality. Certain conditions may alter sexual expression. For example, the presence of an STD may cause fear of transmission to a partner, leading to a decrease in sexual desire.

- Some prescription medications impact sexual functioning (e.g., diuretics decrease vaginal lubrication, cause erectile dysfunction, and decrease sexual desire).

Assessment

Subjective Data	Objective Data
• Cultural background • Quality of relationships • Feelings related to recent body image changes, self-concept, or issues of sexuality • Coping mechanisms used in the past • Expectations	• Posture • Appearance • Demeanor • Eye contact • Grooming • Unusual behaviors

NANDA Nursing Diagnoses

Δ Sexual dysfunction

Δ Anxiety

Δ Ineffective coping

Δ Disturbed body image

Δ Readiness for enhanced self-concept

Interventions

Self-concept	• Suggest a healthier lifestyle (e.g., exercise, diet, stress management). • Encourage the client to verbalize fears or anxieties. • Use therapeutic communication skills to assist the client with self-awareness. • Encourage the use of effective coping skills. • Reinforce successes and strengths.
Body image	• Establish a therapeutic relationship with the client. A caring and nonjudgmental manner puts the client at ease and fosters meaningful communication. • Ensure privacy and confidentiality. Many sensitive issues may be discussed, and the client needs to know that these issues are safe to discuss. • Identify individuals who may be at risk for body image disturbances. • Acknowledge anger, depression, and denial as normal feelings when adjusting to body changes. • Encourage the client to participate in the plan of care. • Arrange for a visit from a volunteer who has experienced a similar body image change.

Sexuality	• Allow the client to discuss issues and/or concerns related to sexuality.
	• Be straightforward with questions, "Are you or have you been concerned about sexual functioning since your surgery?"
	• Health promotion: Determine the client's current knowledge base and provide education as needed.
	• Acute care: Increase awareness through the introduction or clarification of information, and refer the client for counseling if necessary.
	• Inform the client of available resources and support groups.
	• Discuss alternative means of sexual expression if the client experiences a change in body functioning or structure (e.g., hugging, cuddling).

Primary Reference:

Potter, P. A., & Perry, A. G. (2005). *Fundamentals of nursing* (6th ed.). St. Louis, MO: Mosby.

Additional Resources:

Ackley, B. & Ladwig, G. (2005). *Nursing diagnosis handbook* (7th ed.). St. Louis, MO: Mosby.

Berman B., Erb, G., Kozier, B., & Snyder, S. (2004). *Fundamentals of nursing* (7th ed.). Upper Saddle River, NJ: Prentice Hall.

NANDA International (2004). *NANDA nursing diagnoses: Definitions and classification 2005-2006*. Philadelphia: NANDA.

Chapter 62: Self-Concept, Body Image, and Sexuality

Application Exercises

Scenario: A woman had a mastectomy related to breast cancer 6 months ago. She has an appointment for an annual exam today. During the health history, the nurse asks how she is doing, and how she has been coping since her mastectomy. She reluctantly admits that she has not had much of a desire for sex since her surgery, relating "my body is so different now." The nurse encourages her to discuss this in more detail through effective communication skills. The client shares that she does not feel attractive and that she is still mourning the loss of her breast.

1. How do sexual function and psychosocial health impact one another?

2. What are some factors that would influence the nurse's ability to discuss sexual issues with the client?

3. What would be some effective nursing interventions for this client?

4. True or False: In an older adult, problems with sexual response are often affected by illness and medication.

5. Which of the following factors positively affect self-concept? (Select all that apply.)

_____ An amputation

_____ Parental approval

_____ Success at school

_____ Receiving a promotion at work

_____ Excessive use of alcohol

Chapter 62: Self-Concept, Body Image, and Sexuality

Application Exercises Answer Key

Scenario: A woman had a mastectomy related to breast cancer 6 months ago. She has an appointment for an annual exam today. During the health history, the nurse asks how she is doing, and how she has been coping since her mastectomy. She reluctantly admits that she has not had much of a desire for sex since her surgery, relating "my body is so different now." The nurse encourages her to discuss this in more detail through effective communication skills. The client shares that she does not feel attractive and that she is still mourning the loss of her breast.

1. How do sexual function and psychosocial health impact one another?

> **There is a direct relationship between psychosocial health and sexual function. Increased health will increase the likelihood of sexual desire and function.**

2. What are some factors that would influence the nurse's ability to discuss sexual issues with the client?

> **The nurse's therapeutic communication skills**

> **The nurse's thorough self-assessment of his/her sexuality, and a level of comfort in discussing sexuality as an important part of an individual's overall health status**

> **An understanding of how one's health impacts sexuality**

3. What would be some effective nursing interventions for this client?

> **Complete a sexual health history.**

> **Observe for and assist with the grief process related to the mastectomy.**

> **Include other members of the healthcare team in providing care for the client.**

4. True or False: In an older adult, problems with sexual response are often affected by illness and medication.

> **True: Some illnesses and medications affect the ability to respond sexually.**

5. Which of the following factors positively affect self-concept? (Select all that apply.)

_____ An amputation

__X__ **Parental approval**

__X__ **Success at school**

__X__ **Receiving a promotion at work**

_____ Excessive use of alcohol

Parental approval, success at school, and receiving a promotion at work all have a positive impact on the individual's self-concept, as these situations promote good feelings about self-concept. An amputation usually has a negative impact on self-concept requiring the client to adapt to the changes. Excessive use of alcohol is a symptom of a poor self-concept.

Unit 4   Supporting Psychosocial, Family, Cultural, and Spiritual Health

Section: Family Health

Chapter 61:   Assessment of Family Systems and Family Dynamics

Contributor: Ann Schide, MSN, MS, RN, LCCE

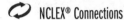 NCLEX® Connections

> **Learning Objective**: Review and apply knowledge within **"Assessment of Family Systems and Family Dynamics"** in readiness for performance of the following nursing activities as outlined by the NCLEX® test plans:
>
> Δ   Develop a therapeutic relationship with families of diverse ages and backgrounds.
>
> Δ   Promote, maintain, and restore the health of families during stressful situations.

 Key Points

Δ   **Family** is defined by the client.

Δ   Five realms of processes involved in family function should be considered during the assessment of a family.

- Interactive

- Developmental

- Coping

- Integrity

- Health

Δ   Assessment of a family can focus on family as a **context**, a **client**, or a **system**.

Δ   Families and clients are not mutually exclusive; thus, **family-centered care** creates a holistic approach to nursing care.

Δ   Family dynamics are constantly evolving due to the processes of family life and developmental stages of the family members.

Key Factors

Δ **Current trends**

• **Family forms**

◊ Nuclear – wife, husband, child(ren)

◊ Extended – nuclear plus relative(s)

◊ Blended – nuclear plus stepchildren; families of divorce with remarriage

◊ Alternative – "skipped" generation households, nonfamilies (single adults living alone), cohabiting partners, and homosexual couples

• **Marital roles**

◊ Single-income families

◊ Dual or greater-income families

• Fastest growing population – those over 65 years old leading to **caregiver** issues

• **Homelessness** – lack of stable environment, financial issues, and inadequate access to health care

• **Family violence** and its endless cycle

• **HIV** with its decreasing death rate but continued disruption of the family unit

Δ **Attributes of Families**

• **Structure** dictates the family's ability to cope.

◊ **Rigid** structure is dictatorial and strict.

◊ **Open** structure includes few or no boundaries or consistent behaviors or consequences.

◊ **Either** structure may provide positive or negative outcomes.

• **Functions**

◊ Communication

◊ Goal setting

◊ Conflict resolution

◊ Caregiving

◊ Nurturing

Assessment

Δ   All clients are assessed within the context of the family.

Δ   A family can be assessed by looking at structure and function.

Δ   Identify who is a family member, what role each family member undertakes, and the dynamic interactions within the family.

Δ   Listen attentively, and use therapeutic communication techniques of reflection and restatement to clarify the family concerns.

Δ   Cultural variables – all of which may vary between and within generations within a family

- Perception of events

- Rites and rituals

- Health beliefs

NANDA Nursing Diagnoses

Δ   Compromised family coping

Δ   Disabled family coping

Δ   Readiness for enhanced family coping

Δ   Dysfunctional family processes: alcoholism

Nursing Interventions

Δ   Identify and adapt family strengths to perceived stressor(s).

- Communication

- Adaptability

- Nurturing

- Crisis as a growth element

- Parenting skills

- Resiliency

Δ   Set goals with the family that are realistic.

Δ   Provide information on support networks.

- Child and adult day care

- Caregiver support groups

Δ   Promote family unity.

Δ   Encourage conflict resolution when it exists.

Δ   Minimize family process disruption effects.

Δ   Remove barriers to health promotion.

Δ   Increase family members' abilities to participate.

Δ   Perform interventions that the family cannot perform.

Δ   Evaluate goals within the context of the family by checking back to ensure that goals were realistic and achievable.

Primary Reference:

Potter, P. A., & Perry, A. G. (2005). *Fundamentals of nursing* (6th ed.). St. Louis, MO: Mosby.

Additional Resources:

NANDA International (2004). *NANDA nursing diagnoses: Definitions and classification 2005-2006*. Philadelphia: NANDA.

Wilkinson, J. M. (2005). *Nursing diagnosis handbook*. Upper Saddle River, NJ: Prentice Hall.

Chapter 61: Assessment of Family Systems and Family Dynamics

Application Exercises

Scenario: A home health nurse performs a 3-day postpartum visit for a first time mother. The household includes her husband, her mother, and her father, all of whom are Hispanic. All of the members of the family, with the exception of the new mother, work outside the home. Upon assessing the newborn, the nurse notes a coin bound to the infant's umbilicus.

1. What type of family form is represented here? Why?

2. What health care issues can be anticipated by the home health nurse?

3. When promoting health in this new family structure, how will this nurse proceed?

4. What should be a priority nursing intervention for a family experiencing violence?

        A. Removing the children from the home

        B. Assessing the family in context

        C. Refining the family communication skills

        D. Using the family's strengths to define them

5. Which of the following interventions is the most beneficial in promoting the health of a caregiver who is providing care to a disabled relative?

        A. Arrange for Meals-on-Wheels.

        B. Refer the disabled client to long-term care.

        C. Provide information on local adult day care.

        D. Mention the good things the caregiver does.

6. Which of the following nursing approaches should work best with a family using an open structure for coping with crisis?

        A. Prescribing tasks unilaterally

        B. Delegating care to one member

        C. Speaking to the primary client privately

        D. Convening a family counsel

Chapter 61: Assessment of Family Systems and Family Dynamics

Application Exercises Answer Key

Scenario: A home health nurse performs a 3-day postpartum visit for a first time mother. The household includes her husband, her mother, and her father, all of whom are Hispanic. All of the members of the family, with the exception of the new mother, work outside the home. Upon assessing the newborn, the nurse notes a coin bound to the infant's umbilicus.

1. What type of family form is represented here? Why?

   This is an extended family because in addition to the nuclear family unit (primary husband, wife, and child), there exists grandparents in the same household.

2. What health care issues can be anticipated by the home health nurse?

   The new mother will provide most of the daily care to the newborn without assistance from her family members, since all adults except the mother of the newborn work outside the home. The new mother may be prone to fatigue, stress, or postpartum depression.

   Culturally accepted practices need to be incorporated into the nurse's plan of care with consideration for potential harm.

3. In promoting health in this new family structure, how will this nurse proceed?

   Identify strengths of each family member and ways these strengths can be used to contribute to the family's health.

   Identify areas of adaptability and successful coping in previous crisis/stressful situations.

4. What should be a priority nursing intervention for a family experiencing violence?

    A. Removing the children from the home

    B. Assessing the family in context

    C. Refining the family communication skills

    D. Using the family's strengths to define them

It is important to assess which family member or members is a victim of abuse and needs assistance to be protected. Removing the children from the home may be an option, but first there needs to be a family assessment to determine if there are safety issues. Refining family communication skills and using family strengths are not the priorities if the safety of a family member is in jeopardy.

5. Which of the following interventions is the most beneficial in promoting the health of a caregiver who is providing care to a disabled relative?

    A. Arrange for Meals-on-Wheels.

    B. Refer the disabled client to long-term care.

    C. Provide information on local adult day care.

    D. Mention the good things the caregiver does.

Providing respite care for a caregiver allows the caregiver to take care of himself. Arranging for Meals-on-Wheels may provide some assistance to the caregiver, and offering verbal support may be beneficial, but this is not as beneficial as respite care. Referring the disabled client to long-term care may not be an option for this family.

6. Which of the following nursing approaches should work best with a family using an open structure for coping with crisis?

    A. Prescribing tasks unilaterally

    B. Delegating care to one member

    C. Speaking to the primary client privately

    D. Convening a family counsel

An open structure is loose, and counseling would give all family members input. Prescribing tasks and delegating care are too rigid for acceptance by a family with an open structure. Speaking to the primary client privately excludes the family.

Unit 4

Section:

Supporting Psychosocial, Family, Cultural, and Spiritual Health

Family Health

Chapter 62:   Situational Role Changes

Contributor: Ann Schide, MSN, MS, RN, LCCE

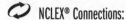 **NCLEX® Connections:**

Learning Objective: Review and apply knowledge within **"Situational Role Changes"** in readiness for performance of the following nursing activities as outlined by the NCLEX® test plans:

Δ Recognize situations that may alter roles for the client and/or family (e.g., illness, loss of a job, move of a close friend).

Δ Assess/monitor the client and family for their ability to adjust to situational role changes.

Δ Offer community resources that assist the client and family in adjusting to new or lost roles.

Δ Encourage the client and family to verbalize their apprehensions concerning role changes.

Δ Evaluate the client and family's adaptation to situational role changes.

 Key Points

Δ A **role** is the function a person adopts within his life. It seldom is limited to one role, but rather is multidimensional and is often relative to the role of others.

- Grandparent

- Parent

- Dependent child

- Employee/employer

- Church member

- Committee member

- Community activist

Δ **Stress** impacts roles in many ways.

- Role conflict

- Sick role

- Role ambiguity

- Role strain

- Role overload

Δ The presence of **stressors** will delay a client's return to health in the same way that the presence of a foreign body or infection will delay the healing of a wound.

Δ One way illness causes role stress is that it creates a **situation** where **roles** may and do **change** simply due to the impact and progression of the illness.

Δ Nurses need to be aware of a client's roles in life, as well as how the situation of illness might change these roles, either temporarily or permanently.

Δ A basic assumption is that a client can either advance or regress in the face of a **situational role change**.

Key Factors

Δ Types of role problems include:

- **Role conflict** – the taking on of two or more roles that are contradictory (e.g., mother of a teen who now must also care for her mother).

- **Sick role** – expectations of society about how one should behave when ill (e.g., caring for oneself while trying to engage in a job role).

- **Role ambiguity** – confusion over role expectations (e.g., introduction of high technology that will cause an employee to question his current role and whether or not he will have a company role in the future).

- **Role strain** – combines ambiguity and conflict when a person feels unsuited for a role that he may not have chosen if given the freedom to do so (e.g., frustration occurring when a role is taken that conflicts with the societal norm – man in a woman's role and vice versa).

- **Role overload** – having more roles than what is manageable (e.g., meeting all the demands of work roles and home roles leaving little time for the personal role).

Δ Situational **Role Changes**

- Encountered by nurses with every client served

- Caused by situations other than normal physical growth and development (e.g., marriage, job changes, divorce)

- Can disrupt one or more of the client's roles in life, such as illness or hospitalization

- With resolution, can attribute to healing in the physical, mental, and spiritual realms

    ◊ Temporary role changes – The client will resume role upon resolution of illness.

    ◊ Permanent role changes – Illness has altered the level of the client's health to a point that previous role(s) are no longer available.

Assessment

Δ Identify what roles the client perceives as owning.

Δ Identify the client roles as perceived by significant others.

Δ Validate any discrepancies.

Δ Identify the impact the loss or addition of a role is having on the client. The client may grieve the loss.

Δ Identify who will now take on the client's role while the client cannot perform.

Δ Questions to consider in assessment phase of care

- Client as primary wage earner in family

    ◊ How does illness influence family finances?

    ◊ Who will provide for family fiscal soundness during illness?

    ◊ Should this role be permanently removed from the client, and how will the family meet fiscal needs?

- Client as caregiver

    ◊ Who will fill this role during the client's illness for the person(s) being cared for?

    ◊ Who will fill this role for the client if the client requires a caregiver?

    ◊ What is happening to those to whom the client gave care now that the client is no longer able to fulfill that role?

NANDA Nursing Diagnoses

Δ Caregiver role strain

Δ Parental role conflict

Δ Ineffective role performance

Nursing Interventions

Δ   Provide short-term care to provide relief for family caregiver.

Δ   Provide encouragement during times of stress.

Δ   Seek congruence among perceived roles.

Δ   Prepare the client for the anticipated situation crisis.

Δ   Anticipate role conflict or overload on the client's part.

Δ   Assist the client to improve relationships by supplementing specific role behaviors.

Δ   Explore which roles the client can relinquish.

Δ   Assist the client to improve personal judgment of self-worth given current situational role change.

Δ   Counsel the client about roles that are permanently altered.

Δ   Refer to community services for outpatient adaptation to lost or new roles.

Δ   Refer to social services for assistance in some roles.

Δ   Evaluate the client after he has accepted the role change(s) to see if adaptation has occurred.

Primary Reference:

Potter, P. A., & Perry, A. G. (2005). *Fundamentals of nursing* (6th ed.). St. Louis, MO: Mosby.

Additional Resources:

NANDA International (2004). *NANDA nursing diagnoses: Definitions and classification 2005-2006*. Philadelphia: NANDA.

Wilkinson, J. M. (2005). *Nursing diagnosis handbook*. Upper Saddle River, NJ: Prentice Hall.

Chapter 62: Situational Role Changes

Application Exercises

Scenario: A mother of two young children who works outside the home part-time is involved in a motor vehicle crash that causes paraplegia.

1. What roles may change for this client given the current situation?

2. What assessments should be performed by the nurse concerning the client's roles?

3. What interventions might the nurse implement?

4. Which of the following is considered a situational role change?

        A. A young adult getting married for the first time

        B. An adolescent experiencing puberty

        C. A middle adult experiencing menopause

        D. A toddler learning to control elimination

5. Once a client has been counseled about her situational role changes and has accepted them, what will be the next step in recovery for her?

        A. Adaptation

        B. Resentment

        C. Tension

        D. Apprehension

Chapter 62: Situational Role Changes

Application Exercises Answer Key

Scenario: A mother of two young children who works outside the home part-time is involved in a motor vehicle crash that causes paraplegia.

1. What roles may change for this client given the current situation?

   Her ability to provide care to her children

   Her ability to earn income

   Her ability to transport her children

2. What assessments should be performed by the nurse concerning the client's roles?

   Relationship with other family members

   Proximity of other family members to the client

   Ability of other family adults to provide care for the children

   Immediate needs of the family

3. What interventions might the nurse implement?

   Connecting directly to other family members to evaluate how they might be able to assist

   Referring to social services for fiscal needs

   Involving community agencies to provide rehabilitation for the client

4. Which of the following is considered a situational role change?

   A. A young adult getting married for the first time
   B. An adolescent experiencing puberty
   C. A middle adult experiencing menopause
   D. A toddler learning to control elimination

   Marriage adds the role of spouse. Puberty, menopause, and elimination control are normal physiologic growth and development occurrences and are not considered situational role changes.

5. Once a client has been counseled about her situational role changes and has accepted them, what will be the next step in recovery for her?

   A. Adaptation
   B. Resentment
   C. Tension
   D. Apprehension

   A client who has accepted role changes will demonstrate adaptation. Resentment, tension, and apprehension are not behaviors/emotions consistent with acceptance.

Unit 4   Supporting Psychosocial, Family, Cultural, and Spiritual Health

Section: Cultural Health

Chapter 63:   Culturally Competent Care

Contributor: Linda Turchin, MSN, RN

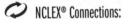 NCLEX® Connections:

Learning Objective: Review and apply knowledge within **"Culturally Competent Care"** in readiness for performance of the following nursing activities as outlined by the NCLEX® test plans:

Δ   Identify the impact of cultural, spiritual, and psychosocial factors when providing care to clients.

Δ   Assess/monitor the client for needs related to culture (e.g., language barriers, education, and personal space).

Δ   Provide written teaching materials in the client/family's language.

Δ   Select appropriate interpreters to assist in helping the client/family/significant others understand health care.

Δ   Serve as interpreter for health care providers per facility policy and state law.

Δ   Respect the client's cultural practices and the impact they have on activities of daily living.

Δ   Plan/provide care that is sensitive to the client's culture (e.g., space and time orientation, and care of the dying).

Δ   Document how care was adapted to meet cultural needs.

 Key Points

Δ   **Culture** is a collection of learned, adaptive, and transmitted social values and beliefs that form the context from which a group interprets the human experience.

Δ   **Communication, dietary preferences, and dress** are influenced by culture.

Δ   Being a multicultural society, nursing in the United States requires **transcultural** nursing care that is **culturally competent**. Effectiveness depends on the nurse's understanding of both her/his personal culture, as well as that of the client.

Δ **Ethnocentrism** is the belief that one's culture is superior to others and interferes with culturally competent care.

Δ Nurses should accommodate the client's cultural beliefs and values whenever possible unless they are in direct conflict with known health practices.

Δ **Acculturation** occurs when a client is living in a new dominant culture and adopts those patterns of behaviors.

Δ In order to meet the client's cultural needs, a nurse must first perform a **cultural assessment** to identify those needs.

Δ When a culturally motivated behavior is in conflict with good client care, the behavior will need to be repatterned.

Key Factors

Δ Culture evolves as:

- Knowledge.

- Values.

  ◊ Values are a set of rules by which individuals in a culture live.

  ◊ Values guide decision making and behavior. For example, health promotion and maintenance are valued, and so monthly self-breast examinations are done.

  ◊ Values are unconsciously developed during childhood.

- Beliefs.

- Art.

- Morals and law.

- Customs and habits.

Δ Culture evolves over time and is shared by a group who has similar needs and life experiences.

Δ While the cultural values are shared among all within the culture, diversity exists, forming **subcultures,** and is based upon the following:

- Age.

- Gender.

- Marital status.

- Family structure.

- Income.

- Education level.

- Religious views.

- Life experiences.

Δ **Transcultural nursing** focuses on the comparison and analysis of cultures and subcultures to respond to individual client values and needs, and not on a predetermined criteria formulated by the culture of the primary care provider.

- It involves the complex integration of knowledge, attitudes, and skills.

- It is achieved through cultural:

  ◊ **Awareness** – appreciation and sensitivity to the culture of others that includes awareness of one's own cultural beliefs, including biases (favoritism) and prejudices (discrimination).

  ◊ **Knowledge** – sufficient comparative data regarding a culture's understanding of health and wellness issues (e.g., client's beliefs regarding what causes illness and how it should be treated).

  ◊ **Skills** – ability to assess the factors related to the care and treatment of individuals within the culture (e.g., health histories and culturally specific assessments).

  ◊ **Encounters** – sufficient interaction with members of the culture.

  ◊ **Desires** – motivation and desire to learn about and from the culture.

Assessment

Δ Perform the cultural assessment in a language that is common to both nurse and client, or employ an interpreter. Assess gestures, vocal tones, and inflections.

Data to be Collected	Example
Cultural background and the amount of acculturation that has occurred	Client was born in Central America and has been a resident of New York for 2 years.
Health and wellness beliefs/practices	There may be a reliance on folk medicine to treat or prevent illness.
Family patterns	The client may be from a patriarchal culture where the oldest male family member makes decisions for all family members.
Verbal and nonverbal communication	In some cultures, it is disrespectful to make direct eye contact.
Space and time orientation	In some cultures, little importance is placed on how past behavior affects future health.
Nutritional patterns	Certain foods may have healing properties.
Meaning of pain	Pain is viewed as a punishment for misbehavior or sin.
Death rituals	In some cultures, suicide is accepted.

Δ   Methods for **assessing culture include**:

- **Observation** – study the client and his environment for examples of cultural relevance.

- **Interview**

  ◊   Establish a **therapeutic relationship** with the client when possible/appropriate. This may be hindered by misinterpretations of communication.

    °   Verbal (language)

    °   Behavior (nonverbal)

  ◊   Use focused, open-ended, and nonjudgmental questions.

- **Participation**

  ◊   Involvement in **culturally related activities** outside the health care setting

  ◊   Awareness of population demographics include:

    °   Number of members in a practice area.

    °   Average educational and economic levels.

    °   Typical occupations.

    °   Commonly practiced religion(s)/spiritual beliefs.

    °   Incidence of most common illnesses/health issues.

    °   Most commonly held health, wellness, and death beliefs.

    °   Social organization.

NANDA Nursing Diagnoses

Δ   Impaired verbal communication

Δ   Relocation stress syndrome

Δ   Risk for relocation stress syndrome

Δ   Social isolation

Δ   Spiritual distress

Nursing Interventions

Δ   **Religion/spirituality/death rituals**

- Respect the religious/spiritual practices of the client.

- Death rituals vary among cultures, and the nurse must be prepared to facilitate such practices whenever possible.

Δ Pain

- Recognize that the way pain is reacted to and displayed varies by culture.

- Use an alterative to the pain scale (1 to 10) as it may not appropriately reflect the pain evaluation of all cultures.

- Explore religious beliefs that may influence the meaning of pain.

Δ Nutrition

- Provide for food choices and preparation that are consistent with cultural beliefs.

- As possible, allow the client to consume foods that may be viewed as a treatment for illness.

- Communicate food intolerances/allergies to dietary staff that are related to ethnicity.

Δ Communication

- Improve the nurse/client communication when cultural variations exist.

- Use interpreters when the communication barrier is great enough to impact the exchange of information between the nurse and client.

- Cautiously use nonverbal communication, as it may have very different meanings for the client and the nurse.

Δ Family patterns and gender roles – Communicate with and include the person who has the authority to make decisions in the family.

Δ Culture and Life Transitions

- Assist families as they mark rituals (rites of passage) that symbolize cultural values.

- Common events that are often expressed with cultural rituals include:

  ◊ Puberty.

  ◊ Pregnancy.

  ◊ Childbirth.

  ◊ Dying and death.

Δ   Repatterning

- Accommodate the client's cultural beliefs and values as much as is in the client's best interest.

- When a cultural value/behavior is a direct hindrance to the client's health/ wellness, the nurse should attempt to **repattern** that belief to one that is compatible with health promotion.

Primary Reference:

Potter, P. A., & Perry, A. G. (2005). *Fundamentals of nursing* (6th ed.). St. Louis, MO: Mosby.

Additional Resources:

Lewis, Heitkemper, and Dirksen (2004). *Medical surgical nursing: Assessment and management of clinical problems* (6th ed.). St. Louis, MO: Mosby.

NANDA International (2004). *NANDA nursing diagnoses: Definitions and classification 2005-2006*. Philadelphia: NANDA.

Chapter 63: Culturally Competent Care

Application Exercises

Scenario: A nurse is caring for a woman who speaks and understands little English and has only recently immigrated to the United States. She appears very anxious and extremely reluctant to accept that the recommended treatment plan will work.

1. Identify several factors that will affect the nurse's cultural assessment of this client.

2. What assessments must be obtained in order for the nurse to provide culturally competent care for this client?

Scenario: A client with limited proficiency in English is hospitalized with abdominal pain. He becomes very agitated when the nurse attempts to remove a religious medallion from around his neck during a bath.

3. How should the nurse respond to the client's behavior?

4. What is the importance of the nurse's behavior?

5. How should the nurse go about determining why the client reacted in such a manner?

6. The belief that one's culture is superior to others is called

        A. ethnocentrism.

        B. competent care.

        C. repatterning.

        D. acculturation.

Chapter 63: Culturally Competent Care

Application Exercises Answer Key

Scenario: A nurse is caring for a woman who speaks and understands little English and has only recently immigrated to the United States. She appears very anxious and extremely reluctant to accept that the recommended treatment plan will work.

1. Identify several factors that will affect the nurse's cultural assessment of this client.

   Language/communication issues

   Cultural beliefs related to health and wellness

   Unfamiliarity with the client's health care customs

2. What assessments must be obtained in order for the nurse to provide culturally competent care for this client?

   Interview and gather data related to the client's cultural values and beliefs related to the following:

   Health and wellness beliefs/practices

   Family patterns

   Verbal and nonverbal communication

   Space and time orientation

   Nutritional patterns

   Meanings of pain

   Death rituals

Scenario: A client with limited proficiency in English is hospitalized with abdominal pain. He becomes very agitated when the nurse attempts to remove a religious medallion from around his neck during a bath.

3. How should the nurse respond to the client's behavior?

The nurse should stop attempting to remove the medallion and apologize.

4. What is the importance of the nurse's behavior?

The nurse insulted/upset the client by attempting to interfere with a cultural or religious practice. This may negatively affect the development of a therapeutic relationship with him.

5. How should the nurse go about determining why the client reacted in such a manner?

If the client is able to understand and communicate in English, the nurse should ask him open-ended questions in a nonthreatening fashion. The questions should be directed at his beliefs regarding the importance of the medallion and how he expects the nurse to address those needs in the future. If communication is a problem, then asking family members or using an interpreter is appropriate.

6. The belief that one's culture is superior to others is called

    A. ethnocentrism.
    B. competent care.
    C. repatterning.
    D. acculturation.

Ethnocentrism is the belief that one's own culture is superior to others. Competent care refers to care that accommodates the client's culture as much as is possible and appropriate. Repatterning refers to working with clients to repattern beliefs to those that are compatible with health promotion. Acculturation refers to the degree to which a client adopts the behaviors of a new dominant culture.

Unit 4
Section:

Supporting Psychosocial, Family, Cultural, and Spiritual Health
Spiritual Health

Chapter 64:   Spiritual Care

Contributor: Ann Schide, MSN, MS, RN, LCCE

 NCLEX® Connections:

> **Learning Objective**: Review and apply knowledge within **"Spiritual Care"** in readiness for performance of the following nursing activities as outlined by the NCLEX® test plans:
>
> Δ   Assess/monitor the client and family's spiritual needs and beliefs.
>
> Δ   Plan/provide care that is respectful and sensitive to the client's spiritual beliefs.
>
> Δ   Evaluate the client and family's achievement of spiritual health.

 Key Points

Δ   Traditional concepts in spiritual health include:

- Spirituality.

- Faith.

- Hope.

- Religion.

Δ   **Spiritual distress** arises when catastrophic events interrupt the individual's sense of being.

Δ   **Spiritual distress** can occur during the following:

- **Acute illnesses.**

  ◊   This poses an immediate threat to an individual.

  ◊   Anger over temporary or long-term loss can be directed toward the higher power.

  ◊   Conflicts center on the perceived meaning of life.

- **Chronic illnesses** – are usually associated with some degree of dependence on others, which can lead to a sense of powerlessness.

582

- **Terminal illnesses.**

    ◊ There is a fear of the unknown.

    ◊ This is a time of reflection and questioning the meaning of life.

- **Near-death experiences.**

    ◊ There is seldom a desire to discuss the event.

    ◊ Any discussion can bring meaning and power to the experience.

- All of these points present an opportunity for a person to question any part of her spiritual self.

Δ Nursing **interventions** are directed at identification, restoration, and/or reconnection of a client and/or family to spiritual strength.

Key Factors

Δ **Congruence**, or the balance of life's patterns and rhythms, is a state that cannot be achieved but is continuously being sought.

Δ Humans attempt to intervene in crises and incongruence through exertion of **control** in the spiritual realm.

Δ Traditional Concepts in Spiritual Health

- **Spirituality** implies connectedness.

    ◊ Intrapersonal – within one's self

    ◊ Interpersonal – with others and the environment

    ◊ Transpersonal – with an unseen higher power

- **Faith**

    ◊ Can be defined by a culture or a religion

    ◊ Can be defined as a relationship with a higher power

    ◊ **An agnostic** – one who believes that a higher power is unknown or does not exist

    ◊ **An atheist** – one who does not believe in the existence of God

- **Hope** is a multidimensional concept that provides comfort during crises.

- **Religion** is a system of beliefs practiced outwardly to express one's spirituality.

Δ   Spiritual rituals and observances include:

Religion	Birth Rituals and Health Care Decisions	Death Rituals	Dietary Rituals
Hinduism	Those practicing Hinduism do not prolong life.	• The client may want to lie on the floor while dying. • Thread is placed around the neck/wrist. • The client pours water in the mouth. • The family bathes the body. • The client may want to be cremated.	Some are vegetarians.
Buddhism	Those practicing Buddhism may refuse care on holy days.	• Call the priest to deliver last rites. • Chanting is common.	• Some are vegetarians. • Those practicing Buddhism avoid alcohol and tobacco. • Client may fast on holy days.
Islam	At birth, a prayer is said in the infant's ear.	• The dying confesses sin. • The body faces east – Mecca. • The body is washed and enveloped in a white clot. • A prayer is said.	• Those practicing Islam avoid alcohol and pork. • Client may fast during Ramadan.
Judaism	On the eighth day after birth, males are circumcised.	• Someone stays with the body. • Burial society prepares the body.	Some may practice a Kosher diet.
Christianity	Some will baptize infants at birth.	Some will give last rites.	• Some avoid alcohol, tobacco, and caffeine. • Client may fast during Lent.
Mormonism	Newborns are baptized.	• Last rites are given. • Communion is offered. • Burial is preferred.	Those practicing Mormonism avoid alcohol, tobacco, and caffeine.
Jehovah's Witnesses	Jehovah's Witnesses do not accept blood transfusions.	The client can choose burial or cremation.	The client will avoid foods having, or prepared with, blood.

Assessment

- Δ Primary – self-reflection (nurse) on personal beliefs and spirituality

- Δ Initial – identifying the client's religion, if any

- Δ Focused – ongoing, as nurse identifies the clients at risk for spiritual distress

- Δ Highly subjective area requiring the development of rapport and trust among the client, family, and healthcare provider(s)

- Δ Assessment of the client includes:

  - Faith/beliefs.

  - Perception of life and self-responsibility.

  - Satisfaction with life.

  - Culture.

  - Fellowship and perceived place in community.

  - Rituals and practices.

  - Incorporation of spirituality within profession/work place.

  - Client expectations for health care in relation to spirituality (e.g., traditional vs alternative paths, such as shamans, priests, prayer).

NANDA Nursing Diagnoses

- Δ Chronic sorrow

- Δ Hopelessness

- Δ Risk for spiritual distress

- Δ Readiness for enhanced spiritual well-being

Nursing Interventions

- Δ Identify the client's perception for the existence of a higher power.

- Δ Facilitate growth in the client's abilities to connect with a higher power.

- Δ Assist the client to feel connected or reconnected to a higher power by

  - allowing time and/or resources for the practice of religious rituals.

  - providing privacy for prayer, meditation, or the reading of religious materials.

- Δ Facilitate development of a positive outcome in a particular situation.

- Δ Provide stability for the person experiencing a dysfunctional spiritual mood.

Δ   Establish a caring presence in "being with" the client and family rather than merely performing tasks for them.

Δ   Support all healing relationships.

- Holistic approach to care – seeing the large picture for the client

- Using client-identified spiritual resources and needs

Δ   Identify and provide for the client's support system.

- Family

- Community

- Pastoral

- Religious artifacts and rituals

Δ   Be aware of diet therapies included in spiritual beliefs.

Δ   Support religious rituals.

- Icons

- Statues

- Prayer rugs

- Devotional reads

- Music

Δ   Support restorative care.

- Prayer

- Meditation

- Grief work

Δ   Evaluation of care is ongoing and continuous, with a need for flexibility as the client and family process the current crisis through their spiritual identity.

Primary Reference:

Potter, P. A., & Perry, A. G. (2005). *Fundamentals of nursing* (6th ed.). St. Louis, MO: Mosby.

Additional Resources:

NANDA International (2004). *NANDA nursing diagnoses: Definitions and classification 2005-2006*. Philadelphia: NANDA.

Wilkinson, J. M. (2005). *Nursing diagnosis handbook*. Upper Saddle River, NJ: Prentice Hall.

Chapter 64: Spiritual Care

Application Exercises

1. A client is observed crying as he reads from his devotional book. What intervention would be the most appropriate?

> A. Contact the hospital's spiritual services.
>
> B. Inquire as to what is making him cry.
>
> C. Provide quiet times for these moments.
>
> D. Turn on the television for a distraction.

2. True or False: A nurse does not need to complete a spiritual assessment on a client who states that she does not belong to any organized religion.

3. A terminally ill client tells the nurse that he believes God has abandoned him. Which of the following nursing diagnoses is most appropriate?

> A. Powerlessness
>
> B. Chronic sorrow
>
> C. Spiritual distress
>
> D. Readiness for enhanced spirituality

4. Match the following terms with the description.

_____ Hope	A. Connectedness with a higher power, one's self, others, and the environment
_____ Congruence	B. Multidimensional concept that provides comfort during crisis
_____ Spirituality	C. The balance of life's patterns and rhythms
_____ Religion	D. System of beliefs practiced outwardly to express one's spirituality

Chapter 64: Spiritual Care

Application Exercises Answer Key

1. A client is observed crying as he reads from his devotional book. What intervention would be the most appropriate?

        A. Contact the hospital's spiritual services.

        B. Inquire as to what is making him cry.

        C. Provide quiet times for these moments.

        D. Turn on the television for a distraction.

Providing privacy and time for the reading of religious materials supports the spiritual health of the client. Contacting the hospital's spiritual services presumes there is a problem. Asking the client about the crying or providing a distraction could be interpreted as discounting or being disrespectful of the client's beliefs.

2. True or False: A nurse does not need to complete a spiritual assessment on a client who states that she does not belong to any organized religion.

False: A client can still have spiritual needs that need to be addressed even when he/she is not a member of an organized religion.

3. A terminally ill client tells the nurse that he believes God has abandoned him. Which of the following nursing diagnoses is most appropriate?

        A. Powerlessness

        B. Chronic sorrow

        C. Spiritual distress

        D. Readiness for enhanced spirituality

The client is expressing disconnectedness to a higher being, which is creating "spiritual distress." Powerlessness and chronic sorrow could be a result of spiritual distress, but neither is the most encompassing diagnosis. Readiness for enhanced spirituality is appropriate for a client who is experiencing spiritual health and is seeking growth.

4. Match the following terms with the description.

__B__	Hope	A. Connectedness with a higher power, one's self, others, and the environment
__C__	Congruence	B. Multidimensional concept that provides comfort during crisis
__A__	Spirituality	C. The balance of life's patterns and rhythms
__D__	Religion	D. System of beliefs practiced outwardly to express one's spirituality

Unit 4   Supporting Psychosocial, Family, Cultural, and Spiritual Health
Section: End of Life

Chapter 65:   Grief, Loss, and End of Life
                Contributor: Ann Schide, MSN, MS, LCCE

 NCLEX® Connections

> **Learning Objective**: Review and apply knowledge within **"Grief, Loss, and End of Life"** in readiness for performance of the following nursing activities as outlined by the NCLEX® test plans:
>
> Δ   Assess/monitor the client and family for ability to cope with grief, loss, and end of life issues.
>
> Δ   Plan/provide for the client and family to have resources related to loss or end of life, such as support groups.
>
> Δ   Instruct the client and family regarding normal feelings, sensations, and thoughts experienced by those experiencing grief and loss.
>
> Δ   Evaluate the effectiveness of end of life or grief interventions.

 Key Points

Δ   Types of Loss

Necessary loss	Part of the cycle of life; anticipated but still may be intensely felt
Actual loss	Any loss of a valued person or item that can no longer be experienced by the client
Perceived loss	Any loss defined by the client but may not be obvious to others
Maturational loss	Losses normally expected due to the developmental processing of life
Situational loss	Unanticipated loss caused by an external event

Δ   **Grief** is the inner emotional response to loss and is exhibited in as many ways as there are individuals.

Δ   Theories of Grief

- **Kübler-Ross**: Five stages of dying

  ◊   Denial – Client has difficulty believing a terminal diagnosis or loss.

  ◊   Anger – Client lashes out at other people or things.

  ◊   Bargaining – Client negotiates for more time or a cure.

  ◊   Depression – Client is saddened over the inability to change the situation.

  ◊   Acceptance – Client recognizes what is happening and plans for the future.

- **Bowlby**: Four stages of mourning

  ◊   Numbing

  ◊   Yearning and searching

  ◊   Disorganization and despair

  ◊   Reorganization

- **Worden**: Four tasks of mourning

  ◊   Accept reality of loss.

  ◊   Work through the pain of grief.

  ◊   Adjust the environment of the missing deceased.

  ◊   Emotionally relocate deceased, and move forward in life.

Δ   Types of Grief

Normal	Includes expected feelings that accompany loss, such as anger, resentment, withdrawal, and crying
Anticipatory	Implies the "letting go" of an object or person before the loss, as in a terminal illness
Complicated • Chronic grief – grief reactions continuing longer than expected • Delayed grief – suppression of normal grieving until a later time that may be due to a desire to avoid the pain of grief • Exaggerated grief – overwhelming emotions causing social dysfunction • Masked grief – occurrence of unwholesome behaviors that survivors do not relate to the loss	Involves difficult progression through the expected stages of grief, making bereavement complicated

Disenfranchised	Entails an experienced loss that cannot be publicly shared or is not socially sanctioned

Δ **Bereavement** includes grief and **mourning** (the outward display of loss).

Δ The issue of **end of life** holds its own unique set of resolutions to be made in its anticipation.

Key Factors

Δ Factors Influencing Loss and Grief

- The stage of **human development** may impact how an individual will grieve.

- **Psychosocial perspectives** include:

  ◊ Valuation of individuals – a learned response per culture and society.

  ◊ The grief response develops as an individual's coping mechanisms mature.

- **Socioeconomic status** influences the options the individual has to express grief and mourning.

- **Personal relationships** prescribe what type of grief will be experienced, as well as the element of support for the grief process.

- **Nature of loss** associates the meaning of and situation surrounding the loss to the type of grief process anticipated.

- **Culture and ethnicity** influences the interpretation of a loss and expression of grief.

- **Spiritual beliefs** affect the individual's ability to cope.

Δ Nurses experience personal grief when caring for clients with whom they have developed rapport and intimacy. Such times require self-reflection and perhaps debriefing for the entire staff by professional grief/mental health counselors.

Δ **End of life** issues include decision making in a highly stressful time during which the nurse must consider the desires of the client and the family. Any decisions must be shared with other health care personnel for smoother transition during this time of stress, grief, and bereavement.

Δ **Advance directives** – legal documents that direct end-of-life issues. Advance directives include:

- **Living wills** – directive documents for medical treatment per client's wishes.

- **Durable power of attorney** for healthcare – an agent appointed by the client or the courts to make medical decisions when the client is no longer able to on his own behalf.

Assessment

Δ Symptoms of Normal Grief

- Feelings range from sadness to anxiety to yearning.
- Thoughts may be confused, hopeless, and preoccupied with the deceased person.
- Difficulties sleeping, eating, and crying are common behaviors.
- Fatigue, muscle tension or weakness, and oversensitivity to stimuli are common physical symptoms.

Δ Determine the stage of grief the client and family are experiencing.

Δ Understand the factors influencing the grieving process.

- Type of loss
- Significance of the loss
- Past coping mechanisms that have been effective
- Availability of support systems
- Prior experience(s) with loss

Δ Understand the desires and expectations of the family for end of life care.

NANDA Nursing Diagnoses

Δ Ineffective coping

Δ Anticipatory grieving

Δ Chronic sorrow

Δ Hopelessness

Δ Spiritual distress

Nursing Interventions

Δ **Set priorities** of the client through collaboration with the client and family.

Δ **Continuity of care**: Keep changes in assigned staff to a minimum so that the client and the family do not have to constantly repeat their wishes.

Δ **Therapeutic communication** is necessary to understand the client's desires and discern the grieving responses of others in an accepting manner.

Δ Keep the client and family informed about diagnosis, treatments, and prognosis.

Δ Assist the client to adapt to perceived or real loss.

Δ   Determine the client's source of strength and hope.

Δ   Assist the client in clarifying her own values in order to facilitate effective decision making.

Δ   Encourage the client to use coping mechanisms that have worked in the past.

Δ   Promote hope in times when hope can be factored into the following dimensions:

- Affective – reinforcement of client strengths.

- Cognitive – evidenced-based information about illness.

- Behavioral – making use of client's external resources.

- Affiliative – creating and maintaining supportive relationships.

- Temporal – focus on short-term goals.

- Contextual – creation of achievable goals given the situation.

Δ   **Facilitate Mourning**

- Assist the client to accept reality of loss.

- Support efforts to "move on" in the face of the loss.

- Encourage the building of new relationships

- Grant time for the grieving process.

- Be mindful of "normal" grieving behaviors.

- Provide continuing support.

- Assess for signs of ineffective coping.

Primary Reference:

Potter, P. A., & Perry, A. G. (2005). *Fundamentals of nursing* (6th ed.). St. Louis, MO: Mosby.

Additional Resources:

NANDA International (2004). *NANDA nursing diagnoses: Definitions and classification 2005-2006*. Philadelphia: NANDA.

Wilkinson, J. M. (2005). *Nursing diagnosis handbook*. Upper Saddle River, NJ: Prentice Hall.

Chapter 65: Grief, Loss, and End of Life

Application Exercises

Scenario: Three adult children place their mother in a residential care facility/agency. Their father died 1 year ago, and their mother is no longer able to care for herself.

1. What assessment data should the nurse collect from the family members?

2. What stage of grieving should the family be experiencing?

3. If the mother's situation overshadows the loss of the father, what type of grief may be expected? What might a nursing intervention be for this outcome?

4. Which stage of dying, per Kübler-Ross, is a terminally ill client displaying when she states that she is going to a clinic for acupuncture?

   A. Anger
   B. Depression
   C. Bargaining
   D. Acceptance

5. Which type of loss is reflected when a client tries to hide any signs of aging?

   A. Actual
   B. Anticipatory
   C. Perceived
   D. Situational

Chapter 65: Grief, Loss, and End of Life

Application Exercises Answer Key

Scenario: Three adult children place their mother in a residential care facility/agency. Their father died 1 year ago, and their mother is no longer able to care for herself.

1. What assessment data should the nurse collect from the family members?

   Previous coping strategies for each member

   Family cultural rituals

   Family religious/spiritual affiliation

   Stage of grief in which each family member is involved in the father's passing and the mother's illness

   Current state of mother's illness and the family's understanding of it

2. What stage of grieving should the family be experiencing?

   Father: depression or acceptance

   Mother: denial and/or anger

3. If the mother's situation overshadows the loss of the father, what type of grief may be expected? What might a nursing intervention be for this outcome?

   Chronic grief with accompanying depression or delayed grief for the father may be expected.

   The nurse will assist the family members in recognizing that this is happening and grant them permission to express their grief in a healthy manner.

4. Which stage of dying, per Kübler-Ross, is a terminally ill client displaying when she states that she is going to a clinic for acupuncture?

    A. Anger

    B. Depression

    C. Bargaining

    D. Acceptance

A client who tries unorthodox treatments is attempting to negotiate a way to lengthen life or find cures. Lashing out at people or things occurs during the anger stage. Being withdrawn and sad occurs during the depression stage. Recognizing the end is near with thoughts for the future occurs during the acceptance stage.

5. Which type of loss is reflected when a client tries to hide any signs of aging?

    A. Actual

    B. Anticipatory

    C. Perceived

    D. Situational

A perceived loss is defined by the client and may not be obvious to others. An actual loss is a loss of a person or item that can no longer be experienced by the client. Anticipatory loss is not an identified type of loss but a stage of dying. A situational loss is one that is unanticipated and caused by an external factor.

Unit 4   Supporting Psychosocial, Family, Cultural, and Spiritual Health
Section: End of Life

Chapter 66:	Palliative Care

Contributor: Ann Schide, MSN, MS, RN, LCCE

 NCLEX® Connections:

Learning Objective: Review and apply knowledge within **"Palliative Care"** in readiness for performance of the following nursing activities as outlined by the NCLEX® test plans:

Δ   Assess/monitor the needs of terminally ill clients and their families.

Δ   Plan and/or provide palliative care for the client and family as desired.

Δ   Respect the religious and cultural practices of the dying client and his family.

Δ   Evaluate the effectiveness of symptom control measures.

 Key Points

Δ   **Palliative care** is a management approach for end-of-life issues that prevent, relieve, reduce, and/or ease the symptoms of the disease without compromising medical interventions.

Δ   It is provided not only for the dying client but also for the family and support network who are intimately involved with the client's life.

Δ   The nurse serves as an advocate of the client's sense of dignity and self-esteem.

Δ   **Hospice** care is a comprehensive care delivery system for the terminally ill.

•   Care is provided for the client, as well as the client's entire family.

•   Hospice care uses an interdisciplinary approach.

•   Controlling symptoms is a priority.

•   Hospice care services are directed by the primary care provider and managed by the nurse.

•   Volunteers are used for nonmedical care.

•   Hospice services may be provided inpatient and/or at home.

- Hospice care can be given within 6 months of the expected death.

- Bereavement services postmortem are offered for the family.

Key Factors

Δ Palliative care is a philosophy of care that includes an interdisciplinary team of:

- Physicians.

- Nurses.

- Social workers.

- Massage therapists.

- Occupational therapists.

- Music/art therapists.

- Touch/energy therapists.

Δ Provides for a "good death" that liberates the client from needless suffering, allows for preparation for life closure, and grants the client's and family's wishes for the end-of-life care.

Δ A caring relationship and "presence" is necessary to provide palliative care.

Δ World Health Organization (WHO) view of palliative care:

- Provides pain/symptom relief.

- Affirms life and death as normal.

- Integrates psychosocial and spiritual aspects of care.

- Allows support system to help the client live as normal of a life as possible.

- Offers coping mechanisms for support systems.

- Enhances the quality of life.

Assessment

Characteristics of Discomfort	Signs and Symptoms of Approaching Death
<ul><li>Pain</li><li>Anxiety</li><li>Dyspnea</li><li>Nausea or vomiting</li><li>Dehydration</li><li>Diarrhea or constipation</li><li>Urinary incontinence</li><li>Inability to perform ADLs</li></ul>	<ul><li>Muscle relaxation</li><li>Labored breathing (e.g., dyspnea, apnea, Cheyne-Stokes respirations)</li><li>Mucus collecting in large airways</li><li>Incontinence of bowel and/or bladder</li><li>Mottling occurring with poor circulation</li><li>Pupils no longer reactive to light</li><li>Pulse weakening and blood pressure dropping</li><li>Cool extremities</li><li>Perspiration</li></ul>

NANDA Nursing Diagnoses

Δ   Anxiety

Δ   Ineffective coping

Δ   Caregiver role strain

Δ   Dysfunctional grieving

Δ   Powerlessness

Δ   Spiritual distress

Nursing Interventions

Δ   Symptom control includes:

• Comfort from distress and anxiety that accompanies disease systems.

• Information about treatment choices.

• Granting choices to clients minimizing anxiety and discomfort.

• Administration of medications that manage pain and air hunger.

• Encouraging the client to participate in religious practices that bring comfort and strength, if appropriate.

Δ   Maintenance of Dignity and Self-esteem

• Definition of dignity varies from individual to individual; therefore, listen to the client's concerns.

• Environmental considerations include:

◊ Cleanliness.

◊ Odor control – remove products of elimination as soon as possible.

◊ Attractive clothing – comfort prevails.

◊ Meticulous grooming – hair, nails, skin.

• Allow the client to make decisions in food selection, activities, and healthcare to permit the client as much control as possible.

• Allow the client to perform ADLs as he is able and desires.

• There should be a continuous flow of information from the primary care provider to the client's family.

• Be sensitive to comments made in the presence of the unconscious client, as hearing is the last sensation lost as a person dies.

Δ   Prevention of Abandonment and Isolation

- Prevent fear of dying alone.

  ◊   Answer call lights immediately.

  ◊   Make contact with the client often.

  ◊   Keep the client informed of procedure/assessment times.

  ◊   Allow family members to spend the night.

  ◊   Place the client close to the nurses' station where he/she can see or hear the staff.

- Provide a peaceful environment with family mementos, cards, fresh flowers, back massages, and relaxation techniques.

Δ   Support for the Grieving Family

- Encourage planned visits to prevent client fatigue.

- Provide a constant flow of information as applicable.

- Provide privacy so family members can speak among themselves to share thoughts and feelings outside the client's hearing.

- Prepare the family.

Primary Reference:

Potter, P. A., & Perry, A. G. (2005). *Fundamentals of nursing* (6ᵗʰ ed.). St. Louis, MO: Mosby.

Additional Resources:

NANDA International (2004). *NANDA nursing diagnoses: Definitions and classification 2005-2006*. Philadelphia: NANDA.

Wilkinson, J. M. (2005). *Nursing diagnosis handbook*. Upper Saddle River, NJ: Prentice Hall.

Chapter 68: Palliative Care

Application Exercises

1. A client is diagnosed with terminal cancer. The nurse observes the client's family assisting with all ADLs. Which of the following rationales for self-care should the nurse communicate to the family?

   A. Allowing the client to function independently will strengthen her muscles and promote healing.

   B. The client needs to be given privacy at times for self-reflection and organizing her life.

   C. Her sense of loss can be lessened through retaining control of certain areas of her life.

   D. Performing ADLs is required prior to discharge from an acute care facility.

2. Which of the following is a sign of impending death?

   A. Elevated blood pressure

   B. Warm extremities

   C. Tense muscles

   D. Labored breathing

3. Identify three nursing interventions that the nurse can use to assist the client to maintain his dignity and self-esteem during end-of-life care.

4. True or False: Palliative care is specialized care that focuses solely on the dying.

5. True of False: Palliative care provides an interdisciplinary approach.

Chapter 68: Palliative Care

Application Exercises Answer Key

1. A client is diagnosed with terminal cancer. The nurse observes the client's family assisting with all ADLs. Which of the following rationales for self-care should the nurse communicate to the family?

    A. Allowing the client to function independently will strengthen her muscles and promote healing.

    B. The client needs to be given privacy at times for self-reflection and organizing her life.

    C. Her sense of loss can be lessened through retaining control of certain areas of her life.

    D. Performing ADLs is required prior to discharge from an acute care facility.

    Allowing the client as much control as possible maintains dignity and self-esteem. The strengthening of muscles is not a priority of palliative care. Privacy for times of self-reflection can be achieved at times apart from performance of ADLs. Performance of ADLs is not a criterion for discharge from an acute care facility.

2. Which of the following is a sign of impending death?

    A. Elevated blood pressure

    B. Warm extremities

    C. Tense muscles

    D. Labored breathing

    Labored breathing, such as dyspnea, apnea, and Cheyne-Stoke respirations, are common in the client approaching death.

3. Identify three nursing interventions that the nurse can use to assist the client to maintain his dignity and self-esteem during end-of-life care.

    Listen to the client's concerns.

    Control physical environment by maintaining cleanliness and controlling odors.

    Allow the client to participate in ADLs as desired.

    Provide personal grooming assistance as necessary.

    Encourage the client to make decisions regarding food selection, activities, and health care.

4. True or False: Palliative care is specialized care that focuses solely on the dying.

False: It is provided not only for the dying client but also for the family and support network who are intimately involved with the client's life.

5. True or False: Palliative care provides an interdisciplinary approach.

True: Members of the interdisciplinary team that can provide palliative care include physicians, nurses, social workers, massage therapists, occupational therapists, music/art therapists, and touch/energy therapists.

Unit 4   Supporting Psychosocial, Family, Cultural, and Spiritual Health
Section: End of Life

Chapter 67:   Death and Postmortem Care
                Contributor: Ann Schide, MSN, MS, RN, LCCE

 NCLEX® Connections:

> **Learning Objective**: Review and apply knowledge within **"Death and Postmortem Care"** in readiness for performance of the following nursing activities as outlined by the NCLEX® test plans:
>
> Δ   Respect the religious and cultural practices of dying clients and their families.
>
> Δ   Plan and/or provide postmortem care.

 Key Points

Δ   The nurse is the staff member who supervises **postmortem**, or after-death, care.

Δ   The care is provided with **dignity** and **sensitivity** while attending to the desires of the client and family per their cultural, religious, and social practices.

Δ   The client's family now becomes the nurse's primary focus.

Key Factors

Δ   Caring long term for clients can create personal attachments for the nurse.

Δ   The need to "let go" is a challenge.

Δ   The ability to "let go" may rely on the presence of:

•   Faith.

•   Memory.

•   Love.

•   One another.

Δ   Nurses can cope through:

•   Attending the funeral process.

- Writing a letter of condolence to the family.

- Seeking out other nurses.

- Stress management techniques.

- Debriefing with a professional counselor.

NANDA Nursing Diagnoses

Δ   Anticipatory grieving

Δ   Dysfunctional grieving

Nursing Interventions

Δ   Care of the Body

- The primary care provider must certify death – pronounce time, document therapies used and any actions taken prior to the death.

- Appropriate and skilled ancillary personnel can be delegated the responsibility for the care.

- Preparing the body for viewing includes:

  ◊   Maintaining privacy.

  ◊   Shaving facial hair if applicable and/or desired by family.

  ◊   Removing all tubes and dirty linens (unless organs are to be donated or this is a coroner's case).

  ◊   Removing all personal belongings to be given to the family.

  ◊   Cleansing and aligning the body with a pillow under the head.

  ◊   Applying fresh linens and a gown.

  ◊   Brushing/combing the client's hair, replacing any hair pieces.

  ◊   Caring for dentures per facility/agency policy.

  ◊   Positioning per facility/agency protocol.

  ◊   Pulling top sheet to below chin with arms outside sheet or per facility/agency protocol.

  ◊   Removing excess equipment and linens from the room.

  ◊   Providing a calm environment by dimming the lights, if possible.

- Viewing considerations include:

  ◊   Asking the family if they would like to visit with the body – any decision is to be honored (do not rush this process).

  ◊   Clarifying where the client's personal belongings should go – with the body or a designated person.

◊ Adhering to the same procedures for newborn viewings with the exception of transport to the family, which include:

  ° Swaddling the infant's body in a clean blanket.

  ° Transporting the cradled infant in the nurse's arms or a special infant carrier.

  ° Collecting mementos of the infant (e.g., identification bracelets, footprints, cord clamp, lock of hair, photos).

- Post Viewing

  ◊ Apply name tags per protocol – usually wrist, right big toe, and shroud.

  ◊ Complete documentation.

  ◊ Remain aware of visitor and staff sensibilities during transport.

Δ Organ Donation

- Maintain ventilatory and cardiovascular support for vital organ retrieval.

- Use private area for any family discussion concerning donation.

- Family may need counseling in what constitutes "brain death."

- Many facilities/agencies have access to transplant coordinators specifically trained in responding to organ donation issues.

Δ Autopsy Considerations

- The primary care provider frequently approaches the family about performing an autopsy.

- The nurse's role is to answer family questions and support choices.

- Autopsies can be conducted to advance scientific knowledge regarding disease processes which can lead to development of new therapies.

Δ Cultural/religious Beliefs

- Identify cultural/religious beliefs of family members.

- Be sensitive to these practices when providing postmortem care.

Δ Documentation and completion of forms following federal and state laws typically includes:

- Person pronouncing the death and at what time.

- Consideration of and preparation for organ donation.

- Disposition of personal articles.

- Names of people notified and any decisions made.

- Location of identification tags.

- Time the body left the facility/agency and the destination.

Primary Reference:

Potter, P. A., & Perry, A. G. (2005). *Fundamentals of nursing* (6th ed.). St. Louis, MO: Mosby.

Additional Resources:

NANDA International (2004). *NANDA nursing diagnoses: Definitions and classification 2005-2006*. Philadelphia: NANDA.

Wilkinson, J. M. (2005). *Nursing diagnosis handbook*. Upper Saddle River, NJ: Prentice Hall.

Chapter 67: Death and Postmortem Care

Application Exercises

Scenario: A nurse is present when a long-term resident at an assisted living facility/agency dies at the age of 95. The client's partner also lives in the facility/agency. The nurse has provided care for both clients for the past 5 years.

1. How should the nurse proceed with the client's remains?

2. What considerations should be made for the partner and the family members of the deceased client?

3. How can the nurse cope effectively with her own sense of loss?

4. A deceased client is a declared organ donor. His heart and lungs will be harvested. What is a priority intervention for the nurse?

    A. Obtain signed permission from the family to harvest.
    B. Contact the region's transplant coordinator.
    C. Continue the ventilator assistance for the client.
    D. Prepare the client's room for family viewing.

5. What is the purpose of reducing the lighting in a deceased client's room prior to family viewing?

    A. The family will be less able to see the medical equipment still attached.
    B. An atmosphere of dim lights is calming and comforting.
    C. A majority of families have a preference for dim lighting.
    D. Dim lighting will hasten the viewing when visitors cannot see as well.

6. What is the best approach for preparing a deceased newborn for viewing?

    A. After cleansing the body, swaddle the infant and cradle in arms.
    B. Leave the cleansing until later and wrap the infant in clean blankets, covering face.
    C. To preserve family dignity, insist that the family not view the newborn.
    D. Suggest funeral homes that specialize in infants, and hold the viewing there.

Chapter 67: Death and Postmortem Care

Application Exercises Answer Key

Scenario: A nurse is present when a long-term resident at an assisted living facility/agency dies at the age of 95. The client's partner also lives in the facility/agency. The nurse has provided care for both clients for the past 5 years.

1. How should the nurse proceed with the client's remains?

   Have a provider certify death.

   Assess and implement any cultural considerations for postmortem care.

   The nurse can delegate the cleansing of the body and immediate environment to assistive personnel (AP).

   The body would be made ready for viewing after giving the partner the option of private time with the deceased client.

   Wash the body, keeping parts not being washed covered to preserve personal dignity.

   If desired by partner, shave the face.

   Replace linens with fresh sheets.

   Position the body per facility/agency protocol.

   Pull top sheet and blanket up to the client's chin, placing arms outside the sheet or per facility/agency protocol.

   Remove soiled linens, trash, and any medical equipment from the room.

   Lower the lighting and pull any window coverings closed.

2. What considerations should be made for the partner and the family members of the deceased client?

   Assess their desires for viewing and at what times.

   Allow family to have as much time with the deceased as they need.

   Determine family wishes for the processing of the remains (funeral arrangements, cremation).

   Grant family access to telephones and paperwork to make final arrangements.

3. How can the nurse cope effectively with her own sense of loss?

Verbally express her regret for the family's loss at the time of death.

Attend any services for the client.

Speak with other members of the healthcare team who had interaction with this couple to share memories and thoughts.

Seek out the employee assistance personnel (EAP) for grief counseling.

Continue caring for the spouse in this long-term situation.

4. A deceased client is a declared organ donor. His heart and lungs will be harvested. What is a priority intervention for the nurse?

    A. Obtain signed permission from the family to harvest.

    B. Contact the region's transplant coordinator.

    C. Continue the ventilator assistance for the client.

    D. Prepare the client's room for family viewing.

Respiratory and cardiovascular support must be continued to support the vital organs until they can be harvested. If respiratory and cardiovascular support is not continued, the organs will not be able to be donated. Preparing the client's room is important, but again, the priority intervention is to maintain the organs for donation.

5. What is the purpose of reducing the lighting in a deceased client's room prior to family viewing?

    A. The family will be less able to see the medical equipment still attached.

    B. An atmosphere of dim lights is calming and comforting.

    C. A majority of families have a preference for dim lighting.

    D. Dim lighting will hasten the viewing when visitors cannot see as well.

The purpose of dimming lights is to create a calm and comfortable atmosphere. The medical equipment should have already been removed. There is no data to support the claim that families prefer dim lighting. Family members need to be given adequate time to view the body.

6. What is the best approach for preparing a deceased newborn for viewing?

A. After cleansing the body, swaddle the infant and cradle in arms.

B. Leave the cleansing until later and wrap the infant in clean blankets, covering face.

C. To preserve family dignity, insist that the family not view the newborn.

D. Suggest funeral homes that specialize in infants, and hold the viewing there.

Swaddling the newborn is the best way to present the body for viewing. Cleansing before the viewing will ensure the elimination of odors. There is no reason to cover the face. Insisting the family not view the newborn and making suggestions regarding types of funeral homes does not allow the family a choice to deal with the death in a way that might be helpful to them.

Unit 5   Supporting Physiologic Needs
Section: Oxygenation needs

Chapter 68:   Oxygenation Assessment and Oxygen Administration
              Contributors: Terri A. Astorino, EdD, MSN, RN
                           Lori A. Budd, BS, RN

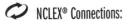 NCLEX® Connections:

> **Learning Objective**: Review and apply knowledge within **"Oxygenation Assessment and Oxygen Administration"** in readiness for performance of the following nursing activities as outlined by the NCLEX® test plans:
>
> Δ   Assess the client's need for oxygen to ensure adequate tissue oxygenation.
>
> Δ   Perform/assist with relevant laboratory, diagnostic, and therapeutic procedures within the nursing role, including:
>
> - Preparation of the client for the procedure.
>
> - Client teaching (before and following the procedure).
>
> - Assessment and evaluation of the client's response (expected, unexpected adverse response, comparison to baseline) to the procedure and appropriate notification of the primary care provider.
>
> - Recognizing signs of potential complications and reporting to the primary care provider.
>
> - Monitoring and taking actions, including client education, to prevent or minimize the risk of complications.
>
> Δ   Document the client's response to nursing interventions.

 Key Points

Δ   Oxygen is a tasteless and colorless gas that accounts for 21% of atmospheric air.

Δ   Oxygen is used to maintain adequate cellular oxygenation. It is used in the treatment of many acute and chronic respiratory problems.

Δ   Oxygen flow rates are varied in an attempt to maintain an $SaO_2 \geq 91\%$ by using the lowest amount of oxygen to achieve the goal without the development of complications.

Δ   Supplemental oxygen may be delivered by a variety of methods that are dependent upon individual client circumstances.

Δ **Hypoxemia** is a condition of inadequate levels of oxygen in the blood. Hypovolemia, hypoventilation, and interruption of arterial flow can lead to hypoxemia.

- Clinical **signs and symptoms** of hypoxemia include:

Early	Late
• Tachypnea • Tachycardia • Restlessness • Pallor of the skin and mucous membranes • Elevated blood pressure • Symptoms of respiratory distress (use of accessory muscles, nasal flaring, tracheal tugging, adventitious lung sounds)	• Confusion and stupor • Cyanosis of skin and mucous membranes • Bradypnea • Bradycardia • Hypotension • Cardiac dysrhythmias

Key Procedural Points

Δ **Respiratory Status**

- Assess/monitor the client's respiratory rate, rhythm, and effort.

- Assess/monitor the client's oxygenation status by arterial blood gases (ABGs) and pulse oximetry (SaO_2).

- Monitor and document the client's response to oxygen therapy.

- Normal values are 95 to 100%. Acceptable levels may range from 91 to 100%. Some disease states may allow for an SaO_2 of 85 to 89%.

- Results less than 91% require nursing intervention to assist the client to regain normal SaO_2 levels. Results < 86% are an emergency. Life-threatening results may start at levels < 80%. The lower the SaO_2 level, the less accurate the value.

Δ **Oxygen Safety**

- Place "No Smoking" or "Oxygen in Use" signs to alert others of fire hazard (Oxygen is combustible.).

- Know where the closest fire extinguisher is located.

- Educate the client and others about the fire hazard of smoking with oxygen use.

- Have the client wear a cotton gown, because synthetics or wools may create sparks of static electricity.

- Ensure that all electric devices (e.g., razors, heating pads) are in good working order.

- Ensure that all electric machinery (e.g., monitors, suction machines) are grounded.

- Do not use volatile, flammable materials (e.g., alcohol, acetone) near clients receiving oxygen.
- Frequently assess the client whose main respiratory drive is hypoxia, such as the client with chronic lung disease, for oxygen-induced hypoventilation.

NANDA Nursing Diagnoses

Δ   Anxiety

Δ   Fatigue

Δ   Activity intolerance

Δ   Imbalanced nutrition: less than body requirements

Nursing Interventions

Δ   Equipment (oxygen delivery systems) – devices that provide a concentration of inhaled oxygen greater than that of room air:

Low-flow oxygen delivery systems – How much oxygen is actually delivered is variable and dependent on the breathing pattern of the client.				
Oxygen Delivery Methods	Definition	Advantages	Disadvantages	Nursing Interventions
Nasal cannula	Nasal cannula delivers oxygen concentrations of 24 to 40% FiO_2 (fraction of inspired oxygen) at a flow rate of 1 to 6 L/min via a disposable plastic tube with two prongs for insertion in the nostrils.	• It is a safe and simple method. • It is easy to apply. • It is comfortable and tolerated well. • The client is able to eat, talk, and ambulate while wearing.	• FiO_2 varies depending on oxygen flow rate, and rate and depth of client breathing. • Nasal cannula may cause skin breakdown and dryness of nasal mucosa if left on for an extended period of time. • It can be easily dislodged.	• Assess the patency of the nares. • Ensure that the prongs fit in the nares properly. • Supply the client with water-soluble jelly if nares are dry. • Provide humidification for flow rates ≥ 4 L/min.

Simple face mask • A simple face mask covers the client's nose and mouth.	• Face mask delivers oxygen concentrations of 40 to 60% FiO$_2$ (at flow rates of 5 to 8 L/min respectively for short-term oxygen therapy. • Minimum flow rate is 5 L/min to ensure flushing of CO$_2$ from the mask.	• Face mask is easy to apply. • It is a simple method for increased oxygen needs. • It is more comfortable than a nasal cannula.	• If flow rates are not > 5 L/min, rebreathing of CO$_2$ can become an issue. • Face mask can be tolerated poorly by anxious clients, or those with claustrophobia. • Eating, drinking, and talking are impaired. • Use with caution in the client with a high risk of aspiration or airway obstruction.	• Assess proper fit to ensure secure fit over nose and mouth. • Request order for nasal cannula use during meals. • Provide emotional support.
Partial rebreather mask • Partial rebreather mask covers the client's nose and mouth.	Partial rebreather mask delivers oxygen concentrations of 60 to 75% FiO$_2$ at flow rates of 6 to 11 L/min respectively.	Mask has a reservoir bag attached with no valve, which allows the client to rebreathe up to 1/3 of exhaled air together with room air.	• Complete deflation of reservoir bag during inspiration causes CO$_2$ build up. • Mask can be tolerated poorly by anxious clients, or those with claustrophobia. • Eating, drinking, and talking are impaired. • Use with caution in the client with a high risk of aspiration or airway obstruction.	• Assess that the reservoir bag does not kink or twist, which will result in bag deflation. • Prevent bag from deflating by adjusting oxygen flow rate to keep the reservoir bag inflated. • The flow rate is based on the client's breathing pattern. • Assess proper fit to ensure secure fit over nose and mouth. • Request order for nasal cannula use during meals. • Provide emotional support.

Nonrebreather mask • Nonrebreather mask covers the client's nose and mouth.	Nonrebreather mask delivers oxygen concentrations of 80 to 95% FiO_2 at flow rates of 10 to 15 L/min in order to maintain reservoir bag to stay 2/3 full during inspiration and expiration.	• Nonrebreather mask delivers the highest O_2 concentration possible (except for intubation). • One-way valve is situated between the mask and reservoir, which allows the client to inhale maximum O_2 from the reservoir bag. The two exhalation ports have flaps covering them that prevent room air from entering the mask.	• Valve and flap on mask must be intact and operating during each breath. • Mask can be tolerated poorly by anxious clients, or those with claustrophobia. • Eating, drinking, and talking are impaired. • Use with caution in the client with a high risk of aspiration or airway obstruction.	• Prepare the client for emergency intubation. • Perform an hourly assessment of valve and flap. • Assess proper fit to ensure secure fit over nose and mouth. • Request order for nasal cannula use during meals. • Provide emotional support.

High-flow oxygen delivery systems – When properly fitted, these devices deliver precise amounts of oxygen.

Venturi mask • Venturi mask covers the client's nose and mouth.	Venturi mask delivers oxygen concentrations of 24 to 55% FiO_2 at flow rates of 2 to 10 L/min respectively via different sized adaptors.	• It delivers the most precise oxygen concentration. • Humidification is not required. • It is best suited for clients with chronic lung disease.	• Use is expensive. • It should be used only when benefits clearly outweigh costs.	• Venturi mask requires frequent assessment to ensure accurate flow rate. • Ensure that tubing is free of kinks. • Provide emotional support.

| Aerosol masks, face tents, (fit loosely around face and neck), and tracheostomy collars (small mask that covers the surgical opening of the trachea) | • These methods deliver oxygen concentration of 24 to 100% FiO$_2$ at flow rates of at least 10 L/min.
• They allow for high humidification of oxygen. | • These methods are used for clients who do not tolerate masks well.
• They are useful for clients with facial trauma, burns, and for clients with thick secretions.
• They are used to deliver high humidity and oxygen to the client with a tracheostomy. | • These methods are difficult to keep intact.
• It is difficult to control oxygen concentration.
• High humidification requires frequent monitoring. | • Frequently empty condensation from tubing.
• Ensure adequate water in humidification canister.
• Position so that the tubing does not pull on the tracheostomy.
• Assess proper fit to ensure secure fit over nose and mouth.
• Request order for nasal cannula use during meals.
• Provide emotional support. |

- **Procedure**

  ◊ Assess/monitor the client for need of supplemental oxygen.

   ° Signs and symptoms of hypoxemia as evidenced by client reports of shortness of breath, anxiety, tachypnea, tachycardia, restlessness, anxiety, skin and mucous membranes from pale to cyanotic, adventitious breath sounds, and confusion

   ° Signs and symptoms of hypercarbia as evidenced by restlessness, hypertension, and headache

  ◊ Monitor and document the client's response to oxygen therapy.

  ◊ Monitor the client's oxygenation status by arterial blood gases (ABGs) and pulse oximetry (SaO$_2$), and notify the primary care provider of abnormal values.

  ◊ Apply the oxygen delivery device as ordered. Assess proper fit of mask to ensure secure fit over the nose and mouth.

  ◊ Place the client in a Fowler's or semi-Fowler's position to facilitate the work of breathing.

  ◊ Promote good oral hygiene and provide as needed.

  ◊ Promote pulmonary toileting to include: turning, coughing, deep breathing, and use of incentive spirometry to prevent atelectasis.

  ◊ Promote rest and decrease environmental stimuli.

  ◊ Provide support for anxious clients.

  ◊ Assess nutritional status. Provide supplements if indicated.

◊ Assess/monitor the client's skin integrity. Provide moisture and pressure relief devices as needed.

◊ Educate the client about the oxygen delivery device and the need for it.

◊ Educate the client and support system to avoid smoking and the use of any open flame in the presence of the oxygen.

◊ Monitor for any deterioration in client status and notify the primary care provider.

◊ For respiratory distress:

○ Position the client for maximum ventilation (Fowler's or semi-Fowler's position).

○ Complete a focused respiratory assessment.

○ Promote adequate oxygenation through deep breathing and provision of supplemental oxygen as prescribed by the primary care provider.

○ Stay with the client and provide emotional support to decrease anxiety.

○ Promote airway clearance through the encouragement of coughing, or oral/oropharyngeal suctioning if necessary, as prescribed by the primary care provider.

Complications and Nursing Implications

Δ **Oxygen Toxicity**

• Oxygen toxicity may result from high concentrations of oxygen (typically > 50%), long duration of oxygen therapy (typically > 24 to 48 hr), and the client's degree of lung disease.

• **Signs and symptoms** include a nonproductive cough, substernal pain, nasal stuffiness, nausea and vomiting, fatigue, headache, sore throat, and hypoventilation.

• **Interventions**

◊ Use the lowest level of oxygen necessary to maintain adequate **SaO_2**.

◊ Monitor ABGs and notify the primary care provider if SaO_2 levels rise above expected parameters.

◊ Use of an oxygen mask with continuous positive airway pressure (CPAP), bilevel positive airway pressure (BiPAP), or positive end-expiratory pressure (PEEP) while a client is on a mechanical ventilator may decrease the amount of needed oxygen.

◊ Oxygen amount should be decreased as soon as the client's condition permits.

Δ   **Oxygen-induced hypoventilation** may occur in **clients with chronic obstructive pulmonary disease (COPD)** who have chronic hypoxemia and hypercarbia (elevated levels of CO_2). Clients with COPD rely on low levels of arterial oxygen as their primary drive for breathing. Providing supplemental oxygen at high levels can decrease or eliminate respiratory drive.

- Monitor for **signs and symptoms** of respiratory depression (e.g., decreased respiratory rate, decreased level of consciousness).

- Provide oxygen therapy at the lowest liter flow that will correct hypoxemia.

- If tolerated, use a Venturi mask to deliver precise oxygen levels.

- Monitor the client's respiratory rate and pattern, level of consciousness, and SaO_2 levels.

- Notify the primary care provider of impending respiratory depression.

Primary Reference:

Potter, P. A., & Perry, A. G. (2005). *Fundamentals of nursing* (6th ed.). St. Louis, MO: Mosby.

Additional Resources:

Ackley, B., & Ladwig, G. (2006). *Nursing diagnosis handbook* (7th ed.). St. Louis, MO: Mosby.

Ignatavicius, D. D., & Workman, M. L. (2006). *Medical-surgical nursing* (5th ed.). St. Louis, MO: Saunders.

NANDA International (2004). *NANDA nursing diagnoses: Definitions and classification 2005-2006*. Philadelphia: NANDA.

Chapter 68: Oxygenation Assessment and Oxygen Administration

Application Exercises

1. Match each of the following oxygen delivery systems with the appropriate description.

_____ Nasal cannula

_____ Simple face mask

_____ Nonrebreather mask

_____ Venturi mask

_____ Face tent

A. Delivers oxygen concentrations of 24 to 55% FiO_2 at flow rates of 2 to 10 L/min respectively via different sized adaptors

B. Delivers oxygen concentration of 24 to 100% FiO_2 at flow rates of at least 10 L/min and allows for high humidification of oxygen

C. Delivers oxygen concentrations of 24 to 40% FiO_2 at a flow rate of 1 to 6 L/min via disposable plastic tube with two prongs for insertion in the nostrils

D. Delivers oxygen concentrations of 40 to 60% FiO_2 at flow rates of 5 to 8 L/min respectively for short-term oxygen therapy

E. Delivers oxygen concentrations of 80 to 95% FiO_2 at flow rates of 10 to 15 L/min in order to maintain reservoir bag to stay 2/3 full during inspiration and expiration

2. Which of the following can cause a low pulse oximetry reading? (Select all that apply.)

_____ Nail polish

_____ Inadequate peripheral circulation

_____ Hyperthermia

_____ Increased hemoglobin level

_____ Edema

3. Differentiate between early (E) and late (L) signs of hypoxemia.

_____ Confusion and stupor

_____ Pallor of skin and mucous membranes

_____ Bradycardia

_____ Hypotension

_____ Elevated blood pressure

_____ Restlessness

_____ Cyanosis of skin and mucous membranes

4. Which of the following positions would be best for the client who is having difficulty breathing?

    A. Supine

    B. Dorsal recumbent

    C. Fowler's

    D. Lateral

5. Which of the following oxygen delivery systems should be used when a precise amount of oxygen needs to be delivered?

    A. Nonrebreather mask

    B. Venturi mask

    C. Nasal cannula

    D. Simple face mask

Chapter 68: Oxygenation Assessment and Oxygen Administration

Application Exercises Answer Key

1. Match each of the following oxygen delivery systems with the appropriate description.

__C__ Nasal cannula

A. Delivers oxygen concentrations of 24 to 55% FiO_2 at flow rates of 2 to 10 L/min respectively via different sized adaptors

__D__ Simple face mask

B. Delivers oxygen concentration of 24 to 100% FiO_2 at flow rates of at least 10 L/min and allows for high humidification of oxygen

__E__ Nonrebreather mask

C. Delivers oxygen concentrations of 24 to 40% FiO_2 at a flow rate of 1 to 6 L/min via disposable plastic tube with two prongs for insertion in the nostrils

__A__ Venturi mask

D. Delivers oxygen concentrations of 40 to 60% FiO_2 at flow rates of 5 to 8 L/min respectively for short-term oxygen therapy

__B__ Face tent

E. Delivers oxygen concentrations of 80 to 95% FiO_2 at flow rates of 10 to 15 L/min in order to maintain reservoir bag to stay 2/3 full during inspiration and expiration

2. Which of the following can cause a low pulse oximetry reading? (Select all that apply.)

__X__ **Nail polish**
__X__ **Inadequate peripheral circulation**
_____ Hyperthermia
_____ Increased hemoglobin level
__X__ **Edema**

Nail polish, inadequate peripheral circulation, and edema can all cause a low reading. Hypothermia rather than hyperthermia and decreased hemoglobin level rather than increased hemoglobin level can lead to a low reading.

3. Differentiate between early (E) and late (L) signs of hypoxemia.

__L__ Confusion and stupor

__E__ Pallor of skin and mucous membranes

__L__ Bradycardia

__L__ Hypotension

__E__ Elevated blood pressure

__E__ Restlessness

__L__ Cyanosis of skin and mucous membranes

4. Which of the following positions would be best for the client who is having difficulty breathing?

    A. Supine

    B. Dorsal recumbent

    C. Fowler's

    D. Lateral

Fowler's position allows for the greatest lung expansion and will optimize breathing.

5. Which of the following oxygen delivery systems should be used when a precise amount of oxygen needs to be delivered?

    A. Nonrebreather mask

    B. Venturi mask

    C. Nasal cannula

    D. Simple face mask

A Venturi mask has an adaptor that allows a precise amount of oxygen to be delivered. The other oxygen delivery systems deliver an approximated amount of oxygen.

Unit 5   **Supporting Physiologic Needs**
Section: Oxygenation Needs

Chapter 69:   **Artificial Airway**
Contributors: Terri Astorino, EdD, MSN, RN
Sharon Kumm, MN, MS, RN, CCRN

 NCLEX® Connections

Learning Objective: Review and apply knowledge within "**Artificial Airway**" in readiness for performance of the following nursing activities as outlined by the NCLEX® test plans:

Δ   Assess the client's need for an artificial airway to ensure adequate tissue oxygenation.

Δ   Perform/assist with relevant laboratory, diagnostic, and therapeutic procedures within the nursing role, including:

   •   Preparation of the client for the procedure.

   •   Client teaching (before and following the procedure).

   •   Assessment and evaluation of the client's response (expected, unexpected adverse response, comparison to baseline) to the procedure and appropriate notification of the primary care provider.

   •   Recognizing signs of potential complications and reporting to the primary care provider.

   •   Monitoring and taking actions, including client education, to prevent or minimize the risk of complications.

Δ   Document the client's response to nursing interventions.

 Key Points

Δ   A **tracheotomy** is a sterile surgical incision into the trachea through the skin and muscles for the purpose of establishing an airway.

Δ   A tracheotomy can be performed as an emergency procedure or as a scheduled surgical procedure; it can be permanent or temporary.

Δ   A **tracheostomy** is the stoma/opening that results from a tracheotomy to provide and secure an open airway.

Δ   Client Indications for a Tracheostomy

- Acute or chronic upper airway obstruction

- Edema (anaphylaxis, burns, trauma, head/neck surgery)

- To facilitate removal of secretions

- To permit long-term mechanical ventilation

- To provide airway reconstruction after laryngeal trauma or laryngeal cancer surgery

- To treat obstructive sleep apnea refractory to conventional therapy

- To permit oral intake and speech in the client who requires long-term mechanical ventilation

Δ   Signs and Symptoms Necessitating Tracheostomy

- Inability to oxygenate through the nasopharynx due to obstruction evidenced by dyspnea, low SaO_2, and abnormal arterial blood gas (ABG) values.

- Inability to wean from mechanical ventilation within 2 weeks.

- Sleep apnea not improved by noninvasive mechanical ventilation (CPAP).

Δ   Advantages of a tracheostomy as the choice for long-term therapy include:

- Less risk of long-term damage to the airway.

- Increased client comfort because no tube is present in the mouth.

- Decreased incidence of pressure ulcers in the oral cavity and upper airway.

- Allows the client to eat because the tube enters lower in the airway.

- Allows the client to talk.

Key Procedural Points

Δ   Air flow in and out of a tracheostomy without air leakage (e.g., a cuffed tracheostomy tube) bypasses the vocal cords resulting in an inability to produce sound or speech.

Δ   Uncuffed tubes and fenestrated tubes that are in place or capped allow the client to speak. Clients with a cuffed tube, who can be off mechanical ventilation and breathe around the tube, can use a special valve to allow for speech. The cuff is deflated, and the valve occludes the opening.

Δ   Swallowing is possible with a tracheostomy tube in place; however, laryngeal elevation is affected, and it is important to assess the client's risk for aspiration prior to intake.

NANDA Nursing Diagnoses

Δ   Risk for infection

Δ   Impaired swallowing

Δ   Deficient knowledge

Δ   Ineffective airway clearance

Nursing Interventions

Δ   Equipment

- Artificial airway or a tracheostomy tube is a device that is inserted into the tracheostomy in order to maintain airway patency.

- They vary in their composition (plastic, steel, silicone), number of parts, size (long vs short), and shape (50 to 90° angles).

- There is no standard tracheostomy sizing system; however, the diameter of the tracheostomy tube must be smaller than the trachea.

- The outside cannula has a flange or neckplate that sits against the skin of the neck and has holes on each side to attach securing ties that go around the client's neck in order to stabilize the tracheostomy tube.

Tubes	Characteristics	Nursing Concerns
Single lumen (cannula)	• Long, single cannula tube • Used for clients with long or thick necks	Do not use with clients with excessive secretions.
Double lumen (cannula)	Has two major parts: • Outer cannula that fits into the stoma and keeps airway open. • Inner cannula that fits snugly into the outer cannula and locks into place.	• This device allows for the inner cannula to be removed, cleaned, and reused or discarded, and a new disposable inner cannula replaced. • It is useful in clients with excessive secretions.
Cuffed tube	Balloon that is inflated around the outside of the distal segment of the tube to protect the lower airway by producing a seal between the upper and lower airway	• Cuffed tube permits mechanical ventilation. • Cuffs do not hold the tube in place. • Cuff pressures must be assessed to prevent tracheal tissue necrosis.

Cuffless tube	No balloon, used for clients with long-term airway management needs	• Client must be at low risk for aspiration. • Cuffless tube is not used for clients on mechanical ventilation. • This device allows the client to speak.
Fenestrated tube – with cuff	• One large or multiple openings (fenestrations) in the posterior wall of the outer cannula with balloon around the outside of the distal segment of the tube • Also has an inner cannula	• Device allows for mechanical ventilation. • Inner cannula must be removed to allow the fenestration to permit air to flow through the openings. • This device allows for the client to speak.
Fenestrated tube – without cuff	• One larger or multiple openings (fenestration) in the posterior wall of the outer cannula with no balloon • Also has an inner cannula	• The device is used to assist with weaning of the client from the tracheostomy because of holes in the tube. • Inner cannula must be removed to allow the fenestration to permit air to flow through the openings. • This device allows for the client to speak.
Obturator	• Thin solid tool placed inside the tracheostomy and used as a guide for insertion of the outer cannula • Removed immediately after outer cannula insertion	• Always stay with the client and at the bedside in case of accidental decannulation and need for reinsertion. • Always stay at the client's bedside in case of accidental tube dislodgement and the need for reinsertion.

Δ Procedure

- Always keep the following at the client's bedside: two extra tracheostomy tubes (one the client's size and one size smaller in case of accidental decannulation), the obturator to the existing tube, oxygen source, suction catheters and suction source, and bag-valve mask.

- Assess/monitor:

  ◊ Oxygenation and ventilation (respiratory rate, effort, SaO$_2$) and vital signs hourly.

  ◊ Thickness, quantity, odor, and color of mucous secretions.

◊ Stoma and skin surrounding stoma for signs of inflammation or infection (redness, swelling, or drainage).

- Provide adequate humidification and hydration to thin secretions and decrease risk of mucus plugging.

- Do not suction routinely, as this causes mucosal damage, bleeding, and bronchospasm.

- Assess/monitor the need for suctioning. Suction on a PRN basis when assessment findings indicate (e.g., audible/noisy secretions, crackles, restlessness, tachypnea, tachycardia, presence of mucus in artificial airway).

- Maintain surgical aseptic technique when suctioning to prevent infection.

- Provide the client with methods to communicate with staff (paper and pen, chalk board, dry erase board). Provide an emergency call system, as well as a call light.

- Provide emotional support to the client and family.

- Provide frequent oral care.

- Provide tracheostomy care every 8 hr to decrease the risk of infection and skin breakdown.

    ◊ Suction the tracheostomy tube, if necessary, using sterile suctioning supplies.

    ◊ Remove old dressings and excess secretions.

    ◊ Apply the oxygen source loosely if the client desaturates during the procedure.

    ◊ Use cotton-tipped applicators and gauze pads to clean exposed outer cannula surfaces. Begin with hydrogen peroxide followed by normal saline. Clean in circular motion from stoma site outward.

    ◊ Using surgical aseptic technique, remove and clean the inner cannula (use hydrogen peroxide to clean the cannula and sterile saline to rinse it). Use new inner cannula if it is disposable.

    ◊ Clean the stoma site and then the tracheostomy plate with hydrogen peroxide followed by sterile saline.

    ◊ Place split 4 x 4 dressing around tracheostomy.

    ◊ Change tracheostomy ties if they are soiled. Secure new ties in place before removing soiled ones to prevent accidental decannulation.

    ◊ If a knot is needed, tie a square knot that is visible on the side of the neck. One or two fingers should be able to be placed between the tie tape and the neck.

    ◊ Document the type and amount of secretions, the general condition of the stoma and surrounding skin, the client's response to the procedure, and any teaching or learning that occurred.

- Change nondisposable tracheostomy tubes every 6 to 8 weeks or per protocol.

- Reposition the client every 2 hr to prevent atelectasis and pneumonia.

- Provide oral hygiene every 2 hr to maintain mucosal integrity.

- Minimize dust in the client's room; do not shake bedding.

- If the client is permitted to eat, position the client in an upright position and tip the client's chin to chest to enable swallowing. Assess for aspiration.

Δ   Administer prescribed medications.

- Anti-inflammatory medications to reduce edema

- Antibiotics as indicated for prophylaxis or infection treatment

- Aerosolized bronchodilators to relieve bronchospasm

- Mucous liquefying agents, such as guaifenesin

Δ   Provide discharge teaching.

- Tracheostomy care

- Signs and symptoms that the client should immediately report to the primary care provider (signs of infection, copious secretions)

Δ   Consider referral of the client to a home healthcare agency and community support groups.

Complications and Nursing Implications

Δ   Accidental Decannulation

- Always keep the tracheostomy obturator and two spare tracheostomy tubes at the client's bedside.

- Accidental decannulation in the first **72 hr** after surgery is an emergency because the tracheostomy tract has not matured, and replacement may be difficult.

  ◊   Ventilate the client with bag-valve mask. Call for assistance.

- If accidental decannulation occurs after the first 72 hr, the nurse should:

  ◊   Immediately open the airway by extending the client's neck.

  ◊   Obtain obturator and spare tracheostomy tube from head of the bed, place the obturator in the outer cannula, insert into the tracheostoma, and then remove the obturator. If unable to reinsert the tube, call for assistance.

  ◊   Secure the tube.

  ◊   Assess tube placement by auscultating for bilateral breath sounds.

- If unable to replace the tracheostomy tube, administer oxygen through the stoma. If unable to administer oxygen through the stoma, occlude the stoma and administer oxygen through the nose and mouth.

Δ   Damage to Trachea

- Tracheal wall necrosis is tissue damage that can occur as a result of the pressure exerted from the inflated cuff that cuts off blood flow to the tracheal wall.

- Tracheal stenosis is the narrowing of the tracheal lumen due to scar formation that forms as a result of irritation to the tracheal mucosa from the tracheal tube cuff.

  ◊   Keep cuff pressure between 14 to 20 mm Hg.

  ◊   Check cuff pressure at least once per shift.

  ◊   Keep the tube in the midline position and prevent pulling or traction on the tracheostomy tube.

Primary Reference:

Potter, P. A., & Perry, A. G. (2005). *Fundamentals of nursing* (6th ed.). St. Louis, MO: Mosby.

Additional Resources:

Ignatavicius, D. D., & Workman, M. L. (2006). *Medical-surgical nursing* (5th ed.). St. Louis, MO: Saunders.

LeMone, P. & Burke, K. (2004). *Medical-surgical nursing: Critical thinking in client care* (3rd ed.). Upper Saddle River, NJ: Prentice-Hall.

NANDA International (2004). *NANDA nursing diagnoses: Definitions and classification 2005-2006*. Philadelphia: NANDA.

Chapter 69: Artificial Airway

Application Exercises

1. Identify indications for placement of a tracheostomy tube.

2. Match the tracheostomy tube with the correct characteristics.

_____ Single lumen (cannula)

_____ Cuffed tube

_____ Cuffless tube

_____ Fenestrated tube (with cuff)

_____ Fenestrated tube (without cuff)

_____ Obturator

A. Balloon that is inflated around the outside of the distal segment of the tube to protect the lower airway by producing a seal between the upper and lower airway (permits mechanical ventilation)

B. One large or multiple opening (fenestration) in the posterior wall of the outer cannula with no balloon – allows for the client to speak and is used to assist with weaning of the client from the tracheostomy because of holes in tube

C. A large or multiple opening (fenestrations) in the posterior wall of the outer cannula with balloon around the outside of the distal segment of the tube – allows for mechanical ventilation and for the client to speak

D. Used for clients with long or thick necks

E. Thin solid tool placed inside the tracheostomy and used as a guide for insertion of the outer cannula – removed immediately after outer cannula insertion

F. No balloon, used for clients with long-term airway management needs

3. A nurse in the ICU is caring for a confused and combative client who is 2 weeks post coronary artery bypass grafting (CABG). The client remains on a mechanical ventilator and is 4 days post tracheotomy, which was completed in attempt to assist with easier weaning. Upon entering the room, the nurse notes that the client is holding the tracheostomy tube in his hand. He is tachypneic, tachycardic, and his pulse oximetry reading is 88%. What are the priority nursing interventions?

4. Which of the following interventions is appropriate when caring for a client with a tracheostomy tube?

    A. Use medical aseptic technique when performing tracheostomy care.

    B. Change tracheostomy ties each time tracheostomy care is given.

    C. Keep cuff pressure between 14 to 20 mm Hg.

    D. Clean stoma site with antibiotic solution.

Chapter 69: Artificial Airway

Application Exercises Answer Key

1. Identify indications for placement of a tracheostomy tube.

   Acute or chronic upper airway obstruction

   Edema (anaphylaxis, burns, trauma, head/neck surgery)

   To facilitate removal of secretions

   To permit long-term mechanical ventilation

   To provide airway reconstruction after laryngeal trauma or laryngeal cancer surgery

   To treat obstructive sleep apnea refractory to conventional therapy

   To permit oral intake and speech in the client who requires long-term mechanical ventilation

2. Match the tracheostomy tube with the correct characteristics.

   D Single lumen (cannula)

   A Cuffed tube

   F Cuffless tube

   C Fenestrated tube (with cuff)

   B Fenestrated tube (without cuff)

   E Obturator

   A. Balloon that is inflated around the outside of the distal segment of the tube to protect the lower airway by producing a seal between the upper and lower airway (permits mechanical ventilation)

   B. One large or multiple opening (fenestration) in the posterior wall of the outer cannula with no balloon – allows for the client to speak and is used to assist with weaning of the client from the tracheostomy because of holes in tube

   C. A large or multiple opening (fenestrations) in the posterior wall of the outer cannula with balloon around the outside of the distal segment of the tube – allows for mechanical ventilation and for the client to speak

   D. Used for clients with long or thick necks

   E. Thin solid tool placed inside the tracheostomy and used as a guide for insertion of the outer cannula – removed immediately after outer cannula insertion

   F. No balloon, used for clients with long-term airway management needs

3. A nurse in the ICU is caring for a confused and combative client who is 2 weeks post coronary artery bypass grafting (CABG). The client remains on a mechanical ventilator and is 4 days post tracheotomy, which was completed in attempt to assist with easier weaning. Upon entering the room, the nurse notes that the client is holding the tracheostomy tube in his hand. He is tachypneic, tachycardic, and his pulse oximetry reading is 88%. What are the priority nursing interventions?

The nurse may be able to reinsert the tube, but if any difficulty arises, the nurse should call for assistance.

Immediately open the airway by extending the client's neck.

Obtain obturator and spare tracheostomy tube from head of the bed, place the obturator in the outer cannula, insert into the tracheostoma, and then remove the obturator. If unable to reinsert the tube, call for assistance.

Secure the tube.

Assess tube placement by auscultating for bilateral breath sounds.

4. Which of the following interventions is appropriate when caring for a client with a tracheostomy tube?

    A. Use medical aseptic technique when performing tracheostomy care.

    B. Change tracheostomy ties each time tracheostomy care is given.

    C. Keep cuff pressure between 14 to 20 mm Hg.

    D. Clean stoma site with antibiotic solution.

Suction pressure should be kept between 14 to 20 mm Hg to prevent tracheal wall necrosis. Use surgical aseptic technique when performing tracheostomy care. Ties only need to be changed when soiled. It is not necessary to clean the stoma site with an antibiotic solution. Hydrogen peroxide and normal saline are routinely used.

Unit 5   **Supporting Physiologic Needs**
Section: Oxygenation Needs

Chapter 70:   Airway Clearance and Specimen Collection
Contributors: Terri Astorino, EdD, MSN, RN
Lori A. Budd, BS, RN

 NCLEX® Connections:

Learning Objective: Review and apply knowledge within "**Airway Clearance and Specimen Collection**" in readiness for performance of the following nursing activities as outlined by the NCLEX® test plans:

Δ   Assess the client's need for suctioning to ensure adequate tissue oxygenation.

Δ   Perform/assist with relevant laboratory, diagnostic, and therapeutic procedures within the nursing role, including:

  •   Preparation of the client for the procedure.

  •   Client teaching (before and following the procedure).

  •   Assessment and evaluation of the client's response (expected, unexpected adverse response, comparison to baseline) to the procedure and appropriate notification of the primary care provider.

  •   Recognizing signs of potential complications and reporting to the primary care provider.

  •   Monitoring and taking actions, including client education, to prevent or minimize the risk of complications.

Δ   Document the client's response to nursing interventions.

 Key Points

Δ   **Mucosal secretion** buildup or aspiration of **emesis** can cause a client's airway to become obstructed or reduced.

  •   Adequate hydration and coughing assist the client to maintain airway patency.

- Clients at risk for developing airway compromise include: infants, clients with neuromuscular disorders, clients who are quadriplegic, and clients with cystic fibrosis.

Δ Indications for obtaining sputum specimens include:

- Cytology to identify aberrant cells or cancer.

- Culture and sensitivity to identify micro-organisms and determine antibiotic sensitivity.

- Acid-fast bacillus (AFB) to diagnose tuberculosis (TB) (requires three consecutive morning samples).

Δ Sputum specimens can be collected during coughing or may necessitate suctioning.

Key Procedural Points

Δ Nursing interventions that mobilize secretions and maintain airway patency include assistance with coughing, hydration, positioning, humidification, nebulizer therapy, chest physiotherapy, and suctioning.

Δ These interventions promote adequate gas exchange and lung expansion.

Δ Indications that the client needs assistance in maintaining airway clearance include signs of hypoxemia (e.g., restlessness, irritability, tachypnea, tachycardia, cyanosis, decreased level of consciousness, decreased SaO_2 levels), adventitious breath sounds, visualization of secretions, and absence of spontaneous cough.

Δ Whenever possible, the client should be encouraged to cough. **Coughing** is more effective than artificial suctioning at moving secretion into the upper trachea or laryngopharynx.

Δ **Humidification** of oxygen moistens the airways, which promotes loosening and mobilizing of pulmonary secretions.

Δ The process of **nebulization** breaks up medications (e.g., bronchodilators, mucolytic agents) into minute particles that are then dispersed throughout the respiratory tract.

Δ **Chest physiotherapy** (CPT) involves the use of chest percussion, vibration, and postural drainage to assist the client to mobilize secretions. Chest percussion and vibration facilitate movement of secretions into the central airways. Postural drainage entails the client assuming one or more positions (9 total) to allow gravity to assist with the removal of secretions from specific areas of the lung.

Δ Early morning postural drainage is best to assist with secretions that have accumulated through the night.

Δ Suctioning can be accomplished **orally, nasally, or endotracheally**. Suctioning is not performed on a routine basis but only when indicated.

Δ   **Surgical aseptic technique** must be maintained when performing any form of **tracheal suctioning** to avoid bacterial contamination of the airway.

Nursing Interventions

Δ   **Sputum Specimen Collection**

- Equipment

  ◊   Obtain all equipment, which includes: a sterile specimen container, client label and laboratory requisition slip, biohazard bag for delivery of specimen to laboratory, clean gloves (mask and goggles if necessary) following the Centers for Disease Control and Prevention's (CDC) standard precautions.

  °   Use container with preservative to obtain specimen for cytology.

  °   Use sterile container for routine culture and acid-fast bacillus (AFB).

- Procedure

  ◊   Check for primary care provider's order.

  ◊   Collect necessary equipment.

  ◊   Wash hands, provide privacy, and explain the procedure and rationale to the client.

  ◊   The client should be placed in Fowler's position.

  ◊   Have the client rinse mouth of any oral contaminant.

  ◊   Assess the client's ability to cough and expectorate secretions.

  ◊   Instruct the client to breathe deeply two to four times, and then cough deeply to raise the sputum from the lung.

  ◊   The sputum (1 to 2 tsp) should be expectorated into the sterile cup without contamination.

  ◊   Maintaining sterility, place the lid on the specimen cup, label it, and place it in the biohazard bag.

  ◊   Specimens should be delivered to the laboratory within 30 min.

  ◊   Document interventions and the client's response.

- Nursing implications

  ◊   **First early morning specimen** provides the best sputum sample.

  ◊   Wait 1 to 2 hr after eating to obtain a specimen in order to decrease the likelihood of emesis or aspiration.

  ◊   Chest physiotherapy may assist with the mobilization of secretions prior to specimen collection.

◊ If an inadequate amount of sputum is collected, repeat the specimen collection after the client takes several deep breaths and coughs.

◊ If client is unable to cough effectively, obtain a provider's order for collection of specimen by endotracheal suctioning. Sputum trap is attached between the suction catheter and the wall unit tubing.

Δ **Postural Drainage**

- Equipment

  ◊ Have emesis basin and tissue available for client to use when expectorating secretions.

- Procedure

  ◊ Wash hands, provide privacy, and explain the procedure and rationale to the client.

  ◊ Ensure proper positioning of client to promote drainage of specific areas of the lungs.

    ° Apical sections of upper lobes – Fowler's position

    ° Posterior sections of upper lobes – side-lying

    ° Right lobe – left side with pillow under the chest wall

    ° Left lobe – Trendelenburg's position

  ◊ Have the client remain in each position for 15 min (typically 5 min in position, 5 min for percussion/vibration/coughing, and 5 min for bronchial drainage).

  ◊ Evaluate the effectiveness of treatment by pre- and postprocedure lung auscultation and assessment of the amount, color, and character of expectorated secretions.

  ◊ Document interventions and repeat procedure as prescribed by the provider (typically 3 to 4 times per day).

- Nursing implications

  ◊ Schedule treatments 1 hr before meals or 2 hr after meals to decrease likelihood of client vomiting or aspiration.

  ◊ Administer bronchodilator medication or nebulizer treatment 30 min to 1 hr prior to postural drainage if ordered by the primary care provider.

  ◊ Postural drainage is often preceded with percussion and vibration.

    ° Percussion – use of cupped hands to rhythmically clap on the chest to break up secretions

    ° Vibration – shaking movement applied during exhalation to assist with removal of secretions

◊ Postural drainage is contraindicated for clients who are pregnant; clients with a rib, chest, head or neck injury; clients who have had recent abdominal surgery; and clients with a pulmonary embolism.

◊ Postural drainage should be discontinued on any client who reports feeling dizzy or faint.

◊ Those clients who are too weak to effectively expectorate secretions following postural drainage should have a provider's order for tracheobronchial suctioning.

◊ Postural drainage may induce hypoxia and dyspnea; therefore, continuous respiratory assessment during treatment is essential.

Δ **Suctioning** – If suctioning is indicated, it is best to begin with oropharyngeal suctioning, since it is better tolerated by clients.

- Equipment (for all types of suctioning)

    ◊ Collect suction kit with appropriate size catheter, sterile water/normal saline, extra gloves, towel or drape and protective clothing, and a sputum trap if obtaining a sputum specimen has been ordered.

- Procedure (for all types of suctioning)

    ◊ Wash hands, provide privacy, and explain the procedure (to ALL clients, conscious or unconscious) and rationale to the client.

    ◊ Don necessary protective clothing.

    ◊ Place the client in **Fowler's or semi-Fowler's position** for suctioning, if possible.

    ◊ Encourage the client to **deep breathe and cough** in an attempt to clear the secretions without artificial suction.

    ◊ If secretions remain, continue with the procedure.

    ◊ Obtain baseline breath sounds and vital signs, including oxygen saturation (SaO_2) by pulse oximeter prior to procedure. Continue to monitor SaO_2 during and after.

    ◊ Use **surgical aseptic technique** when **opening suction catheter kits.**

    ◊ **Medical aseptic technique** can be used to suction the mouth (oropharyngeal), whereas **surgical aseptic technique** must be used for all other types of suctioning.

    ◊ Open sterile suction package.

    ◊ Place sterile drape or towel on the client's chest.

    ◊ Set up container, touching only the outside.

    ◊ Pour approximately 100 mL of sterile water or normal saline into container.

◊ Don sterile gloves.

◦ Clean hand/nondominant hand holds the connecting tube; glove protects the nurse.

◦ Sterile hand/dominant hand holds the sterile catheter; glove protects the client.

◊ Connect suction catheter to wall unit tubing.

◊ Set suction pressure at 80 to 120 mm Hg.

◊ **Test the suction setup** by aspirating sterile water/normal saline from the cup. If the unit is operating properly, continue with the procedure.

◊ Limit each suction attempt to **no longer than 10 to 15 sec** to avoid hypoxemia and the vagal response. Limit suctioning to two to three attempts.

◊ Once suctioning is complete, **clear the suction tubing** by aspirating sterile water/normal saline solution.

◊ Document pre- and postassessment data (e.g., vital signs, SpO_2, breath sounds); how the client tolerated the procedure; and color, consistency, and amount of secretions.

• Procedure

◊ **Oropharyngeal suctioning**

◦ Oropharyngeal suctioning is most often performed using a Yankauer or tonsil-tipped rigid suction catheter.

◦ Insert the catheter into the client's mouth.

◦ **Apply suction** and move the catheter around the mouth, gum line, and pharynx.

◦ Clear the catheter and tubing.

◦ Repeat as needed.

◦ Replace oxygen mask, if applicable.

◦ Store the catheter in a clean, dry place for reuse.

◦ Allow the client to perform own suctioning if possible.

◦ Document the client's response.

◊ **Nasopharyngeal and nasotracheal suctioning**

◦ Suctioning is performed with a flexible catheter.

◦ **Catheter size** is based upon the diameter of the client's nostrils and the thickness of the secretions.

◦ **Hyperoxygenate** the client during equipment preparation with 100% FiO_2.

- ° Lubricate the distal end 6 to 8 cm (2 to 3 in) of the suction catheter with a **water-soluble lubricant**.

- ° Remove the oxygen delivery device with the nondominant hand, if applicable.

- ° **Insert** the catheter into the nare **during inhalation**.

- ° Do not apply suction while inserting the catheter.

- ° **Follow the natural course of the nare** and slightly slant the catheter downward as it is advanced.

- ° Advance the catheter the approximate distance from nose tip to base of earlobe.

- ° **Apply suction intermittently** by covering and releasing the suction port with the thumb for 10 to 15 sec.

- ° **Only** apply suction while **withdrawing the catheter** and rotating it with the thumb and forefinger.

- ° Allow the client time for recovery between sessions, 20 to 30 sec.

- ° Repeat as necessary, hyperoxygenating the client before each suctioning pass.

- ° **Document** client response.

- ° Do not reuse the suction catheter.

◊ **Endotracheal suctioning (ETS)**

- ° ETS is performed through a tracheostomy or endotracheal tube.

- ° This procedure may require an assistant.

- ° **Sterility must be maintained** during endotracheal suctioning.

- ° The outer diameter of the suction catheter should be less than ½ the internal diameter of the endotracheal tube.

- ° **Hyperoxygenate** the client using a bag-valve-mask (BVM) or specialized ventilator function with 100% FiO_2.

- ° Immediately after the BVM or ventilator is removed from the tracheostomy or endotracheal tube, **insert the catheter into the lumen of the airway. Advance until resistance is met.** The catheter should reach the level of the carina (location of bifurcation into the main stem bronchi).

- ° Pull catheter back 1 cm prior to applying suction to prevent mucosal damage.

- ° **Apply suction intermittently** by covering and releasing the suction port with the thumb for 10 to 15 sec.

- ° **Only** apply suction while **withdrawing the catheter** and rotating it with the thumb and forefinger.

- ° **Reattach the BVM or ventilator** and supply the client with 100% inspired oxygen.
- ° Clear the catheter and tubing.
- ° Allow time for client recovery between sessions.
- ° Repeat as necessary.
- ° Many mechanical ventilators have **in-line suction devices**. This may eliminate the need for an assistant. Follow institution protocols for these systems. Always maintain sterile technique.

Complications and Nursing Implications

Δ **Hypoxemia**

- Limit each suction attempt to **no longer than 10 to 15 sec.**
- Limit suctioning to two to three attempts.
- Allow the client time for recovery between sessions, 20 to 30 sec.
- Hyperoxygenate the client before and after each suctioning pass.

Δ **Anxiety**

- Explain the procedure prior to suctioning to all clients.
- Provide reassurance before, during, and after the procedure.
- Maintain calm manner.

Primary Reference:

Potter, P. A., & Perry, A. G. (2005). *Fundamentals of nursing* (6th ed.). St. Louis, MO: Mosby.

Additional Resources:

Harkreader, H., & Hogan, M. A. (2004). *Fundamentals of nursing: Caring and clinical judgment*. Philadelphia: Elsevier.

Ignatavicius, D. D., & Workman, M. L. (2006). *Medical-surgical nursing* (5th ed.). St. Louis, MO: Saunders.

NANDA International (2004). *NANDA nursing diagnoses: Definitions and classification 2005-2006*. Philadelphia: NANDA.

Chapter 70: Airway Clearance and Specimen Collection

Application Exercises

1. Place the following steps for obtaining a sputum specimen in the correct order.

    _____ Place the client in Fowler's position.

    _____ Have the client expectorate the sputum into sterile cup without contamination.

    _____ Check for a provider's order.

    _____ Deliver specimen to the laboratory within 30 min.

    _____ Have the client rinse mouth.

    _____ Maintaining sterility, place the lid on the specimen cup, label it, and place it in the biohazard bag.

    _____ Assess the client's ability to cough and expectorate secretions.

    _____ Obtain necessary equipment.

    _____ Instruct the client to breathe deeply two to four times and then cough deeply to raise the sputum from the lung.

    _____ Wash hands, provide privacy, and explain the procedure and rationale to the client/family.

2. A client is unable to produce a sputum specimen. Identify nursing interventions that may be instituted to assist the client with sputum production.

3. Which of the following client assessments indicates that the nurse needs to perform suctioning? (Select all that apply.)

    _____ Client resting comfortably

    _____ Adventitious breath sounds

    _____ Absence of spontaneous cough

    _____ SaO_2 87%

    _____ Respirations even, unlabored, 16/min

4. A nurse is preparing to perform endotracheal suctioning. Which of the following are appropriate guidelines to be followed? (Select all that apply.)

    _____ Only apply suction while withdrawing the catheter.

    _____ Suctioning should be performed on a routine basis, every 2 to 3 hr.

    _____ Maintain medical aseptic technique.

    _____ Use a new tube each time suctioning is performed.

    _____ Limit suctioning to two to three attempts.

Chapter 70: Airway Clearance and Specimen Collection

Application Exercises Answer Key

1. Place the following steps for obtaining a sputum specimen in the correct order.

   __4__ Place the client in Fowler's position.

   __8__ Have the client expectorate the sputum into sterile cup without contamination.

   __1__ Check for a provider's order.

   __10__ Deliver specimen to the laboratory within 30 min.

   __5__ Have the client rinse mouth.

   __9__ Maintaining sterility, place the lid on the specimen cup, label it, and place it in the biohazard bag.

   __6__ Assess the client's ability to cough and expectorate secretions.

   __2__ Obtain necessary equipment.

   __7__ Instruct the client to breathe deeply two to four times and then cough deeply to raise the sputum from the lung.

   __3__ Wash hands, provide privacy, and explain the procedure and rationale to the client/family.

2. A client is unable to produce a sputum specimen. Identify nursing interventions that may be instituted to assist the client with sputum production.

   Attempt the procedure in the early morning when mucus has accumulated, and the client has more energy to expectorate it.

   Perform postural drainage to mobilize secretions prior to attempting sputum collection.

   Increase fluid intake to liquidize secretions and allow for greater ease of expectoration.

   Notify the primary care provider and request an order for a nebulizer/bronchodilator to allow for greater sputum production.

   Notify the primary care provider and request an order for oropharyngeal or nasotracheal suctioning to obtain the sputum specimen.

3. Which of the following client assessments indicates that the nurse needs to perform suctioning? (Select all that apply.)

_____ Client resting comfortably

__X__ **Adventitious breath sounds**

__X__ **Absence of spontaneous cough**

__X__ **SaO$_2$ 87%**

_____ Respirations even, unlabored, 16/min

Adventitious breath sounds, absence of spontaneous cough, and an SaO$_2$ 87% are signs of respiratory distress and indications of the need for suctioning. The client is usually restless with labored respirations.

4. A nurse is preparing to perform endotracheal suctioning. Which of the following are appropriate guidelines to be followed? (Select all that apply.)

__X__ **Only apply suction while withdrawing the catheter.**

_____ Suctioning should be performed on a routine basis, every 2 to 3 hr.

_____ Maintain medical aseptic technique.

__X__ **Use a new tube each time suctioning is performed.**

__X__ **Limit suctioning to two to three attempts.**

Suctioning should only be applied while the catheter is being withdrawn. Endotracheal suctioning is performed using surgical aseptic technique, so the catheter should not be reused. Each suctioning session is limited to two to three attempts to prevent hypoxemia. Suctioning should only be performed when indicated, not on a routine basis.

Unit 5   Supporting Physiologic Needs
Section: Circulatory Needs

Chapter 71:   **Cardiopulmonary Resuscitation**
                  Contributor: Linda Turchin, MSN, RN

NCLEX® Connections:

Learning Objective: Review and apply knowledge within "**Cardiopulmonary Resuscitation (CPR)**" in readiness for performance of the following nursing activities as outlined by the NCLEX® test plans:

Δ   Recognize life-threatening situations and intervene appropriately.

Δ   Perform CPR according to current newborn/infant/child/adult guidelines.

Δ   Notify the primary care provider of the client's medical emergency.

Δ   Evaluate and document the client's response to emergency intervention.

Key Points

Δ   A **cardiac arrest,** the sudden cessation of breathing and adequate circulation of blood, results in the termination of **cardiac output** and is characterized by the **absence of spontaneous respirations and a pulse**.

Δ   Management of a cardiac arrest depends on prompt recognition of signs and symptoms and the introduction of therapeutic interventions directed at artificially sustaining circulation and ventilation.

Δ   Ventricular fibrillation is the cause of sudden, nontraumatic cardiac arrest in 80 to 90% of victims.

Δ   Without sufficient cardiac output, the brain will suffer **cell anoxia** (cell death) within 4 to 6 min, with **death** following shortly thereafter.

Δ   An interdisciplinary team will provide care during in-hospital cardiac arrests. This team should include nurses, physicians, respiratory therapists, laboratory personnel, and chaplain services.

Δ   **CPR** is the process of externally supporting the circulation and respirations of an individual who has experienced a cardiac arrest. CPR significantly increases the chances of survival when initiated immediately.

Δ   Prehospital care greatly improves the chance of survival of cardiac arrest victims.

Key Procedural Points

Δ   Basic interventions can be delivered by trained citizens, but advanced interventions require more sophisticated training, certification, and the use of emergency equipment.

Δ   CPR is a series of emergency procedures directed at artificially providing a client with circulation (chest compressions) and oxygenation (ventilations) in the absence of cardiac output.

Δ   CPR is a component of basic life support (BLS) and advanced cardiac life support (ACLS).

Δ   The goal of BLS is to provide oxygen to the vital organs until appropriate advanced resuscitation measures can be initiated or until resuscitative efforts are ordered to be stopped. BLS involves the ABCs of CPR:

- **Airway**

  ◊   Confirm the absence of spontaneous respirations.

  ◊   Establish a patent airway.

  ◊   If the airway is obstructed with a foreign object, use the Heimlich maneuver for a conscious client, and use abdominal thrusts for unconscious clients.

- **Breathing**

  ◊   Check for breathing.

  ◊   Provide artificial respirations (ventilations) to deliver oxygen into the blood in an attempt to prevent cell anoxia.

- **Circulation**

  ◊   Confirm the absence or presence of a pulse.

  ◊   Provide external support of circulation (chest compressions) to transport oxygenated blood to the brain.

Δ   The goal of ACLS is the return of spontaneous breathing and circulation. In addition to the ABCs of BLS, ACLS involves:

- Diagnosis of underlying cardiac dysrhythmias.

- Defibrillation as required. This involves delivering a premeasured shock to the heart in order to interrupt the aberrant rhythm and to allow the natural pacemaker of the heart to initiate beats.

- Insertion of an oropharyngeal or endotracheal airway with bag ventilation and supplemental oxygen.

- Administration of IV fluids.

- Administration of IV antidysrhythmic medications based on the dysrhythmias identified.

Δ The chain of survival is a series of interventions directed at the resuscitation of the cardiac arrest victim. It involves:

- Early activation of the emergency medical services.

- **Look**, **Listen**, and **Feel** for:

    ◊ Unresponsiveness (no signs of movement).

    ◊ No spontaneous respirations (Apnea).

    ◊ No palpable pulse (Asystole).

- Early CPR/early defibrillation.

- Early ACLS care.

Nursing Interventions

Δ The nurse assisting during a cardiac arrest must:

- Use the current BLS and ACLS guidelines from the American Heart Association (AHA).

- Be knowledgeable about institutional policies/procedures and the location and operation of emergency equipment (crash cart).

- Have current certification for BLS. ACLS certification may be required by facility/agency policy for specific practice settings.

Δ Nursing responsibilities include:

- Maintaining airway patency.

- Assessing the depth and rate of respirations.

- Providing chest compressions at the appropriate rate and depth for age (*Refer to the chart on the following page.*).

- Assessing vital signs for effectiveness of chest compressions and ventilations.

- Defibrillating the client when indicated.

- Obtaining and maintaining IV access.

- Providing medications as ordered.

- Monitoring laboratory values (e.g., ABGs, CBC, electrolytes).

- Documenting all interventions and medications.

AHA Guidelines: BLS for Infants, Children, and Adults

Maneuver	Adult (adolescent and up)	Child (1 year to adolescent)	Infant (under 1 year)
Activate Emergency Response Number	Activate when victim found unresponsive. If asphyxial arrest is likely, call after 5 cycles (2 min) of CPR.	Activate after performing 5 cycles of CPR. For sudden, witnessed collapse, activate after verifying that the victim is unresponsive.	
Airway	Head tilt chin lift (For suspected trauma, use jaw thrust.)		
Breaths Initial	2 breaths at 1 sec/breath	2 effective breaths at 1 sec/breath	
Rescue Breaths without chest compressions	10 to 12 breaths/min (approx. 1 breath every 5 to 6 sec)	12 to 20 breaths/min (approx. 1 breath every 3 to 5 sec)	
Rescue Breaths for CPR with advanced airway	8 to 10 breaths/min (approx. 1 breath every 6 to 8 sec)		
Foreign-Body Airway Obstruction	Abdominal thrusts		Back slaps and chest thrusts
Circulation	Carotid	Carotid or femoral	Brachial or femoral
Compression Landmarks	Center of chest, between nipples		Just below nipple line
Compression Method	2 hands: heel of one hand, other hand on top	2 hands: heel of one hand, other hand on top 1 hand: heel of one hand only	1 rescuer: 2 fingers 2 rescuers: 2 thumb-encircling hands
Compression Depth	1 ½ to 2 inches	Approx. ⅓ to ½ the depth of the chest	
Compression Rate	Approx. 100/min		
Compression-Ventilation Ratio	30:2 (1 or 2 rescuers)	30:2 (1 rescuer) 15:2 (2 rescuers)	

*Table based on AHA guidelines for healthcare providers.

Source: American Heart Association. American Heart Association 2005 Guidelines for CPR and ECC. Retrieved May 10, 2006, from: *http://www.americanheart.org/presenter.jhtml?identifier=3035517*

Primary Reference:

Potter, P. A., & Perry, A. G. (2005). *Fundamentals of nursing* (6th ed.). St. Louis, MO: Mosby.

Additional Resources:

American Heart Association. (Winter 2005-2006). Currents in Emergency Cardiovascular Care. *Table 2. Summary of BLS ABCD Maneuvers for Infants, Children, and Adults.* Retrieved October 16, 2006, from *http://www.americanheart.org/downloadable/heart/1132621842912Winter2005.pdf*

Ignatavicius, D. and Workman, M. (2006). *Medical-surgical nursing* (5th ed.). St. Louis: MO, Saunders.

Lewis, Heitkemper, & Dirksen (2004). *Medical surgical nursing: Assessment and management of clinical problems* (6th ed.). St. Louis, MO: Mosby.

NANDA International (2004). *NANDA nursing diagnoses: Definitions and classification 2005-2006.* Philadelphia: NANDA.

Chapter 71: Cardiopulmonary Resuscitation

Application Exercises

Scenario: A 62-year-old client has been hospitalized for abdominal pain. He has a history of hypertension and coronary artery disease and is currently taking a medication for a sinus infection. The client is found by the nurse on the floor next to his bed.

1. Which of the following immediate actions should the nurse take?

        A. Confirm presence or absence of spontaneous respirations.

        B. Check for unresponsiveness.

        C. Check the client's oxygen saturation.

        D. Assist the client to stand up.

2. What client findings would indicate the need for BLS?

3. Identify the order in which the nurse should perform the following interventions when performing CPR on an adult or a child older than age 8.

    _____ Perform ventilations.

    _____ Open the airway.

    _____ Start compressions.

    _____ Check for breathing.

    _____ Check for spontaneous pulse.

    _____ Check for unresponsiveness.

    _____ Call for help.

    _____ Check circulation (carotid pulse/signs of circulation).

4. A child is found unconscious and without spontaneous respirations or a pulse beneath a swing at a local park. What concern should the rescuer have regarding positioning the child for ventilation? How should the rescuer position the child before delivering ventilations?

5. Which of the following are nursing responsibilities while assisting during a cardiac arrest? (Select all that apply.)

_____ Maintain a patent airway.

_____ Assess respirations.

_____ Perform chest compressions.

_____ Administer medications as ordered.

_____ Decide when to stop interventions.

Chapter 71: Cardiopulmonary Resuscitation

Application Exercises Answer Key

Scenario: A 62-year-old client has been hospitalized for abdominal pain. He has a history of hypertension and coronary artery disease and is currently taking a medication for a sinus infection. The client is found by the nurse on the floor next to his bed.

1. Which of the following immediate actions should the nurse take?

   A. Confirm presence or absence of spontaneous respirations.
   B. Check for unresponsiveness.
   C. Check the client's oxygen saturation.
   D. Assist the client to stand up.

2. What client findings would indicate the need for BLS?

   The client is nonresponsive.

   The client is not breathing spontaneously.

   The client does not have a pulse.

3. Identify the order in which the nurse should perform the following interventions when performing CPR on an adult or a child older than age 8.

   5 Perform ventilations.
   3 Open the airway.
   7 Start compressions.
   4 Check for breathing.
   8 Check for spontaneous pulse.
   1 Check for unresponsiveness.
   2 Call for help.
   6 Check circulation (carotid pulse/signs of circulation).

4. A child is found unconscious and without spontaneous respirations or a pulse beneath a swing at a local park. What concern should the rescuer have regarding positioning the child for ventilation? How should the rescuer position the child before delivering ventilations?

Due to the possibility of cervical trauma, the jaw thrust rather than the head tilt – chin lift, should be used.

5. Which of the following are nursing responsibilities while assisting during a cardiac arrest? (Select all that apply.)

  X   **Maintain a patent airway.**

  X   **Assess respirations.**

  X   **Perform chest compressions.**

  X   **Administer medications as ordered.**

  _____   Decide when to stop interventions.

Maintaining a patent airway, assessing respirations, performing chest compressions, and administering medications are all within the scope of practice for the nurse. The primary care provider usually decides when interventions should be stopped.

Unit 5	Supporting Physiologic Needs
Section:	Circulatory Needs

Chapter 72:   Promoting Venous Return
Contributor: Wendy Buenzli, MN, RN

 NCLEX® Connections

Learning Objective: Review and apply knowledge within "**Promoting Venous Return**" in readiness for performance of the following nursing activities as outlined by the NCLEX® test plans:

Δ   Assess/monitor the client for impaired venous return.

Δ   Identify clients at risk for poor venous return, and initiate interventions.

Δ   Plan and/or provide care to prevent the development of deep vein thrombosis and pulmonary embolism.

Δ   Plan and/or provide for elastic and compression stockings, positioning, and leg exercises to improve venous return.

Δ   Evaluate and document care given to clients to prevent the development of deep vein thrombosis and pulmonary embolism.

 Key Points

Δ   **Elastic stockings or TED hose** aid in the maintenance of external pressure on the muscles of the lower extremities and cause the blood to return to the heart.

Δ   **Sequential Compression Devices (SCDs) and Intermittent Pneumatic Compression (IPC)** are plastic or fabric sleeves that wrap around the leg and secure with Velcro™. The sleeves are then attached to an electric pump that alternately inflates and deflates the sleeve around the leg. These machines are set to cycle, and a normal cycle is inflation 10 to 15 sec and deflation 45 to 60 sec.

Δ   **Positioning** techniques reduce compression of leg veins.

Δ   **Range-of-motion exercises** cause skeletal muscle contractions, which promote blood return. Specific exercises that help prevent thrombophlebitis include ankle pumps, foot circles, and knee flexion.

Key Procedural Points

Δ Elastic stockings, sequential compression devices, and intermittent pneumatic compression require a primary care provider's order.

Δ The nurse should encourage immobile clients to perform leg exercises, increase fluid intake, and change positions frequently. These interventions can be implemented without a primary care provider's order.

Δ If at any time the nurse suspects poor venous return or possible thrombus, the primary care provider must be notified. Make sure no pressure is applied to a thrombus as not to dislodge it.

NANDA Nursing Diagnoses

Δ Ineffective tissue perfusion (peripheral)

Δ Impaired gas exchange

Δ Risk for injury

Nursing Interventions

Δ **Elastic Stockings or TED Hose**

- Equipment

  ◊ Tape measure

  ◊ TED hose

- Procedure

  ◊ Wash hands.

  ◊ Assess the condition of the skin and circulation of the client's legs.

  ◊ Measure the client's calf and/or thigh circumference and length of leg and select the correct fitting stocking.

  ◊ Turn stockings inside to the heel.

  ◊ Put stocking on the foot.

  ◊ Pull remaining part of the stocking over the heel and on up the leg.

  ◊ Remove any creases or wrinkles.

  ◊ Stockings must be removed and reapplied at least twice a day. It is important to make sure the client has the necessary support to accomplish this task.

  ◊ Make sure the toes are not too tight at the end of the stockings.

  ◊ The stockings must always be clean and dry. A postsurgical client or a client with special needs may need a second pair of hose.

  ◊ Document application and removal of stockings.

Δ   **SCDs and IPC**

- Equipment
  - ◊ Tape measure
  - ◊ Sequential stockings
  - ◊ Stockinette

- Procedure
  - ◊ Wash hands.
  - ◊ Assess circulation and skin prior to application.
  - ◊ Measure around the largest part of the client's thigh to obtain proper stocking size.
  - ◊ Place stockinette on first.
  - ◊ Apply sleeves.
  - ◊ Attach the sleeves to the inflator.
  - ◊ Turn on device.
  - ◊ Monitor circulation and skin after application.
  - ◊ Document application and removal of stockings.

Δ   Positioning techniques reduce compression of leg veins.

- Equipment – none

- Procedure – Teach the client to avoid:
  - ◊ Crossing legs.
  - ◊ Sitting for long periods of time.
  - ◊ Wearing restrictive clothing on the lower extremities.
  - ◊ Putting pillows behind knees.
  - ◊ Massaging the legs.

Δ   Range-of-motion exercises are performed hourly while the client is awake.

- Equipment – none

- Procedure – Teach the client to perform:
  - ◊ Ankle pumps – Point toes toward the head and then away from the head.
  - ◊ Foot circles – Rotate the feet in circles at the ankles.
  - ◊ Knee flexion – Flex and extend the legs at the knees.

Complications and Nursing Implications

Δ **Thrombophlebitis/deep vein thrombosis** is an inflammation of a vein (usually in the lower extremities) that results in clot formation.

- Signs and symptoms are pain, edema, warmth, and erythema at the site.

- Nursing implications:

  ◊ Notify the primary care provider immediately.

  ◊ Place the client in bed with the leg elevated.

  ◊ No pressure should be applied to the site of the inflammation.

  ◊ Anticipate giving anticoagulants as ordered.

Δ **Pulmonary embolism** is the occlusion of blood flow to one or more of the pulmonary arteries by a clot. The condition can be life threatening. The clot or embolus often originates in the venous system of the lower extremities.

- Signs and symptoms are shortness of breath, chest pain, coughing up blood, decreased blood pressure, and rapid pulse.

- Nursing implications

  ◊ Prepare to give thrombolytics or anticoagulants depending on the severity.

Primary Reference:

Potter, P. A., & Perry, A. G. (2005). *Fundamentals of nursing* (6th ed.). St. Louis, MO: Mosby.

Additional Resources:

NANDA International (2004). *NANDA nursing diagnoses: Definitions and classification 2005-2006*. Philadelphia: NANDA.

Chapter 72: Promoting Venous Return

Application Exercises

1. An 82-year-old client presents to the surgical unit following a total hip replacement. The client's vital signs are stable. Prior to surgery, she walked with a cane because of her hip. She has significant varicose veins in her lower extremities and has a history of blood clots. Identify the priority nursing diagnoses for this client.

2. A nurse has just started an admission assessment for a client with limited mobility. The nurse notes that there is no medical order for a sequential compression device. Which of the following nursing interventions should the nurse take next?

    A. Apply the compression devices as no primary care provider's order is required.

    B. Contact the primary care provider to get an order.

    C. Complete the assessment before taking any other action.

    D. Apply the compression devices and then call the primary care provider.

3. Sequential compression devices are used on clients to

    A. prevent bed sores.

    B. promote venous return.

    C. prevent muscular atrophy.

    D. increase joint mobility.

4. Identify the order in which the following steps of elastic stocking application should be completed.

    _____ Wash hands.

    _____ Remove any creases or wrinkles.

    _____ Pull remaining part of the stocking over the client's heel and on up his leg.

    _____ Turn stockings inside to heel.

    _____ Assess the condition of the client's skin and circulation of his legs.

    _____ Put stocking on the client's foot.

    _____ Measure the client's calf and/or thigh circumference and length of the leg, and select the correctly-fitted stocking.

Chapter 72: Promoting Venous Return

Application Exercises Answer Key

1. An 82-year-old client presents to the surgical unit following a total hip replacement. The client's vital signs are stable. Prior to surgery, she walked with a cane because of her hip. She has significant varicose veins in her lower extremities and has a history of blood clots. Identify the priority nursing diagnoses for this client.

   Risk for injury due to immobility

   Ineffective (peripheral) tissue perfusion

2. A nurse has just started an admission assessment for a client with limited mobility. The nurse notes that there is no medical order for a sequential compression device. Which of the following nursing interventions should the nurse take next?

   A. Apply the compression devices as no primary care provider's order is required.

   B. Contact the primary care provider to get an order.

   C. Complete the assessment before taking any other action.

   D. Apply the compression devices and then call the primary care provider.

   An assessment is the first step. The assessment will provide information regarding the client's need for a compression device (e.g., The client may be able to follow positioning advice, perform range-of-motion exercises, and be taking an anticoagulant medication.). A medical order is required for a compression device, so applying the device prior to getting an order is not appropriate practice. Before contacting the primary care provider, it is important for the nurse to collect all necessary data.

3. Sequential compression devices are used on clients to

   A. prevent bed sores.

   B. promote venous return.

   C. prevent muscular atrophy.

   D. increase joint mobility.

   The purpose of sequential compression devices is to promote venous return. Sequential compression devices do not prevent bed sores or muscular atrophy, and they do not increase joint mobility.

4. Identify the order in which the following steps of elastic stocking application should be completed.

  1   Wash hands.

  7   Remove any creases or wrinkles.

  6   Pull remaining part of the stocking over the client's heel and on up his leg.

  4   Turn stockings inside to heel.

  2   Assess the condition of the client's skin and circulation of his legs.

  5   Put stocking on the client's foot.

  3   Measure the client's calf and/or thigh circumference and length of the leg, and select the correctly-fitted stocking.

Unit 5   Supporting Physiologic Needs
Section: Fluid, Electrolyte, and Acid-Base Balance

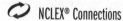

Chapter 73:   Fluid Balance

Contributor: Linda Turchin, MSN, RN

 NCLEX® Connections

Learning Objective: Review and apply knowledge within **"Fluid Balance"** in readiness for performance of the following nursing activities as outlined by the NCLEX® test plans:

Δ   Recognize signs and symptoms associated with fluid imbalances.

Δ   Interpret data that needs to be reported to the primary care provider immediately.

Δ   Perform and document appropriate assessments based upon the client's problem – fluid imbalances.

Δ   Plan and provide care for the client with a fluid imbalance.

Δ   Evaluate the client's response to interventions to correct fluid imbalances.

Key Points

Δ   Body fluids are distributed between **intracellular (ICF)** and **extracellular (ECF) fluid compartments**.

Δ   Fluid can move between compartments (through **selectively permeable membranes**) by a variety of methods (**diffusion, active transport, filtration, and osmosis**) in order to maintain homeostasis.

Δ   **Assessment** of fluid and electrolytes is a nursing responsibility that includes:

•   Nursing history.

•   Physical assessment.

◊   Mental status, behavior

◊   Skin and mucous membranes

◊   Breath and heart sounds

◊   Neurological status

- Measurement of I&O.

- Daily weight.

- Specific laboratory data.

Key Factors

Δ **Maintaining Balance**

- Homeostasis requires that fluid I&O be in balance, and the volumes and chemical composition of the fluid compartments be maintained within narrow limits

- Regulation is achieved through:

  ◊ Fluid intake that is primarily regulated by thirst and stimulated by the **increase** of plasma osmolality (**concentration of solutes in a solution**) and the **decrease of blood volume.**

  ◊ Fluid output occurs through the kidneys, skin, lungs, and the gastrointestinal tract.

Δ **Hormonal Regulation**

- **Antidiuretic hormone** is responsible for the reduction of urine production.

- **Renin** is released in response to decreased blood flow or decreased renal pressure (sensed by receptors in the nephrons).

- **Aldosterone** is produced by the adrenal cortex (in response to stimulation by angiotensin II) causing the tubules to excrete K$^+$ while retaining Na^{2+}, adding to the reabsorption of water back into the vascular system.

Fluid Volume Deficits

 Key Points

Δ **Fluid volume deficits (FVDs)** include **hypovolemia** (body loses both water and electrolytes from the ECF) and **dehydration** (water is lost from the body, but there is no loss of electrolytes).

Δ **Hypovolemia** can lead to **hypovolemic shock.**

Key Factors

△ **Risk Factors/Causes**

Hypovolemia	Dehydration
• **Gastrointestinal (GI) losses** – vomiting, nasogastric suctioning, diarrhea • **Skin losses** – diaphoresis • **Renal losses** – diuretic therapy, diabetes insipidus, renal disease, adrenal insufficiency, osmotic diuresis • **Third spacing** – peritonitis, intestinal obstruction, ascites, burns • **Hemorrhage** • **Altered intake**, such as nothing by mouth (NPO)	• Hyperventilation • Diabetic ketoacidosis • Enteral feeding without sufficient water intake

Assessment

• **Hemoglobin (Hgb) and hematocrit (Hct)**	• Hypovolemia – ↓ **Hgb and Hct** • Dehydration – ↑ **Hgb and Hct (hemoconcentration)**
• **Serum osmolarity**	• Dehydration – ↑ **(hemoconcentration)**
• **Urine specific gravity and osmolarity**	• Dehydration – ↑ **(concentration)**
• **Serum sodium**	• Dehydration – ↑ **(hemoconcentration)**
• **Vital signs**	• Hyperthermia, **tachycardia**, thready pulse, **hypotension**, orthostatic hypotension, decreased central venous pressure
• **Neuromusculoskeletal**	• Dizziness, **syncope**, **confusion**, **weakness**, fatigue
• **GI**	• Thirst, dry furrowed tongue, nausea/vomiting, anorexia, acute weight loss
• **Renal**	• **Oliguria**
• **Other signs**	• Diminished capillary refill, cool clammy skin, diaphoresis, sunken eyeballs, flattened neck veins

NANDA Nursing Diagnoses

△ Decreased cardiac output

△ Ineffective tissue perfusion

△ Deficient fluid volume

△ Potential for dysrhythmias

△ Risk for injury

Nursing Interventions

Δ   Place client in **shock position** (on back with legs elevated).

Δ   **Fluid replacement** – Administer oral and IV fluids (crystalloid solutions such as Ringer's lactate solution; blood transfusions) as ordered.

Δ   Monitor I&O. Alert the primary care provider to urine output less than 30 mL/hr for 2 consecutive hr.

Δ   Monitor vital signs and heart rhythm.

Δ   Monitor level of consciousness and maintain client safety.

Δ   Treat underlying cause of fluid volume deficit.

Δ   Encourage the client to change positions slowly.

Complications and Nursing Implications

Δ   **Hypovolemic Shock**

- This can lead to **vital organ hypoxia/anoxia – decreased** hemoglobin, **oxygen saturation**, and **pulse pressure** (systolic-diastolic blood pressure).

- Administer **oxygen.**

- Provide **fluid replacement.**

- Administer **vasoconstrictors**, **coronary** vasodilators, and/or **positive inotropes.**

- Perform hemodynamic monitoring.

Fluid Volume Excess

 Key Points

Δ   **Fluid volume excesses (FVEs)** include **hypervolemia** (occurs when both water and sodium are retained in abnormally high proportions) and **overhydration** (occurs when more water is gained than electrolytes).

Key Factors

Δ   Risk Factors/Causes

Hypervolemia	Overhydration
• **Chronic stimulus** to the kidney to **conserve sodium and water** (heart failure, cirrhosis, glucocorticosteroids) • **Abnormal renal function** with ↓ excretion of sodium and water (renal failure) • Interstitial to plasma **fluid shifts** (hypertonic fluids, burns) • **Age-related changes** in cardiovascular and renal function • **Excessive sodium intake**	• Water replacement without electrolyte replacement such as strenuous exercise with profuse diaphoresis

Assessment

• **Hemoglobin (Hgb) and hematocrit (Hct)**	• Overhydration – ↓ (**hemodilution**)
• **Serum osmolarity**	• Overhydration – ↓ (**hemodilution**) osmolarity (< 270 mOsm/L) – ↓ **protein and electrolytes**
• **Serum sodium**	• Overhydration – ↓ (**hemodilution**)
• **Electrolytes, BUN, and creatinine**	• Hypervolemia – ↑ **electrolytes, BUN, and creatinine**
• **Vital signs**	• **Tachycardia**, bounding pulse, **hypertension, tachypnea**, increased central venous pressure
• **Neuromusculoskeletal**	• **Confusion**, muscle weakness
• **GI**	• **Weight gain**, ascites
• **Respiratory**	• **Dyspnea, orthopnea, crackles**
• **Other signs**	• **Edema, distended neck veins**

NANDA Nursing Diagnoses

Δ   Excess fluid volume

Δ   Impaired gas exchange

Δ   Impaired skin integrity

Nursing Interventions

Δ   Assess/monitor for signs of respiratory distress, including breath sounds and arterial blood gases (ABGs).

Δ   Position the client in **semi-Fowler's** position.

Δ   Administer **oxygen** as needed.

Δ   **Reduce IV flow rates.**

Δ   Administer **diuretics** (osmotic, loop) as ordered.

Δ   Monitor daily I&O and weight.

Δ   **Limit fluid and sodium** intake as ordered.

Δ   Assess/monitor and document peripheral vascular system including skin color, presence of edema (pretibial, sacral, periorbital), and circulation to extremities.

Δ   Turn and position the client at least every 2 hr.

Δ   Support arms and legs to **decrease dependent edema and promote venous return** as appropriate.

Δ   Monitor for/treat skin breakdown.

Complications and Nursing Implications

Δ   **Pulmonary Edema**

- Signs and symptoms include **ascending crackles, dyspnea at rest,** and confusion.

- Position the client in **Fowler's position**.

- Administer **IV morphine**.

- Administer IV diuretic.

- Prepare for **possible intubation** and mechanical ventilation.

Primary Reference:

Potter, P. A., & Perry, A. G. (2005). *Fundamentals of nursing* (6th ed.). St. Louis, MO: Mosby.

Additional Resources:

Heitz, U., & Horne, M. M. (2005). *Pocket guide to fluid, electrolyte, and acid-base balance* (5th ed.). St. Louis, MO: Mosby.

Ignatavicius, D. D., & Workman, M. L. (2006). *Medical-surgical nursing* (5th ed.). St. Louis, MO: Saunders.

NANDA International (2004). *NANDA nursing diagnoses: Definitions and classification 2005-2006*. Philadelphia: NANDA.

Chapter 73: Fluid Balance

Application Exercises

1. A client admitted to the acute care facility/agency with hyperemesis is at risk for which of the following?

        A. Hypervolemia

        B. Hypovolemia

        C. Dehydration

        D. Overhydration

2. Which of the following places the client at a risk for dehydration?

        A. Excessive diaphoresis

        B. Hemorrhage

        C. Enteral feeding without sufficient water intake

        D. Diarrhea

3. A client experiencing hypovolemic shock should be placed in which of the following positions?

        A. On the side with the head elevated

        B. On the side with the legs elevated

        C. On the back with the head elevated

        D. On the back with the legs elevated

4. A long-distance runner is running a marathon and is frequently drinking bottled water along the run. He develops severe muscle weakness and becomes very confused. He is taken to the emergency department for evaluation. The client is found to have low hemoglobin and hematocrit levels, tachycardia, and hypertension. Which of the following is the most likely cause of his signs and symptoms?

        A. Overhydration

        B. Dehydration

        C. Hypervolemia

        D. Hypovolemia

5. Which of the following findings on physical assessment is most consistent with laboratory values showing increased electrolytes, BUN, and creatinine?

    A. Poor skin turgor

    B. Dependent edema

    C. Weight loss

    D. Decreased blood pressure

Chapter 73: Fluid Balance

Application Exercises Answer Key

1. A client admitted to the acute care facility/agency with hyperemesis is at risk for which of the following?

    A. Hypervolemia

    B. Hypovolemia

    C. Dehydration

    D. Overhydration

Hypovolemia is a fluid volume deficit in which the body loses both water and electrolytes (isotonic losses) from the extracellular fluid. This occurs during hyperemesis. Hypervolemia is a fluid volume excess in which the body retains both excess water and sodium. Dehydration occurs when water is lost from the body, but there is no loss of electrolytes. Overhydration occurs when more water is gained than electrolytes.

2. Which of the following places the client at a risk for dehydration?

    A. Excessive diaphoresis

    B. Hemorrhage

    C. Enteral feeding without sufficient water intake

    D. Diarrhea

Enteral feeding without sufficient water intake places a client at risk for dehydration. Diaphoresis, hemorrhage, and diarrhea place the client at risk for hypovolemia.

3. A client experiencing hypovolemic shock should be placed in which of the following positions?

    A. On the side with the head elevated

    B. On the side with the legs elevated

    C. On the back with the head elevated

    D. On the back with the legs elevated

A client in hypovolemic shock should be placed in the shock position, on his back with legs elevated to promote the return of blood flow to the vital organs.

4. A long-distance runner is running a marathon and is frequently drinking bottled water along the run. He develops severe muscle weakness and becomes very confused. He is taken to the emergency department for evaluation. The client is found to have low hemoglobin and hematocrit levels, tachycardia, and hypertension. Which of the following is the most likely cause of his signs and symptoms?

> **A. Overhydration**
> B. Dehydration
> C. Hypervolemia
> D. Hypovolemia

These are signs and symptoms of overhydration. The client is strenuously exercising and replacing water without electrolyte replacement. The client's laboratory values show hemodilution with low hemoglobin and hematocrit. The client's vital signs show tachycardia and hypertension, findings consistent with overhydration.

5. Which of the following findings on physical assessment is most consistent with laboratory values showing increased electrolytes, BUN, and creatinine?

> A. Poor skin turgor
> **B. Dependent edema**
> C. Weight loss
> D. Decreased blood pressure

Increased electrolytes, BUN, and creatinine are laboratory findings that occur with hypervolemia. Dependent edema in the lower extremities is consistent with hypervolemia. Poor skin turgor, weight loss, and decreased blood pressure are consistent with hypovolemia and dehydration.

Unit 5   Supporting Physiologic Needs
Section: Fluid, Electrolyte, and Acid-Base Balance

Chapter 74:   Electrolyte and Acid-Base Balance
                 Contributor: Linda Turchin, MSN, RN

 NCLEX® Connections

> **Learning Objective**: Review and apply knowledge within "**Electrolyte and Acid-Base Balance**" in readiness for performance of the following nursing activities as outlined by the NCLEX® test plans:
>
> Δ   Recognize signs and symptoms associated with electrolyte and acid-base imbalances.
>
> Δ   Interpret data that needs to be reported to the primary care provider immediately.
>
> Δ   Perform and document appropriate assessments based upon the client's problem – electrolyte and acid-base imbalances.
>
> Δ   Plan and provide care for the client with an electrolyte or acid-base imbalance.
>
> Δ   Evaluate the client's response to interventions to correct fluid imbalances.

Electrolytes

 Key Points

Δ   Electrolytes are **minerals** (sometimes called salts) that are present in all body fluids. They **regulate fluid balance**, hormone production, and strengthen skeletal structures, as well as act as **catalysts in nerve response, muscle contraction**, and the metabolism of nutrients.

Δ   When dissolved in water or other solvent, electrolytes separate into ions and then conduct either a positive (cations – magnesium, potassium, sodium, calcium) or negative (anions – phosphate, sulfate, chloride, bicarbonate) electrical current.

Δ   Electrolytes are distributed between **intracellular (ICF)** and **extracellular (ECF) fluid compartments**. While laboratory tests can accurately reflect the electrolyte concentrations in plasma, it is **not possible to directly measure** electrolyte concentrations **within cells.**

Δ **Sodium Imbalances**

- **Sodium (Na⁺)** is the major electrolyte found in extracellular fluid.

- Sodium is essential for the maintenance of acid-base balance, active and passive transport mechanisms, and maintaining irritability and conduction of nerve and muscle tissue.

- **Normal serum sodium levels** are **135 to 145 mEq/L.**

Δ **Potassium Imbalances**

- **Potassium (K⁺)** is the major cation in the intracellular fluid (ICF).

- Potassium plays a vital role in cell metabolism, transmission of nerve impulses, **functioning of cardiac**, lung, and muscle tissues, and **acid-base balance.**

- Potassium has **reciprocal** action with sodium.

- **Normal serum potassium levels** are **3.5 to 5 mEq/L.**

Δ **Other Serum Electrolytes**

- **Normal serum calcium levels** are **9.0 to 10.5 mEq/L.**

- **Normal serum magnesium levels** are **1.3 to 2.1 mEq/L.**

Hyponatremia

 Key Points

Δ **Hyponatremia** is a serum sodium level **< than 135 mEq/L.**

Δ Hyponatremia is a **net gain of water** or **loss of sodium**-rich fluids.

Δ Hyponatremia delays and **slows the depolarization** of membranes.

Δ Water moves from ECF into the ICF, which causes **cells to swell** (e.g., cerebral edema).

Key Factors

Δ **Risk factors/causes** include:

- Deficient ECF volume.

- **Abnormal gastrointestinal (GI) losses** – vomiting, nasogastric suctioning, diarrhea, and tap water enemas.

- **Renal losses** – diuretics, kidney disease, adrenal insufficiency.

- **Skin losses** – burns, wound drainage, gastrointestinal obstruction, peripheral edema, ascites.

- **Increased or normal ECF volume** – excessive oral water intake, syndrome of inappropriate antidiuretic hormone (SIADH).

- **Edematous states** – heart failure, cirrhosis.

- Excessive **hypotonic IV fluids.**

- **Inadequate sodium** intake – NPO status.

- **Age-related risk factors** – older adult clients at greater risk due to **increased incidence of chronic illnesses,** use of **diuretic medications,** and risk for **insufficient sodium intake.**

Assessment

Δ   Clinical indicators depend on whether it is associated with a normal, decreased, or increased ECF volume.

Serum sodium	**Decreased**: < 135 mEq/L
Serum osmolarity	**Decreased**: < 270 mOsm/L
Vital signs	Hypothermia, **tachycardia**, thready pulse, **hypotension**, orthostatic hypotension
Neuromusculoskeletal	**Headache**, confusion, lethargy, **muscle weakness** leading to respiratory compromise, fatigue, **decreased deep tendon reflexes (DTR)**
GI	**Increased motility, hyperactive** bowel sounds, abdominal cramping, nausea

NANDA Nursing Diagnoses

Δ   Excess fluid volume

Δ   Deficient fluid volume

Δ   Impaired memory

Nursing Interventions

Δ   Fluid overload: Restrict water intake as ordered.

Δ   Acute Hyponatremia

- Administer hypertonic oral and IV fluids as ordered.

- Encourage foods and fluids high in sodium (cheese, milk).

Δ   Restoration of normal ECF volume: Administer isotonic IV therapy (0.9% normal saline, Ringer's lactate solution).

Δ   Monitor I&O and daily weight.

Δ   Monitor vital signs and level of consciousness – report abnormal findings.

Δ   Encourage the client to change positions slowly.

Complications and Nursing Implications

Δ   Seizures, Coma, and Respiratory Arrest

- Seizure precautions and management

- Life support interventions

Hypernatremia

 Key Points

Δ   **Hypernatremia** is a serum sodium **greater than 145 mEq/L.**

Δ   Hypernatremia is a serious electrolyte imbalance. It can cause significant neurological, endocrine, and cardiac disturbances.

Δ   Increased sodium causes **hypertonicity** of the serum. This causes a shift of water out of the cells, making the **cells dehydrated.**

Key Factors

Δ   **Risk factors/causes** include:

- Water deprivation – NPO status.

- **Excessive sodium intake** – dietary sodium intake, hypertonic IV fluids, sodium bicarbonate intake.

- **Excessive sodium retention** – renal failure, Cushing's syndrome, some medications (glucocorticosteroids).

- **Fluid losses – fever,** diaphoresis, burns, respiratory infection, diabetes insipidus, hyperglycemia, watery diarrhea.

- **Age-related changes – Altered thirst mechanism** can lead to **decreased total body water content** and **inadequate fluid intake.**

Assessment

Serum sodium	• **Increased**: > 145 mEq/L
Serum osmolarity	• **Increased**: > 300 mOsm/L
Vital signs	• Hyperthermia, tachycardia, orthostatic hypotension
Neuromusculoskeletal	• Restlessness, **irritability,** seizures, and possibly coma, **muscle twitching** leading to muscle weakness, **diminished or absent DTRs** with more severe hypernatremia
GI	• **Thirst**, dry mucous membranes, ↑ **motility,** **hyperactive** bowel sounds, abdominal cramping, nausea
Other signs	• Edema, warm flushed skin, oliguria

NANDA Nursing Diagnoses

Δ   Deficient fluid volume

Δ   Impaired memory

Δ   Risk for injury

Δ   Impaired oral mucous membrane

Nursing Interventions

Δ   Fluid Loss

•   Based on serum osmolarity

◊   Administer hypotonic IV fluids (0.45% sodium chloride).

◊   Administer isotonic IV fluids (0.9% sodium chloride).

Δ   Excess Sodium

•   Encourage water intake and discourage sodium intake.

•   Administer diuretics, such as loop diuretics.

Δ   Monitor level of consciousness and maintain client safety.

Δ   Provide oral hygiene and other comfort measures to decrease thirst.

Δ   Monitor I&O, and alert the primary care provider of inadequate renal output.

Complications and Nursing Implications

Δ   Cellular Dehydration, Convulsions, and Death

- Seizure precautions and management
- Life support interventions

Hypokalemia

 Key Points

Δ   **Hypokalemia** is a serum potassium **less than 3.5 mEq/L**.

Δ   Hypokalemia is the result of **increased loss of potassium** from the body or **movement of potassium into the cells.**

Key Factors

Δ   **Risk Factors/Causes**

Risk Factors/Causes	Examples
Decreased total body potassium	• Abnormal GI losses – vomiting, nasogastric suctioning, diarrhea, inappropriate laxative use • Renal losses – excessive use of diuretics such as furosemide (Lasix), corticosteroids • Skin losses – diaphoresis, wound losses
Insufficient potassium	• Inadequate dietary intake (rare) • Prolonged administration of nonelectrolyte-containing IV solutions such as D_5W
Intracellular shift	Metabolic alkalosis, during periods of tissue repair (burns, trauma, starvation), total parenteral nutrition
Age-related risk factors	Older adult clients are at a greater risk due to **increased use of diuretics and laxatives**

Assessment

Serum potassium	**Decreased**: < 3.5 mEq/L
Arterial blood gases (ABGs)	Metabolic **alkalosis**: pH > 7.45
Electrocardiogram	Dysrhythmias
Vital signs	Hyperthermia, **weak irregular pulse**, hypotension, respiratory distress
Neuromusculoskeletal	**Weakness** to the point of respiratory collapse and paralysis, **muscle cramping**, decreased muscle tone and **hypoactive reflexes**, **paresthesias, mental confusion**
GI	**Decreased motility**, abdominal distention, **constipation**, ileus, nausea, vomiting, anorexia
Other signs	Polyuria (dilute urine)

Nursing Diagnoses

Δ   Decreased cardiac output

Δ   Ineffective breathing pattern

Δ   Risk for injury

Δ   Constipation

Nursing Interventions

Δ   Treat underlying cause.

Δ   **Replacement of Potassium:**

- Encourage foods high in potassium (e.g., avocados, broccoli, dairy products, dried fruit, cantaloupe, bananas).

- Provide oral potassium supplementation.

- IV potassium supplementation

    ◊   **Never IV push** (high risk **cardiac arrest**).

    ◊   Monitor for **phlebitis** (tissue irritant).

    ◊   Monitor for and maintain adequate urine output.

Δ   Monitor for shallow ineffective respirations and diminished breath sounds.

Δ   Monitor the client's cardiac rhythm, level of consciousness, and bowel function.

Complications and Nursing Implications

Δ **Respiratory Failure**

- Monitor for hypoxemia and hypercapnia.

- Intubation and mechanical ventilation may be required.

Δ **Cardiac Arrest**

- Perform continuous cardiac monitoring.

- Treat life-threatening dysrhythmias.

Hyperkalemia

 Key Points

Δ **Hyperkalemia** is a serum potassium **greater than 5.0 mEq/L.**

Δ Hyperkalemia is the result of **increased intake** of potassium, **movement of potassium out of the cells,** or **inadequate renal excretion**.

Key Factors

Δ **Risk Factors/Causes**

Increased total body potassium	IV potassium administration, salt substitute
Extracellular shift	Decreased insulin, acidosis, such as diabetic ketoacidosis, tissue catabolism (sepsis, trauma, surgery, fever, myocardial infarction)
Decreased excretion of potassium	Renal failure, severe dehydration, potassium-sparing diuretics, ACE inhibitors, NSAIDs, adrenal insufficiency
Age-related risk factors	Older adult clients at a greater risk due to **increased use of salt substitutes, ACE inhibitors,** and potassium-sparing diuretics

Assessment

Serum potassium	**Increased**: > 5.0 mEq/L
ABGs	Metabolic **acidosis**: pH < 7.35
Electrocardiogram	**Dysrhythmias**
Vital signs	**Slow, irregular pulse, hypotension**
Neuromusculoskeletal	Restlessness, irritability, **weakness** to the point of ascending flaccid paralysis, **paresthesias**
GI	Nausea, vomiting, **increased motility, diarrhea, hyperactive bowel sounds**
Other signs	Oliguria

Nursing Diagnoses

Δ   Decreased cardiac output

Δ   Risk for injury

Δ   Diarrhea

Nursing Interventions

Δ   **Decrease potassium intake.**

- Stop infusion of IV potassium.

- Withhold oral potassium.

- Provide potassium-restricted diet. Avoid foods high in potassium (e.g., avocados, broccoli, dairy products, dried fruit, cantaloupe, bananas).

Δ   **Increase potassium excretion.**

- Administer potassium-losing diuretics, such as furosemide (Lasix), if renal function is adequate.

- Administer cation exchange resins such as sodium polystyrene sulfonate (Kayexalate).

- Perform dialysis.

Δ   **Promote movement of potassium from ECF to ICF.**

- Administer IV fluids with dextrose (glucose) and regular insulin.

- Administer sodium bicarbonate (reverse acidosis).

Δ   Monitor the client's cardiac rhythm, and notify primary care provider of abnormal findings.

Complications and Nursing Implications

Δ **Cardiac Arrest**

- Perform continuous cardiac monitoring.

- Treat life-threatening dysrhythmias.

Other Electrolyte Imbalances

 Key Points and Factors

Δ **Hypocalcemia**

- Hypocalcemia is a **serum calcium** level **less than 9.0 mg/dL**.

- **Risk factors/causes** of hypocalcemia

◊ Malabsorption syndromes such as Crohn's disease

◊ End-stage renal disease

◊ Post thyroidectomy

Assessment

Δ Neuromuscular

- Muscle twitches/tetany

- Frequent painful muscle spasms at rest

- Hyperactive deep tendon reflexes

- Positive Chvostek's sign (tap on facial nerve triggers facial twitching)

- Positive Trousseau's sign (hand/finger spasms with sustained blood pressure cuff inflation)

Δ Cardiovascular

- Decreased myocardial contractility – decreased heart rate and hypotension

- Dysrhythmias

Δ GI – hyperactive bowel sounds, diarrhea, abdominal cramping

Nursing Interventions

Δ Administer oral or IV calcium supplements.

Δ Encourage foods high in calcium including dairy products and dark green vegetables.

Δ Be aware of seizure precautions.

Δ Keep emergency equipment on standby.

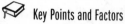 **Key Points and Factors**

Δ **Hypomagnesemia**

- Hypomagnesemia is a **serum magnesium** level **less than 1.2 mg/dL.**
- **Risk factors/causes** of hypomagnesemia
  ◊ Malnutrition (insufficient magnesium intake)
  ◊ Alcohol ingestion (magnesium excretion)

Assessment

Δ Neuromuscular – increased nerve impulse transmission (hyperactive deep tendon reflexes, paresthesias, muscle tetany), positive Chvostek's and Trousseau's signs

Δ GI – hypoactive bowel sounds, constipation, abdominal distention, paralytic ileus

Nursing Interventions

Δ Discontinue magnesium-losing medications, such as loop diuretics.

Δ Administer oral or IV magnesium sulfate following safety protocols.

Δ Encourage foods high in magnesium, including dairy products and dark green vegetables.

Acid-Base Balance

 Key Points

Δ In order for cells to function optimally, metabolic processes must maintain a steady balance between the acids and the bases found in the body.

Δ **Acid-base balance** represents homeostasis of **hydrogen (H⁺)** ion concentration in body fluids. Hydrogen shifts between the extracellular and intracellular compartments to compensate for acid-base imbalances.

Δ Minor changes in hydrogen concentration have major effects on normal cellular function.

Δ **Arterial pH** is an indirect measurement of hydrogen ion concentration and is a result of respiratory and renal compensational function. **ABGs** are most commonly used to evaluate acid-base balance.

Δ The **pH** is the expression of the balance between **carbon dioxide (CO_2)**, which is regulated by the lungs, and **bicarbonate (HCO_3^-)**, a base regulated by the kidneys.

- The **greater the concentration of hydrogen ions**, the more **acidic** the body fluids and the **lower the pH.**

- The **lower the concentration of hydrogen**, the more **alkaline** the body fluids and the **higher the pH.**

Δ **Compensation** refers to the process by which the **body attempts to correct changes and imbalances in pH levels.**

- **Full compensation** occurs when the **pH level of the blood returns to normal (7.35 to 7.45).**

- If the pH is not able to normalize, then it is referred to as **partial compensation.**

Δ **Respiratory alkalosis, respiratory acidosis, metabolic alkalosis and metabolic acidosis** are examples of acid-base imbalances.

Key Factors

Δ **Acid-base imbalances are a result of insufficient compensation. Respiratory** and **renal** function play a large role in the body's ability to effectively compensate for acid-base alterations. Organ dysfunction negatively affects acid-base compensation.

Δ   Risk factors/causes of acid-base imbalances:

Respiratory Acidosis	Respiratory Alkalosis
• **Respiratory depression** from poisons, anesthetics, trauma, or neurological diseases, such as myasthenia gravis or Guillain-Barré • **Inadequate chest expansion** due to muscle weakness, pneumothorax/hemothorax, flail chest, obesity, tumors, or deformities • **Airway obstruction** that occurs in laryngospasm, asthma, and some cancers • **Alveolar-capillary blockage** *secondary to a pulmonary embolus, thrombus, cancer, or pulmonary edema* • **Inadequate mechanical ventilation**	• **Hyperventilation** due to fear, anxiety, intracerebral trauma, salicylate toxicity, or excessive mechanical ventilation • **Hypoxemia** from asphyxiation, high altitudes, shock, or early-stage asthma or pneumonia
Metabolic Acidosis	**Metabolic Alkalosis**

• **Excess production of hydrogen ions**
  ◊ DKA
  ◊ Salicylate intoxication
  ◊ Starvation
  ◊ Heavy exercise
  ◊ Seizure activity
  ◊ Fever
  ◊ Hypoxia
• **Inadequate elimination of hydrogen ions**
  ◊ Renal failure
• **Inadequate production of bicarbonate**
  ◊ Renal failure
  ◊ Pancreatitis
  ◊ Liver failure
  ◊ Dehydration
• **Excess elimination of bicarbonate**
  ◊ Diarrhea, ileostomy
	• **Base excess**
	  ◊ Oral ingestion of bases (antacids)
	  ◊ Venous administration of bases (blood transfusions, TPN, or sodium bicarbonate)
	• **Acid deficit**
	  ◊ **Loss of gastric secretions** due to prolonged vomiting or NG suction
	  ◊ **Potassium depletion** due to thiazide diuretics, laxative abuse, Cushing's syndrome

Assessment

Δ   To determine the type of imbalance, follow these steps:

- **Step 1**
    - ◊   Look at pH. If < 7.35, diagnose as acidosis.
    - ◊   If > 7.45, diagnose as alkalosis.

- **Step 2**
    - ◊   Look at $PaCO_2$ and HCO_3^- simultaneously.
    - ◊   Determine which one is in the normal range.

◊   Then, conclude that the other is the indicator of imbalance.

◊   Diagnose < 35 or > 45 $PaCO_2$ as respiratory in origin.

◊   Diagnose < 22 or > 26 HCO_3^- as metabolic in origin.

- **Step 3** – Combine diagnoses of Steps 1 and 2 to name the type of imbalance.

The following are the five classic types of ABG results demonstrating balance and imbalance.

Step 1	Step 2		Step 3
If	Determine which is in normal range.		Combine names.
pH	$PaCO_2$	HCO_3^-	Diagnosis
7.35 to 7.45	35 to 45	22 to 26	Homeostasis
< 7.35	> 45	22 to 26	Respiratory acidosis
< 7.35	35 to 45	< 22	Metabolic acidosis
> 7.45	< 35	22 to 26	Respiratory alkalosis
> 7.45	35 to 45	> 26	Metabolic alkalosis

- **Step 4**

  ◊   Evaluate the PaO_2 and the SaO_2.

  ◊   If the results are below the normal range, the client is hypoxic.

- **Step 5**

  ◊   Determine compensation as follows:

    °   **Uncompensated** – The pH will be abnormal and either the HCO_3^- or the $PaCO_2$ will be abnormal.

    °   **Partially compensated** – The pH, HCO_3^-, and $PaCO_2$ will be abnormal.

    °   **Fully compensated** – The pH will be normal, but the $PaCO_2$ and HCO_3^- will both be abnormal. Then, looking back at the pH will provide a clue as to which system initiated the problem – respiratory or metabolic. If the pH is < 7.40, think "acidosis" and determine which system has the acidosis value. If the pH is > 7.40, think "alkalosis" and determine which system has the alkalosis value.

Δ   **Assessment findings of acid-base imbalances:**

	Respiratory Acidosis Hypoventilation	Respiratory Alkalosis Hyperventilation
Vital signs	• **Tachycardia** • **Tachypnea**	**Tachypnea**
Cardiovascular	Dysrhythmias	• Palpitations • Chest pain • Dysrhythmias
Neurological	• Anxiety • Irritability • Confusion, coma	• Anxiety • **Tetany** • **Convulsions** • Tingling, numbness

	Metabolic Acidosis	Metabolic Alkalosis
Vital signs	**Bradycardia**, tachypnea, hypotension	**Tachycardia**, hypotension
Cardiovascular	Dysrhythmias	Dysrhythmias
Neurological	Fatigue, weakness, lethargy, confusion	Numbness, tingling, **tetany, muscle weakness**, hyporeflexia, confusion, convulsion
Other	GI – anorexia, nausea, vomiting, diarrhea	GU – polyuria, polydipsia

Nursing Diagnoses

Δ   Respiratory Acidosis/Alkalosis

- Impaired gas exchange

- Ineffective breathing pattern

Δ   Metabolic Acidosis/Alkalosis

- Decreased cardiac output related to dysrhythmias

Nursing Interventions

Δ   For all acid-base imbalances, it is imperative to treat the underlying cause.

- Respiratory acidosis

  ◊ Oxygen therapy

  ◊ Maintenance of a patent airway

  ◊ Enhancing gas exchange (positioning and breathing techniques, ventilatory support, bronchodilators, and mucolytics)

- Respiratory alkalosis
  ◊ Oxygen therapy
  ◊ Anxiety-reduction interventions
  ◊ Rebreathing techniques
- Metabolic acidosis – varies with causes
  ◊ DKA, administration of insulin
  ◊ Related to GI losses – administration of antidiarrheals and provision of rehydration
  ◊ Administration of sodium bicarbonate (1 mEq/kg) due to low serum bicarbonate
- Metabolic alkalosis – varies with causes
  ◊ GI losses – administration of antiemetics, fluids, and electrolyte replacements
  ◊ Potassium depletion – discontinuation of the causative agent, treatment of the cause

Primary Reference:

Potter, P. A., & Perry, A. G. (2005). *Fundamentals of nursing* (6th ed.). St. Louis, MO: Mosby.

Additional Resources:

Heitz, U., & Horne, M. M. (2005). *Pocket guide to fluid, electrolyte, and acid-base balance* (5th ed.). St. Louis, MO: Mosby.

Ignatavicius, D. D., & Workman, M. L. (2006). *Medical-surgical nursing* (5th ed.). St. Louis, MO: Saunders.

NANDA International (2004). *NANDA nursing diagnoses: Definitions and classification 2005-2006.* Philadelphia: NANDA.

Chapter 74: Electrolyte and Acid-Base Balance

Application Exercises

1. Match the abnormality with the correct laboratory value.

_____ Hyperkalemia	A. Serum sodium 125 mEq/L
_____ Hypomagnesemia	B. Serum sodium 152 mEq/L
_____ Hyponatremia	C. Serum potassium 2.9 mEq/L
_____ Hypokalemia	D. Serum potassium 6.2 mEq/L
_____ Hypercalcemia	E. Serum calcium 11.0 mg/dL
_____ Hypernatremia	F. Serum magnesium 0.9 mEq/L

2. Which of the following client findings is most consistent with a serum sodium level of 125 mEq/L and a serum osmolarity of 230 mOsm/L? (Select all that apply.)

_____ Orthostatic hypotension

_____ Constipation

_____ Bradycardia

_____ Decreased DTRs

_____ Lethargy

3. Which of the following medications places an older adult client at a higher risk for hyperkalemia?

A. Lisinopril (Prinivil)

B. Verapamil (Calan)

C. Furosemide (Lasix)

D. Hydrochlorothiazide (HCTZ)

4. Identify the acid-base imbalance caused by the following disorders.

_____ Respiratory acidosis	A. Seizure activity
_____ Respiratory alkalosis	B. Blood transfusion
_____ Metabolic acidosis	C. Mechanical ventilation
_____ Metabolic alkalosis	D. Myasthenia gravis

5. For the following laboratory values, determine the correct acid-base imbalance.

pH 7.30; $PaCO_2$ 47; HCO_3^- 23	
pH 7.50; $PaCO_2$ 37; HCO_3^- 30	
pH 7.52; $PaCO_2$ 42; HCO_3^- 33	
pH 7.51; $PaCO_2$ 30; HCO_3^- 25	
pH 7.28; $PaCO_2$ 41; HCO_3^- 18	

Chapter 74: Electrolyte and Acid-Base Balance

Application Exercises Answer Key

1. Match the abnormality with the correct laboratory value.

D Hyperkalemia   A. Serum sodium 125 mEq/L

F Hypomagnesemia   B. Serum sodium 152 mEq/L

A Hyponatremia   C. Serum potassium 2.9 mEq/L

C Hypokalemia   D. Serum potassium 6.2 mEq/L

E Hypercalcemia   E. Serum calcium 11.0 mg/dL

B Hypernatremia   F. Serum magnesium 0.9 mEq/L

2. Which of the following client findings is most consistent with a serum sodium level of
   125 mEq/L and a serum osmolarity of 230 mOsm/L? (Select all that apply.)

   X **Orthostatic hypotension**

   _____ Constipation

   _____ Bradycardia

   X **Decreased DTRs**

   X **Lethargy**

   These laboratory values indicate hyponatremia. Orthostatic hypotension, decreased DTRs,
   and lethargy are clinical indicators of hyponatremia. The client also experiences increased
   GI motility and tachycardia.

3. Which of the following medications places an older adult client at a higher risk for hyperkalemia?

   A. Lisinopril (Prinivil)

   B. Verapamil (Calan)

   C. Furosemide (Lasix)

   D. Hydrochlorothiazide (HCTZ)

   ACE inhibitors promote excretion of sodium and water and retention of potassium.
   Verapamil has no effect on the serum potassium level. Furosemide and hydrochlorothiazide
   can result in hypokalemia.

4. Identify the acid-base imbalance caused by the following disorders.

  D   Respiratory acidosis   A. Seizure activity

  A   Respiratory alkalosis   B. Blood transfusion

  C   Metabolic acidosis   C. Mechanical ventilation

  B   Metabolic alkalosis   D. Myasthenia gravis

5. For the following laboratory values, determine the correct acid-base imbalance.

pH 7.30; $PaCO_2$ 47; HCO_3^- 23	**Respiratory acidosis**
pH 7.50; $PaCO_2$ 37; HCO_3^- 30	**Metabolic alkalosis**
pH 7.52; $PaCO_2$ 42; HCO_3^- 33	**Metabolic alkalosis**
pH 7.51; $PaCO_2$ 30; HCO_3^- 25	**Respiratory alkalosis**
pH 7.28; $PaCO_2$ 41; HCO_3^- 18	**Metabolic acidosis**

Unit 5   Supporting Physiologic Needs
Section: Gastroenteral Needs

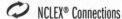

Chapter 75:   Glucose Monitoring
                  Contributor: Peggy Mossholder, MSN, RN, CHPN

 NCLEX® Connections

> **Learning Objective**: Review and apply knowledge within **"Glucose Monitoring"** in readiness for performance of the following nursing activities as outlined by the NCLEX® test plans:
>
> Δ   Assess/monitor the client's blood glucose levels and compare them to desired target range.
>
> Δ   Perform blood glucose monitoring.
>
> Δ   Evaluate and document effectiveness of insulin administration based on glucose monitoring.
>
> Δ   Assess/monitor the client for signs and symptoms of hypoglycemia or hyperglycemia.

Key Points

Δ   **Urine testing** is **NOT** an adequate measure of glucose level. Urine testing is usually performed at home by the client with diabetes at times of acute illness, stress, or consistent blood glucose levels > 300 mg/dL to test for ketones.

Δ   Blood **glucose** testing is the preferred method of monitoring blood glucose levels.

Δ   The client can learn how to self-monitor blood glucose (SMBG) levels, providing the client is able and willing to independently continue monitoring. Abilities should include:

   •   Alertness or the ability to comprehend and return demonstrate the process.

   •   Adequate finger dexterity.

   •   Adequate visual acuity.

Key Procedural Points

Δ   Check the client's record for:

- Frequency and type of test. Testing times will vary based on the goals of management and the complexity of the hypoglycemic medication schedule.

- Results from previous tests – norms and ranges.

Δ   If testing urine, evaluate client's ability to urinate.

Δ   If testing blood, evaluate puncture site for:

- Integrity of the skin.

- Circulation or compromised condition.

Δ   Review medication profile.

- Note anticoagulant usage.

- Note the time and dose of hypoglycemic agents.

- Note the use of steroids or medications that may elevate blood glucose levels.

Δ   The nurse **may delegate** to assistants who are educated in glucose strip testing.

Δ   It is the responsibility of the nurse to be aware of the test results.

NANDA Nursing Diagnoses

Δ   Risk for infection

Δ   Ineffective health maintenance

Nursing Interventions

Δ   **Urine Glucose Testing**

- Equipment
    ◊   Sterile urine sample bottle
    ◊   Urinalysis strips and container with glucose reading scale
    ◊   Gloves

- Procedure
    ◊   Verify the order for frequency and actions to be taken based on results.
    ◊   Gather materials and prepare equipment.
    ◊   Check strip for expiration dates.
    ◊   Inform client of intent of test and rationale.

◊   Sanitize hands and put on gloves.

◊   Instruct or assist the client with sample collection of urine.

◊   Dip reagent strip into fresh urine sample.

◊   Compare the strip color change with the ranges on the bottle within the instructed time (1 to 5 sec in most cases).

◊   Document results.

◊   Dispose of remaining urine sample, test strip, and gloves.

◊   Perform hand hygiene.

◊   Check orders for medication or treatment actions.

∆   **Blood Glucose Monitoring**

•   Equipment

◊   Blood glucose meter

◊   Meter and reagent strip compatible with the meter

◊   Washcloth and soap

◊   Gloves

◊   Sterile lancet

◊   Cotton ball

•   Procedure

◊   Verify the order for frequency and actions to be taken based on results.

◊   Gather materials and prepare equipment.

◊   Review the meter and manufacturer's instructions.

◊   Check strip solution expiration date.

◊   Calibrate the meter and run a control sample per facility/agency protocol. This is usually performed when a new bottle of test strips is opened.

◊   Inform the client of the intent of test and rationale.

◊   Perform hand hygiene and put on gloves.

◊   Select a site to collect blood sample.

°   Outer edge of finger tip (most common site)

°   Ear lobe (alternate site)

°   Rotate sites with each testing to avoid tender area development.

°   Wrap site in warm moist towel to enhance circulation if indicated.

◊ Cleanse the site with warm water and soap and allow to dry. If appropriate, ask the client to wash hands. Alcohol can interfere with results and should be avoided.

◊ Pierce the skin using sterile lancet (may use lancet injector device).

◊ Drop or draw a fresh blood drop onto the check strip

° Follow procedure specific to each blood glucose meter for applying blood to strip.

° The nurse may need to gently milk finger to squeeze out a drop. Do not touch direct site to stimulate bleeding.

° Do not smear blood onto the strip, as this can cause an inaccurate reading.

◊ Allow meter to process reading (Time will vary with each machine.).

◊ Hold cotton ball over puncture site.

◊ Turn off the meter and dispose of cotton ball, test strip, and gloves.

◊ Perform hand hygiene.

◊ Document the meter reading.

◊ Check orders for medication or treatment actions.

◊ Implement interventions as indicated.

Complications and Nursing Implications

Δ Hypoglycemia

- Hypoglycemia is a blood glucose level < 70 mg/dL.

- Signs and symptoms usually have an acute onset and include shakiness, irritability, confusion, diaphoresis, anxiety, and fatigue.

- Causes of hypoglycemia include taking too much insulin or too much of an oral hypoglycemic, not eating enough food when insulin/oral hypoglycemic agent is peaking, and/or exercising without adequate glucose stores.

- Nursing implications

  ◊ Evaluate the client's level of orientation/alertness.

  ◊ Perform blood glucose testing.

  ◊ Administer 10 to 15 g of glucose orally, if possible.

  ◊ Recheck in 15 to 20 min.

  ◊ Repeat if necessary.

  ◊ Review recent nutritional intake history.

  ◊ Notify primary care provider if blood glucose remains low or symptoms worsen.

Δ   Hyperglycemia

- Hyperglycemia is a blood glucose level > 120 mg/dL.

- Brief elevations may go undetected unless blood glucose monitoring is being done.

- Causes of hyperglycemia include taking inadequate amounts of insulin or oral hypoglycemic agent, infection, and stress.

- Signs and symptoms may be slower to manifest and include blurred vision, polyuria, polydipsia, fatigue, dry mucous membranes, and weakness.

- Nursing implications

    ◊   Review recent nutritional intake history.

    ◊   Assess client for possible signs and symptoms.

    ◊   Perform blood glucose testing.

    ◊   Check for sliding scale insulin orders.

    ◊   Notify primary care provider if sliding scale is not ordered or the order indicates.

Primary Reference:

Potter, P. A., & Perry, A. G. (2005). *Fundamentals of nursing* (6th ed.). St. Louis, MO: Mosby.

Additional Resources:

Ignatavicius, D. D., & Workman, M. L. (2006). *Medical-surgical nursing* (5th ed.). St. Louis, MO: Saunders.

Kozier, B., Erb, G., Berman, A., & Snyder, S. (2004). *Fundamentals of nursing*. New Jersey: Prentice Hall.

NANDA International (2004). *NANDA nursing diagnoses: Definitions and classification 2005-2006*. Philadelphia: NANDA.

Chapter 75: Glucose Monitoring

Application Exercises

1. Which of the following tests is the most effective in monitoring blood glucose levels?

      A. Urinalysis

      B. Blood sampling

      C. Client report of symptoms

      D. Sputum specimen

2. Which of the following directions should the nurse give to the client who is learning how to perform self-monitoring of blood glucose (SMBG)? (Select all that apply.)

      _____ Perform SMBG once daily at bedtime.

      _____ Warm hand before puncturing finger.

      _____ Calibrate the glucose monitor each time a new bottle of strips is started.

      _____ Wipe hand with an alcohol swab.

      _____ Prick outer edge of fingertip for blood sample.

3. Which of the following medications potentially influences the results of blood glucose testing?

      A. Amoxicillin

      B. Dexamethasone

      C. Morphine

      D. Acetaminophen

4. A client has an admission blood glucose reading of 350 mg/dL. The client has no prior history of elevated blood glucose, and there is no sliding scale insulin order. Which of the following actions should the nurse take first?

      A. Assess the client for level of consciousness.

      B. Check dietary orders.

      C. Review recent nutritional intake history.

      D. Notify the primary care provider.

Chapter 75: Glucose Monitoring

Application Exercises Answer Key

1. Which of the following tests is the most effective in monitoring blood glucose levels?

>   A. Urinalysis
>   **B. Blood sampling**
>   C. Client report of symptoms
>   D. Sputum specimen

Blood samples give the most accurate information. Urinalysis is not a recommended method of monitoring blood glucose but is used in times of acute illness and stress. Client report of symptoms is especially not effective for hyperglycemia, as symptoms do not appear until glucose levels are consistently high. Sputum does not reflect blood glucose levels.

2. Which of the following directions should the nurse give to the client who is learning how to perform self-monitoring of blood glucose (SMBG)? (Select all that apply.)

>   _____ Perform SMBG once daily at bedtime.
>   __X__ **Warm hand before puncturing finger.**
>   __X__ **Calibrate the glucose monitor each time a new bottle of strips is started.**
>   _____ Wipe hand with an alcohol swab.
>   __X__ **Prick outer edge of fingertip for blood sample.**

Warming the hand prior to obtaining a blood sample will increase circulation and facilitate adequate amount of blood for the sample. The monitor should be calibrated each time a new bottle of strips is started. The outer edge of the fingertip is an appropriate site to obtain the blood sample. SMBG should be performed based on medication schedule. It may be done as often as before each meal and at bedtime. Once a day at bedtime monitoring will not give information necessary to monitor blood glucose control. The hand should be washed with warm water and soap. Alcohol can interfere with blood glucose reading.

3. Which of the following medications potentially influences the results of blood glucose testing?

    A. Amoxicillin

    B. Dexamethasone

    C. Morphine

    D. Acetaminophen

Dexamethasone is a steroid that may raise blood glucose. Amoxicillin, morphine, and acetaminophen should not affect blood glucose levels.

4. A client has an admission blood glucose reading of 350 mg/dL. The client has no prior history of elevated blood glucose, and there is no sliding scale insulin order. Which of the following actions should the nurse take first?

    A. Assess client for level of consciousness.

    B. Check dietary orders.

    C. Review recent nutritional intake history.

    D. Notify the primary care provider.

Even though the level of consciousness is more likely to be altered with a low blood glucose reading or a very high blood glucose reading (> 450 mg/dL), it is important to assess prior to notifying the primary care provider. Next, the primary care provider should be notified of the abnormal blood glucose. Dietary interventions and nutritional history are important to perform at some point, but they are not the priority nursing intervention.

Unit 5 Supporting Physiologic Needs

Section: Gastroenteral Needs

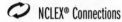

Chapter 76: Gastroenteral Feedings

Contributor: Peggy Mossholder, MSN, RN, CHPN

 NCLEX® Connections

Learning Objective: Review and apply knowledge within **"Gastroenteral Feedings"** in readiness for performance of the following nursing activities as outlined by the NCLEX® test plans:

Δ   Plan and/or provide care to the client requiring enteral feedings.

Δ   Evaluate the patency and placement of the client's feeding tube.

Δ   Assess/monitor the client for side effects of tube feedings (e.g., dehydration, nausea, vomiting, diarrhea).

Δ   Ensure adequate nutritional intake through use of enteral feedings.

Key Points

Δ   Indications for enteral nutrition include:

•   Critical illness/trauma.

•   **Neurological and muscular disorders** – brain neoplasm, cerebrovascular accident, dementia, myopathy, Parkinson's disease.

•   **Gastrointestinal disorders** – enterocutaneous fistula, inflammatory bowel disease, mild pancreatitis.

•   **Respiratory failure with prolonged intubation.**

•   **Inadequate oral intake.**

Δ   Enteral Formulas

•   Polymeric – (1.0 to 2.0 kcal/mL) milk-based blenderized foods

◊   Whole-nutrient formulas prepared by hospital dietary staff or commercially prepared

◊   Only used if GI tract able to absorb whole nutrients

- Modular formulas – (3.8 to 4.0 kcal/mL) single macronutrient preparation
  ◊ Not nutritionally complete
  ◊ Added to other foods for supplemental nutrition
- Elemental formulas – (1.0 to 3.0 kcal/mL) predigested nutrients
  ◊ Not nutritionally complete
  ◊ Easier for a partially dysfunctional gastrointestinal tract to absorb
- Specialty formulas – (1.0 to 2.0 kcal/mL) designed to meet specific nutritional needs
  ◊ Not nutritionally complete
  ◊ Primarily for liver failure, pulmonary disease, or HIV infection

Δ Enteral access tubes – Gastroparesis, esophageal reflux, or a history of aspiration pneumonia generally requires that tubes be placed into the intestine.

- **Nasogastric or nasointestinal**
  ◊ Therapy less than 4 weeks
  ◊ Inserted via nose
- **Gastrostomy or jejunostomy**
  ◊ Therapy greater than 4 weeks
  ◊ Inserted surgically
- **Percutaneous endoscopic gastrostomy (PEG) or jejunostomy (PEJ)**
- Therapy greater than 4 weeks
- Inserted endoscopically

Key Procedural Points

Δ All tube feedings should be monitored with I&O with 24-hr totals.

Δ Monitor capillary blood glucose every 6 hr until maximum administration rate is reached and maintained for 24 hr.

Δ An infusion pump is required for intestinal tube feedings.

Δ The type of tube feeding formula is usually determined by the primary care provider in consultation with dietary staff.

Δ Follow manufacturer recommendations for formula hang time. Unused formula should be refrigerated and discarded after 24 hr.

Δ Residuals should be checked every 4 to 8 hr. Facility/agency protocol will determine what actions should be taken based on amount of residual obtained.

Δ Delegation of this skill to assistive personnel is inappropriate.

NANDA Nursing Diagnoses

Δ   Diarrhea

Δ   Imbalanced nutrition: less than body requirements

Δ   Impaired swallowing

Δ   Risk for imbalanced fluid volume

Nursing Interventions

Δ   Equipment

- Feeding bag

- Tubing

- 30 to 60 mL syringe (tip should match the tubing)

- Stethoscope

- pH indicator strip

- Infusion pump (if not a gravity drip)

- Appropriate enteral formula

- Gloves

- Supplies for blood glucose (if protocol or orders indicate)

Δ   Procedure

- **Insertion of a nasogastric feeding tube** is done by:

  ◊   Performing hand hygiene.

  ◊   Placing the client in Fowler's position.

  ◊   Measuring the length of the tubing required to reach the stomach.

  ◊   Lubricating the tip.

  ◊   Inserting the tube through one nare and asking the client to swallow once the tube reaches the back of the throat.

  ◊   Advancing the tube with each swallow until the measured length has been reached.

  ◊   Checking for position by looking at the back of the throat for coiled tubing, checking for stomach aspirates, auscultating breath sounds, and confirming with an x-ray prior to administering the feeding.

  ◊   Taping the tube to the client's nose.

- **Prepare formula, tubing, and infusion device.**

  ◊   Check expiration dates and observe content of formula.

◊ Assure that formula is at room temperature.

◊ Set up the feeding system to gravity or pump.

◊ Mix or shake formula, fill container, and prime tubing and clamp.

- **Position client in a Fowler's position or at a minimum of 30° elevation of head.**

- **Monitor for tube placement.**

  ◊ Initial placement is confirmed with x-ray.

  ◊ Monitor gastric contents for pH. A good indication of appropriate placement is obtaining gastric contents with a pH between 0 to 4.

  ◊ Injecting air into the tube and listening over the abdomen is not an acceptable practice.

  ◊ Aspirate for residual volume – note: intestinal residual < 10 mL, gastric residual < 100 mL.

  ◊ Observe aspiration appearance.

  ◊ Return aspirated contents or follow facility/agency protocol.

- **Flush tubing with 30 to 60 mL water.**

- **Administer formula.**

  ◊ Intermittent feeding

    ° Have formula and 60 mL syringe prepared.

    ° Remove plunger from the syringe.

    ° Hold tubing above infusion site.

    ° Open stopcock on tubing, and insert the barrel of the syringe with the end up.

    ° Fill syringe with 40 to 50 mL of formula.

    ° If feeding bag is used, fill bag with total amount of ordered formula for one feeding, and hang to empty via gravity until complete (about 30 min).

    ° Hold syringe high enough for the formula to empty gradually via gravity.

    ° Continue to refill syringe until formula amount for the feeding is infused.

    ° Follow with 60 to 100 mL of water (Check for specific order.) to flush the tube and prevent clogging.

  ◊ Continuous-drip feeding

    ° Connect the feeding bag system to the feeding tube.

    ° If using a pump, program infusion rate per order, and set total volume to infuse.

     °   Start infusion.

     °   Flush enteral tubing with 30 to 60 mL of water every 4 to 6 hr, and repeat check of tube placement.

Complications and Nursing Implications

Δ   **Gastric residual exceeding 100 mL (10 mL for intestinal placement) includes:**

- Holding the feeding.

- Notifying the provider.

- Maintaining semi-Fowler's position.

- Rechecking residual in 1 hr or per primary care order.

Δ   **Diarrhea Three Times or More in a 24-hr Period**

- Notify the provider.

- Confer with the dietitian.

- Provide skin care protection.

Δ   **Nausea or Vomiting**

- Hold feeding.

- Notify the provider.

- Check the patency of the tubing.

- Aspirate for residual.

- Auscultate for bowel sounds.

Δ   **Aspiration of Formula**

- Hold feeding.

- Position client to the side.

- Suction airway.

- Provide oxygen if indicated.

- Monitor the client's vital signs for elevated temperature.

- Auscultate breath sounds for increased congestion.

- Notify the provider.

- Obtain a chest x-ray.

Δ   **Skin Irritation Around Tubing Site**

- Provide skin barrier from any drainage at site.

- Monitor placement of tube.

Primary Reference:

Potter, P. A., & Perry, A. G. (2005). *Fundamentals of nursing* (6th ed.). St. Louis, MO: Mosby.

Additional Resources:

Kozier, B., Erb, G., Berman, A., & Snyder, S. (2004). *Fundamentals of nursing.* New Jersey: Prentice Hall.

NANDA International (2004). *NANDA nursing diagnoses: Definitions and classification 2005-2006.* Philadelphia: NANDA.

Chapter 76: Gastroenteral Feedings

Application Exercises

1. Which of the following formulas is nutritionally complete?

      A. Polymeric formulas

      B. Modular formulas

      C. Elemental formulas

      D. Specialty formulas

2. The enteral access tube best suited for short-term use (less than 4 weeks) is a

      A. nasogastric tube.

      B. gastrostomy tube.

      C. jejunostomy tube.

      D. PEG tube.

3. The purpose of flushing a tube after an enteral feeding is given is to

      A. provide adequate fluid intake.

      B. dilute the concentration of the formula.

      C. clear the tubing and prevent clogging.

      D. ensure that the placement of the tube is maintained.

4. The highest priority nursing assessment prior to initiating an enteral feeding is determining

      A. if the client is alert and oriented.

      B. tube placement.

      C. how long the feeding has been opened.

      D. when the client last voided.

5. Which of the following nursing interventions is/are appropriate when aspiration of tube feeding is suspected? (Select all that apply.)

_____ Auscultate for bowel sounds.

_____ Auscultate breath sounds for increased congestion.

_____ Flush tubing.

_____ Hold feeding.

_____ Maintain semi-Fowler's position.

_____ Obtain baseline vital signs and monitor for elevated temperature.

_____ Notify primary care provider.

_____ Obtain chest x-ray.

_____ Provide oxygen if indicated.

_____ Suction airway.

Chapter 76: Gastroenteral Feedings

Application Exercises Answer Key

1. Which of the following formulas is nutritionally complete?

    A. Polymeric formulas
    B. Modular formulas
    C. Elemental formulas
    D. Specialty formulas

Polymeric formulas are nutritionally complete. Modular formulas provide a single macronutrient. Elemental formulas have predigested nutrients, and specialty formulas are designed to meet specific nutritional needs and are not nutritionally complete.

2. The enteral access tube best suited for short-term use (less than 4 weeks) is a

    A. nasogastric tube.
    B. gastrostomy tube.
    C. jejunostomy tube.
    D. PEG tube.

Nasogastric tubes are used short-term and can be inserted through the nose. Insertion of a gastrostomy or jejunostomy tube is done by surgical procedure and a PEG tube is inserted endoscopically. Surgical and endoscopic insertion presents an increased risk for injury and infection; therefore, they are only indicated for long-term use.

3. The purpose of flushing a tube after an enteral feeding is given is to

    A. provide adequate fluid intake.
    B. dilute the concentration of the formula.
    C. clear the tubing and prevent clogging.
    D. ensure that the placement of the tube is maintained.

Flushing the tube after the feeding has been given will help maintain patency by clearing any excess formula from the tube. If the client requires additional fluids, the small amount used for flushing will not be adequate. If formula is to be diluted, it should be done prior to administration of the feeding. Flushing the tube does not maintain placement of the tube.

4. The highest priority nursing assessment prior to initiating an enteral feeding is determining

        A. if the client is alert and oriented.

        B. tube placement.

        C. how long the feeding has been opened.

        D. when the client last voided.

The tube must be in the proper place before enteral feedings can be initiated. The client does not need to be alert and oriented. It is important to determine how long a feeding has been opened, but tube placement must be determined. When the client last voided is not a necessary assessment for administering enteral tube feedings.

5. Which of the following nursing interventions is/are appropriate when aspiration of tube feeding is suspected? (Select all that apply.)

    _____ Auscultate for bowel sounds.

    __X__ **Auscultate breath sounds for increased congestion.**

    _____ Flush tubing.

    __X__ **Hold feeding.**

    _____ Maintain semi-Fowler's position.

    __X__ **Obtain baseline vital signs and monitor for elevated temperature.**

    __X__ **Notify primary care provider.**

    __X__ **Obtain chest x-ray.**

    __X__ **Provide oxygen if indicated.**

    __X__ **Suction airway.**

If aspiration is suspected, the priority nursing intervention is to hold the feeding. The nurse should next turn the client to his side, suction the airway, provide oxygen if indicated, obtain baseline vital signs, continue to monitor for elevated temperature, notify the primary care provider, and prepare the client for a chest x-ray. It is not necessary to auscultate for bowel sounds, because the client should be turned to his side and nothing should be administered through the tube.

Unit 5   Supporting Physiologic Needs
Section: Gastroenteral Needs

Chapter 77:	Nasogastric Tubes

Contributor: Peggy Mossholder, MSN, RN, CHPN

 NCLEX® Connections

Learning Objective: Review and apply knowledge within **"Nasogastric Tubes"** in readiness for performance of the following nursing activities as outlined by the NCLEX® test plans:

Δ   Plan and/or provide care to initiate, maintain, and discontinue nasogastric tube therapy.

Δ   Evaluate the placement and patency of the client's nasogastric tube.

Δ   Assess/monitor the client's nasogastric tube output for changes from the expected findings.

Δ   Document the client's nasogastric tube output.

 Key Points

Δ   **Nasogastric tube (NG tube)** is a hollow lumen inserted through the nasopharynx into the stomach.

Δ   **Types of Nasogastric Intubations and Indications**

•   **Decompression**

◊   Removal of gases or stomach contents to relieve distention, nausea, or vomiting

◊   Tube types – Salem sump, Miller-Abbott, Levin

•   **Feeding**

◊   Route of administering nutritional supplements when oral/esophageal passageways are contraindicated

◊   Tube types – Duo, Levin, Dophoff

•   **Lavage**

◊   Washing out of the stomach to treat overdose or ingestion of poison

◊   Tube types – Ewald, Levin, Salem sump

- **Compression**

  ◊   Applied pressure using an internal balloon to prevent hemorrhage

  ◊   Tube types – Sengstaken-Blakemore

Key Procedural Points

Δ   The nurse may require assistance for the confused or disoriented client.

Δ   If the client has emesis, clear airway and provide comfort prior to continuing.

Δ   Salem sump tubing has a blue pigtail for negative air release. Do not insert any substance into the blue pigtail, as it will break the seal and the tubing will leak.

Δ   Auscultation is considered the least reliable method for verification of placement.

Δ   Assess whether or not the client has had any nasopharyngeal surgery or septal deviation to determine which nares to use.

Δ   Evaluate the client's ability to assist and/or cooperate.

Δ   Review orders, purpose, identify appropriate materials, plan for drainage or suction, any laboratory samples, and need for placement for diagnostic purposes.

Δ   The insertion and maintenance of a nasogastric tube is the responsibility of the nurse, but measuring output, providing comfort, and giving oral care can be delegated.

NANDA Nursing Diagnoses

Δ   Altered elimination

Δ   Pain

Δ   Altered nutrition

Δ   Fluid volume excess

Δ   Risk for imbalanced fluid volume

Nursing Interventions

Δ   Equipment

- Nasogastric tube – choose according to indication

- Solution basin with warm water or ice – warm water for plastic tubing to make it more pliable, ice for rubber tubing to stiffen and decrease curling

- Tape/secure dressing

- Gloves

- Water-soluble lubricant

- Glass of water and straw

- Catheter-tipped syringe, usually 30 to 60 mL

- Basin – preparation for gag-induced nausea

- pH test strip or meter – measurement of gastric secretion for acidity

- Stethoscope – to check placement

- Disposable towel – to maintain a clean environment

- Clamp or plug – to close tubing after insertion

- Suction apparatus – if continuous or intermittent suction is needed

- Gauze square – to cleanse external tubing after insertion

- Safety pin and elastic band – to secure tubing and prevent erroneous removal

Δ   Procedure

- **Insertion**

    ◊   Wash hands.

    ◊   Identify the client and inform of procedure.

    ◊   Set up equipment.

    ◊   Position the client in Fowler's position (if possible).

    ◊   Position disposable towel and basin.

    ◊   Provide privacy.

    ◊   Assess nares for best position/route.

    ◊   Prepare tube (place tube in ice/warm water).

    ◊   Measure tubing – tip of nose to tip of ear lobe to tip of xiphoid, and mark tubing with adhesive tape.

    ◊   Put on gloves.

    ◊   Lubricate the tip of the tubing.

    ◊   If able, have the client hold the glass of water with a straw in place, and tell the client that she will be instructed when to drink.

    ◊   Have the client hyperextend the head back.

    ◊   Gradually insert the tube.

    ◊   When resistance is met, apply gentle pressure downward, and proceed beyond the curve of the nasopharynx.

◊ Have the client lean her head forward and begin sipping as continued insertion occurs. Swallowing will feed the tubing downward toward the stomach.

◊ When the tubing reaches the mark, anchor the tube using tape or a nasogastric clamp.

◊ Placement check

  ○ Ask the client to talk.

  ○ Inspect posterior pharynx for coiled tube.

  ○ Aspirate gently to collect gastric content and observe color.

  ○ Test pH (Four or less is expected.).

  ○ If ordered, follow up with an x-ray confirmation.

  ○ Injecting air into the tube and listening over the abdomen is not acceptable practice.

◊ If not in stomach, advance the tube 5 cm and repeat placement check.

◊ When placement is confirmed, secure the tube to the nose using tape.

◊ Secure the lower end of the tube by wrapping a rubber band around the tube and pinning it to the client's gown.

◊ Clamp the nasogastric tube or connect to appropriate suction device.

- **Discontinuation/removal**

◊ Inform the client of order, process, and emphasize that removal is less stressful than placement.

◊ Sanitize hands and apply gloves.

◊ Remove safety pin from gown, and remove the tape anchoring the tube to the nose.

◊ Disconnect from suction and clamp tubing.

◊ Provide tissues to the client.

◊ Instruct the client to take and hold a deep breath.

◊ Remove tubing with steady continuous pull while the client is holding breath.

◊ Measure and record drainage.

◊ Clean nares and provide oral care.

◊ Ensure the client's comfort.

◊ Dispose of equipment.

◊ Document all relevant information to include:

   ° Tubing removal and condition of tube.

   ° Volume and description of drainage solution.

   ° Assessment of abdomen distention and tenderness.

   ° Presence or absence of bowel sounds.

   ° Record of last and next bowel movement and urine output.

Complications and Nursing Implications

Δ **Excoriation** of Nares and Stomach

- Apply lubricant to nares as needed.

- Assess color of the nasogastric tube drainage – Dark "coffee ground" or blood-streaked drainage should be reported to the primary care provider immediately.

Δ **Discomfort**

- Rinse mouth with water for dryness.

- Throat lozenges may be helpful.

- Provide frequent oral hygiene.

Δ **Occlusion** of the NG Tube Leading to Distension

- Irrigate the tube with normal saline to unclog blockages per facility/agency protocol.

- Have the client change positions in case the tube is up against the stomach wall.

Primary Reference:

Potter, P. A., & Perry, A. G. (2005). *Fundamentals of nursing* (6th ed.). St. Louis, MO: Mosby.

Additional Resources:

Kozier, B., Erb, G., Berman, A., & Snyder, S. (2004). *Fundamentals of nursing.* (6th ed.) New Jersey: Prentice Hall.

NANDA International (2004). *NANDA nursing diagnoses: Definitions and classification 2005-2006.* Philadelphia: NANDA.

Chapter 77: Nasogastric Tubes

Application Exercises

Scenario: A client arrives to the unit with brown emesis with the odor of stool. The client's vital signs are: temperature 38.9° C (102° F), pulse rate 98/min, and BP 134/82 mm Hg. The client's abdomen is distended and firm to the touch. His last bowel movement was more than 3 days ago. The primary care provider orders placement of a Salem sump nasogastric tube.

1. Explain the rationale for nasogastric tube placement and the expected outcome.

2. What nursing diagnoses are appropriate for this client?

3. Which of the following assessments gathered postinsertion of a Salem sump tube gives information that the placement is correct?

    A. Gag reflex
    B. Vital signs
    C. Mental status
    D. pH $\leq$ 4

4. Prior to insertion, a plastic nasogastric tube is placed in

    A. warm water.
    B. ice.
    C. sterile saline.
    D. room temperature sterile water.

5. The proper way to secure a nasogastric tube is to apply

    A. tape from the client's nose to the nasogastric tube.
    B. a safety pin through the nasogastric tube to the client's gown.
    C. tape to the client's cheek and loop a small amount of tubing at the nose.
    D. tape around the connection of the nasogastric tube and suction tubing.

Chapter 77: Nasogastric Tubes

Application Exercises Answer Key

Scenario: A client arrives to the unit with brown emesis with the odor of stool. The client's vital signs are: temperature 38.9° C (102° F), pulse rate 98/min, and BP 134/82 mm Hg. The client's abdomen is distended and firm to the touch. His last bowel movement was more than 3 days ago. The primary care provider orders placement of a Salem sump nasogastric tube.

1. Explain the rationale for nasogastric tube placement and the expected outcome.

Based on the situation, the likely purpose of this placement is for decompression of the client's abdomen due to his potential for bowel obstruction/constipation. Expected outcome includes resting the abdomen, removal of excess solution, treatment of the causative problem, and comfort to the client.

2. What nursing diagnoses are appropriate for this client?

Altered elimination

Pain

Altered fluid volume excess

Altered nutrition

3. Which of the following assessments gathered postinsertion of a Salem sump tube gives information that the placement is correct?

    A. Gag reflex
    B. Vital signs
    C. Mental status
    D. pH $\leq$ 4

A pH of 4 or less is expected of gastric content. The gag reflex, vital signs, and mental status do assess gastric placement.

4. Prior to insertion, a plastic nasogastric tube is placed in

A. warm water.

B. ice.

C. sterile saline.

D. room temperature sterile water.

Warm water makes a plastic tube more pliable and easier to insert. Ice is used for rubber tubing. Sterile saline and sterile water are not used for nasogastric tube insertion.

5. The proper way to secure a nasogastric tube is to apply

A. tape from the client's nose to the nasogastric tube.

B. a safety pin through the nasogastric tube to the client's gown.

C. tape to the client's cheek and loop a small amount of tubing at the nose.

D. tape around the connection of the nasogastric tube and suction tubing.

Tape from the client's nose to the nasogastric tube secures the placement. Safety pins pose a risk for piercing the tubing. The tubing is too bulky to loop around. Applying tape to the connection of the nasogastric tube and suction tubing does not secure the tube.

Unit 5   Supporting Physiologic Needs
Section: Elimination Needs

Chapter 78:   Bowel Elimination Needs and Specimen Collection
                Contributor: Ann Schide, MSN, MS, LCCE

 NCLEX® Connections

> **Learning Objective**: Review and apply knowledge within **"Bowel Elimination Needs and Specimen Collection"** in readiness for performance of the following nursing activities as outlined by the NCLEX® test plans:
>
> Δ   Assess/monitor the client for changes in bowel elimination pattern.
>
> Δ   Identify factors that affect the client's bowel elimination.
>
> Δ   Instruct the client on methods of preventing or managing incontinence or constipation.
>
> Δ   Plan and/or provide care for the client with alterations in bowel elimination.
>
> Δ   Plan and/or provide for skin care when the client has incontinence.
>
> Δ   Assist the client undergoing diagnostic evaluation of the bowel.
>
> Δ   Plan and/or provide stoma care as appropriate.
>
> Δ   Evaluate and document care given to promote bowel elimination.

 Key Points

Δ   Interventions such as surgery, immobility, medications, and therapeutic diets may affect a client's bowel elimination.

Δ   Collect stool specimens for **fecal occult blood testing** three times from three different defecations.

Δ   **Bowel diversions** through ostomies are temporary or permanent openings in the abdominal wall to allow fecal matter to pass.

Δ   End stomas are a result of colorectal cancer or types of bowel disease. **Colostomies** end in the colon, and **ileostomies** end in the ileum.

Δ   Loop colostomies are performed as a medical emergency and are temporary.

Δ   Double-barrel colostomies consist of two abdominal stomas – one proximal and one distal.

Key Procedural Points

Δ   Factors Affecting Normal Bowel Elimination

Age	• Infants:
	  ◊ Breastfed stools – watery and yellow brown
	  ◊ Formula stools – pasty and brown
	• Toddlers: bowel control at 2 to 3 years old
	• Older adult: decreased peristalsis, relaxation of sphincters

Diet	• Fiber: 25 to 30 g/day • Lactose intolerance: difficulty in digesting milk products
Fluids	• 1,500 to 2,000 mL/day
Physical activity	• Promotes peristalsis
Psychosocial factors	• Emotional distress exacerbating chronic conditions (e.g., colitis, Crohn's disease, ulcers)
Personal habits	• Use of public toilets, false perception of "one-a-day" being mandatory, lack of privacy in hospitalized situation
Positioning	• Normal: squatting • Immobilized client: difficulty defecating
Pain	• Suppression of the defecation urge • Opioid use contributing to constipation
Pregnancy	• Growing fetus compromising intestinal space • Slower peristalsis • Straining increasing the incidence of hemorrhoids
Surgery and anesthesia	• Temporary cessation of peristalsis • Paralytic ileus • Primary rationale for auscultating bowel sounds before advancing a client's diet
Medications	• Laxatives – to soften stool • Cathartics – to promote peristalsis • Laxative abuse leading to diarrhea that leads to dehydration

Δ   Diagnostic Tests

• Visualization of the bowel

◊   Colonoscopies – the large colon and sometimes a portion of the lower small bowel are visualized and may be biopsied.

◊   Sigmoidoscopies – the sigmoid colon and rectum are visualized and may be biopsied.

- Preparation
  - ◊ All require the client to be NPO for 12 hr prior to the procedure and to eat nothing but clear liquids 24 hr prior.
  - ◊ A bowel prep using laxatives is commonly prescribed.
  - ◊ Conscious sedation with a benzodiazepine and an opioid is commonly used, and the client is not able to drive himself home afterwards.

NANDA Nursing Diagnoses

- Δ Bowel incontinence
- Δ Perceived constipation
- Δ Risk for constipation
- Δ Risk for impaired skin integrity
- Δ Diarrhea

Nursing Interventions

- Δ Promoting Healthy Bowel Elimination

Equipment	Procedure

• Bedpans
  ◊ Fracture pan – for supine clients and clients in body casts or leg casts
  ◊ Regular pan – for seated clients
• Beside commode
• Toilet
• Adequate fiber in the diet
• Adequate fluid intake – minimum of 1,500 mL/day of water and/or juices
• Adequate activity – walking 15 to 20 min/day if mobile and exercises in bed or chair (e.g., pelvic tilt, single leg lifts, and lower trunk rotation)
	• Encourage the client to set aside time to defecate – sometimes after a meal works the best.
	• If not contraindicated or restricted, encourage the client to drink plenty of fluids and to consume a diet high in fiber to prevent constipation.
	• Wear gloves when caring for toileting needs.
	• Assist the client to the sitting position whether using a regular bedpan, commode, or toilet.
	• For clients using a fracture pan, the head of the bed should be raised to 30°.
	• If the client cannot lift his hips to get the bedpan under him, the client can be rolled onto one side, the bedpan positioned over the buttocks, and the client rolled back onto the bedpan.
	• Decrease stress when sitting or rising by using an elevated toilet seat or a footstool.
	• Provide privacy.
	• Never leave a client lying flat on a regular bedpan.
	• After defecation, provide skin care to the perianal area.

Δ   Specimen Collection

Equipment	Procedure

• Appropriate nonsterile specimen container
• Soap/cleansing solution or towel
• Gloves
• Specimen label
• Hemoccult slide
• Wooden applicator or tongue depressor
• Hemoccult developer solution
• Stool collection container (e.g., bedside commode, bedpan, receptacle in toilet)
	• Fecal occult blood testing (Guaiac test)
	◊ Explain the procedure to the client.
	◊ If able, ask the client to collect specimen in the toilet receptacle, bedpan, or bedside commode.
	◊ Apply gloves, and with wooden applicator, place small amounts of stool on part A and part B of the Hemoccult slide.
	◊ Follow facility procedures for developing.
	  ° Apply label to the slide and send to the laboratory for processing.
	  ° Place a couple of drops of developer on the opposite side of the slide, and if blue color appears, the test is positive for blood.
	◊ Remove gloves and perform hand hygiene.
	• Stool for culture, parasites, and ova
	◊ Explain the procedure to the client.
	◊ If able, ask the client to collect the specimen in the toilet receptacle, bedside commode, or bedpan.
	◊ Put on gloves.
	◊ Use wooden tongue depressor to transfer to a specimen container.
	◊ Label container with the client's identifying information.
	◊ Remove gloves.
	◊ Perform hand hygiene.
	◊ Transport specimen to the laboratory.

Δ   Cleansing enema – The height of the bag above the rectum determines the depth
of cleansing.

Equipment	Procedure

• Gloves
• Lubricant
• Absorbent, waterproof pads
• Bedpan, beside commode, or toilet
• IV pole
• Enema bag with tubing or prepackaged enema
• Solutions and additives – dependent on the type of enema given
  ◊ Tap water or hypotonic
    ° Stimulates evacuation
    ° Never repeated due to potential water toxicity
  ◊ Soap suds
    ° Pure Castile soap in tap water or normal saline
    ° Acts as an irritant to promote bowel peristalsis
  ◊ Normal saline
    ° Safest due to equal osmotic pressure
    ° Volume stimulates peristalsis
  ◊ Low-volume hypertonic
    ° Good for clients who cannot tolerate high-volume enemas
    ° Fleets® – a commercially prepared hypertonic enema
  ◊ Oil retention – lubricates the rectum and colon for easier passage of stool
  ◊ Medicated enemas – contains medications that need to be retained
	• Perform hand hygiene.
	• Prepare enema solution.
	• Pour solution in enema bag allowing it to fill the tubing, and then close the clamp.
	• Explain the procedure to the client.
	• Provide privacy.
	• Provide quick access to commode or bedpan.
	• Place absorbent pads under the client to protect the bed.
	• Position the client on the left side with right leg flexed forward.
	• Put on gloves.
	• Lubricate the rectal tube or nozzle.
	• Slowly insert rectal tube 6 to 8 cm.
	• With bag at the level of the client's hip, open the clamp.
	• Raise the bag 30 to 45 cm above the anus, depending on the level of cleansing desired.
	• Discontinue the flow of solution if the client reports clamping, or if fluid leaks around the tube at the anus.
	• If a prepackaged solution is used, insert the lubricated tip into the rectum and squeeze the container until the solution is administered.
	• Ask the client to retain the solution for the prescribed amount of time, or until the client is no longer able to hold it.
	• Discard the enema bag and tubing.
	• Assist the client to a position to defecate.
	• Remove gloves.
	• Perform hand hygiene.
	• Should the client have little or no sphincter control, the nurse should administer the enema on a bedpan.
	• Document results.

Δ   Ostomy Care

Equipment	Procedure
• Pouch system (skin barrier and pouch) • Pouch closure clamp • Barrier pastes (optional) • Gloves • Washcloths • Towel • Warm water • Scissors • Pen	• Educate the client in the care of the stoma. • Often there is an enterostomal therapist (RN) available. • Perform hand hygiene. • Put on gloves. • Remove previous pouch. • Inspect the stoma. It should appear moist, shiny, and pink. The peristomal area should be intact, and the skin should appear healthy. • Use mild soap and water to cleanse the skin with thorough drying. • Apply paste if used. • Measure and draw where the skin barrier should be cut, allowing only the stoma to appear through the opening. • Cut the opening in the skin barrier. • If necessary, apply barrier pastes to creases. • Apply skin barrier and pouch. • Fold bottom of the pouch and place closure pouch. • Dispose of old pouch. Dispose of gloves and perform hand hygiene.

Complications and Nursing Implications

Δ   **Constipation**

- Signs and symptoms – bowel pattern of difficult and infrequent evacuation of hard, dry feces

- Fiber and water consumption is increased prior to treating constipation with laxatives.

- Bulk-forming products are used prior to stool softeners, stimulants, or suppositories to promote bowel elimination.

- Enemas are a last resort used to bring about defecation.

Δ   **Impaction**

- Signs and symptoms – stool that is wedged into the rectum with leaking diarrhea fluid from around the impacted stool

- Digital removal of the stool is done using a lubricated, gloved index finger.

- The stool is loosened around the edges and then removed in small pieces, allowing the client to rest as necessary.

- When evacuating the rectum, care needs to be taken not to stimulate the vagus nerve.

Δ   **Diarrhea**

- Signs and symptoms – frequent, liquid stools caused by various disorders.

- The cause needs to be determined and treated.

- Medications to slow peristalsis may also be prescribed.

- Provide good perineal care after each stool and apply moisture barrier if indicated.

- The client and caregivers should use good hand hygiene.

Δ   **Fecal Incontinence**

- Signs and symptoms – the inability to control defecation that is often caused by diarrhea

- Assess the client for causes, such as medications, infections, or impaction.

- Provide good perineal care after each stool and apply moisture barrier if indicated.

Δ   **Flatulence**

- Signs and symptoms – the distension of the bowel from gas accumulation (may cause cramping or feeling of fullness)

  ◊ Assess the client for abdominal distension and the ability to pass the gas through the anus.

  ◊ If mobile, encourage the client to ambulate to encourage the passage of flatus.

  ◊ Notify the primary care provider if the problem continues.

Δ   **Hemorrhoids**

- Signs and symptoms – engorged, dilated blood vessels in the rectal wall caused by difficult defecation, pregnancy, liver disease, and heart failure

  ◊ Hemorrhoids may be itchy, painful, and bloody after defecation.

  ◊ When cleansing the perianal area, moist wipes may be more comfortable.

  ◊ Application of prescribed ointments or creams may be prescribed.

Primary Reference:

Potter, P. A., & Perry, A. G. (2005). *Fundamentals of nursing* (6th ed.). St. Louis, MO: Mosby.

Additional Resources:

Wilkinson, J. M. (2005). *Nursing diagnosis handbook*. Upper Saddle River, NJ: Prentice Hall.

NANDA International (2004). *NANDA nursing diagnoses: Definitions and classification 2005-2006*. Philadelphia: NANDA.

Chapter 78: Bowel Elimination Needs and Specimen Collection

Application Exercises

Scenario: A client with a broken tibia and fibula is administered opiates to control his pain. Prior to his injury, the client tells the nurse he ran 2 to 3 miles most days of the week and expected a daily, pain-free bowel movement, "regular as clockwork."

1. Based on this initial data, what should be a priority nursing diagnoses for this client pertaining to bowel function?

2. List possible ways to support normal bowel function for this client.

3. A tap water enema is ordered for a client to be repeated until the return is clear. What is the nurse's next action?

        A. Clarify the order with the primary care provider.

        B. Explain the procedure to the client.

        C. Insure that the tap water is not too hot.

        D. Keep the amount per enema to less than 1,000 mL.

4. Which of the following foods should be encouraged for a client experiencing constipation?

        A. Macaroni and cheese

        B. Fresh fruit and whole wheat toast

        C. Beef tips and noodles

        D. Mashed potatoes and gravy

Chapter 78: Bowel Elimination Needs and Specimen Collection

Application Exercises Answer Key

Scenario: A client with a broken tibia and fibula is administered opiates to control his pain. Prior to his injury, the client tells the nurse he ran 2 to 3 miles most days of the week and expected a daily, pain-free bowel movement, "regular as clockwork."

1. Based on this initial data, what should be a priority nursing diagnoses for this client pertaining to bowel function?

   Risk for constipation related to the use of opiates and decreased physical activity

2. List possible ways to support normal bowel function for this client.

   Encourage him to drink plenty of fluids.

   Monitor frequency of bowel movements.

   Assist the client to a sitting position to defecate at certain times of the day.

   When able, increase activity.

   Consider consulting with the primary care provider for a bulk-forming laxative if needed.

   When pain lessens, switch the client to a nonopiate form of pain medication.

3. A tap water enema is ordered for a client to be repeated until the return is clear. What is the nurse's next action?

   A. Clarify the order with the primary care provider.
   B. Explain the procedure to the client.
   C. Insure that the tap water is not too hot.
   D. Keep the amount per enema to less than 1,000 mL.

   Tap water is a hypotonic solution and can cause water toxicity. It should not be repeated. The order should be clarified. Explaining the procedure to the client, ensuring the tap water is not too hot, and keeping the amount to less than 1,000 mL is not pertinent if the enema should not be repeated.

4. Which of the following foods should be encouraged for a client experiencing constipation?

    A. Macaroni and cheese

    B. Fresh fruit and whole wheat toast

    C. Beef tips and noodles

    D. Mashed potatoes and gravy

A high-fiber diet promotes normal bowel elimination. The choice of fruit and toast is the highest fiber option. Macaroni and cheese, beef tips, noodles, and mashed potatoes and gravy are lower-fiber options.

Unit 5   Supporting Physiologic Needs
Section: Elimination Needs

Chapter 79:   Urinary Elimination Needs and Specimen Collection
Contributor: Ann Schide, MSN, MS, RN, LCCE

 NCLEX® Connections

Learning Objective: Review and apply knowledge within **"Urinary Elimination Needs and Specimen Collection"** in readiness for performance of the following nursing activities as outlined by the NCLEX® test plans:

Δ   Assess/monitor the client for changes in urinary elimination pattern.

Δ   Identify factors that affect the client's urinary elimination.

Δ   Instruct the client on methods of preventing or managing incontinence.

Δ   Plan and/or provide care for the client with alterations in urinary elimination.

Δ   Plan and/or provide for skin care when the client has incontinence.

Δ   Evaluate and document care given to promote urinary elimination.

 Key Points

Δ   Interventions such as surgery, immobility, medications, and therapeutic diets may affect a client's urinary elimination.

Δ   **Urinary diversions** – temporary and permanent; stoma necessary for drainage of urine

- Ureterostomy – one or both ureters to abdominal surface

- Nephrostomy – tube from renal pelvis to abdominal surface

- Pouched system similar to bowel diversions with similar body image concerns

Δ   Urinary diversions may be needed for a client with cancer of the bladder, trauma, or injury to the bladder.

Key Procedural Points

Δ   Factors Affecting Normal Urinary Elimination

- Age

  ◊   Full bladder control at 4 to 5 years

  ◊   Enlargement of the prostate after 40 years leading to urinary frequency, hesitancy, and retention

  ◊   Childbirth and gravity weakening the pelvic floor, allowing prolapse of the bladder, which leads to **stress incontinence** – can be managed with pelvic floor (Kegel) exercises.

  ◊   Older adult clients

    ○   Decreased number of nephrons

    ○   Loss of muscle tone of the bladder – incontinence/frequency

    ○   Bladder not emptied as efficiently – residual urine

    ○   Increase in the incidence of **nocturia**

- Pregnancy

  ◊   **Growing fetus** compromises bladder space and compresses the bladder.

  ◊   There is a 30 to 50% increased circulatory volume, which increases renal workload and output.

  ◊   The hormone relaxin causes relaxation of sphincter.

- **Poor abdominal and pelvic muscle tone**

- Disease conditions

- **Immobility**

- Psychosocial factors

  ◊   Emotional stress and anxiety

  ◊   Having to use public toilets, lack of privacy in hospitalized situation

  ◊   Not having enough time to void – predetermined "potty" breaks in elementary schools

- Pain

  ◊   Suppression of the urge to void in the presence of pain in the urinary tract

  ◊   Delayed micturition due to painful musculoskeletal joints, such as with arthritis

- Surgical procedures

  ◊ Anesthesia/opioid analgesics alter glomerular filtration rate resulting in decreased urine output.

  ◊ Lower abdominal surgeries can create obstructing edema and inflammation.

- Medications

  ◊ **Diuretics** prevent reabsorption of water.

  ◊ **Antihistamines and anticholinergics** may cause urinary retention.

  ◊ Some medications change urine color.

    ° Pyridium – orange

    ° Amitriptyline – green/blue

    ° Levodopa – brown/black

  ◊ Chemotherapy may create a toxic environment for the kidneys.

Δ Diagnostic Tests

- **KUB** – x-ray to determine size, shape, and position of kidneys

- **IVP** (intravenous pyelogram) – contrast used to view ducts, renal pelvis, ureters, bladder, and urethra. Iodine is used; therefore, it is important to determine if the client has an allergy to shellfish.

- **Renal scan** – view of renal blood flow and anatomy of kidneys – no contrast

- **Renal ultrasound** – view of gross renal structures

- **Cystoscopy** – use of endoscope to visualize bladder and urethra

- **Urodynamic testing** – to test bladder muscle function by filling the bladder with CO_2 or saline and comparing pressure readings with the client's reported sensations

NANDA Nursing Diagnoses

Δ Urinary incontinence (functional, reflex, stress, total, urge)

Δ Risk for infection

Δ Self-care deficit, toileting

Δ Impaired urinary elimination

Δ Urinary retention

Nursing Interventions

Δ   Promoting Healthy Urinary Elimination

Equipment	Procedure

• Urinal for men
• Toilet, bedpan, or commode
   ◊ Fracture pan – for supine clients and clients in body or leg casts
   ◊ Regular pan – for seated clients
	• Position the client in a sitting position when possible.
	• Provide for privacy needs with adequate time for urinating (generally, at least 30 min).

Δ   I&O

Equipment	Procedure
• Hard plastic urometer on Foley sets is a reliable measuring tool on catheter bags. • Graduated cylinders, urinal, or toilet receptacle	• Measure output from a bedpan, commode, or Foley bag into a graduated container. • Use receptacle to measure urine voided in the toilet. • Use markings on the side of the urinal to measure voided urine. • Less than 30 mL/hr for more than 2 hr is cause for concern.

Δ   Bladder Retraining

Equipment	Procedure
• Clock	• Use timed voidings to increase intervals between voidings/decrease voiding frequency. • Perform pelvic floor (Kegel) exercises. • Perform relaxation techniques. • Offer undergarments while client is retraining. • Teach client not to ignore urge to void. • Provide positive reinforcement as client maintains continence.

Δ   Specimen Collection

- Equipment

  ◊ Appropriate specimen container

    ° Nonsterile for urinalysis

    ° Sterile for clean catch midstream

  ◊ Soap/cleansing solution or towel

  ◊ Gloves

  ◊ Specimen label

  ◊ Urine collection container (e.g., Foley catheter, urinal, receptacle in toilet, commode)

Urinalysis – unsterile specimen	<ul><li>Explain procedure to the client.</li><li>Ask the client to void.</li><li>Put on gloves.</li><li>Pour urine into specimen container.</li><li>Apply label on the container with the client's identifying information.</li><li>Remove gloves and wash hands.</li><li>Transport specimen to the laboratory.</li></ul>
Clean catch midstream (CCMS) for culture and sensitivity (C&S)	<ul><li>Teach the client the technique for obtaining specimen.</li><li>Urine sample "caught" midstream of urine.</li><li>Requires thorough cleansing of urethral meatus.</li><li>The client voids a bit of urine into commode, bedpan, and/or urinal, and then the rest of the void is caught in a sterile cup.</li><li>The client needs to understand not to place fingers in cup or to touch the lid.</li></ul>
Catheter urine specimen for C&S	<ul><li>Sterile specimen</li><li>Straight catheter under sterile technique</li><li>Foley catheter under sterile technique<ul><li>◊ Drain catheter tubing of urine.</li><li>◊ Clamp catheter tubing below "port" for 20 min.</li><li>◊ Use sterile technique to withdraw required specimen amount from the port with a syringe.</li><li>◊ Unclamp the catheter.</li></ul></li></ul>
Timed urine specimens	<ul><li>These are usually done for 24 hr but can be ordered for varying times.</li><li>Discard first void.</li><li>Collect all other voids in a container placed on ice.</li><li>Education of the client, family, and visitors is required to prevent collecting urine other than the client's, or missing a void (Timing for specimen would begin again in either scenario.).</li></ul>

Δ Straight or Indwelling Catheter Insertion

- Equipment

  ◊ Correct size and type of catheters. In general, 8 to 10 Fr for children, 14 to 16 Fr for women, and 16 to 18 Fr for men (use silicon or teflon products for clients with latex allergies).

  ◊ Catheterization kit – with sterile drainage bag for Foley catheter insertion

◊ Soap and water

◊ Collection container for straight catheterization

- Procedure

◊ Explain procedure to the client.

◊ Wash hands.

◊ Establish a location in the room to set up a sterile field.

◊ Provide privacy.

◊ Lower side rail, raise bed to a comfortable height, and establish a good light source on the perineal area.

◊ Position the client.

  ° Female – supine with knees bent and apart

  ° Male – supine position and thighs abducted slightly

◊ Put on gloves and wash perineal area.

◊ Remove gloves.

◊ Open sterile package.

◊ Put on sterile gloves.

◊ Put antiseptic solution on cotton balls.

◊ Inflate the balloon of an indwelling catheter with the syringe to check its performance and integrity.

◊ Lubricate the lower portion of catheter.

◊ Apply sterile drape exposing the urinary meatus.

◊ Cleanse meatus.

  ° Female – spread labia with one hand while wiping front-to-back with the antiseptic cotton balls held in the forceps. The hand on the labia is now contaminated and holds this position for the rest of the procedure.

  ° Male – hold the penis with one hand and wipe in a circular motion starting at the meatus and working down the glans. Repeat three more times.

◊ Insert the catheter into the meatus using the sterile hand.

◊ Advance the catheter until urine returns and then continue to advance another 2.5 to 5 cm.

◊ Release labia/penis and stabilize catheter with nondominant hand.

◊ Inflate the balloon, if the catheter is to be indwelling. Release hand and pull back gently.

◊ Secure catheter to the client's leg.

◊ Place drainage bag below the level of the client's bladder.

    ◊   If a straight catheterization, remove catheter after the flow of urine has ceased.

    ◊   Dispose of drapes, equipment, and gloves.

    ◊   Replace side rail and lower bed.

    ◊   Wash hands.

Δ   Closed intermittent irrigation

- Prepare sterile syringe with irrigant.

- Clamp the catheter between the injection port and the extension tubing.

- Cleanse the injection port with an antiseptic swab or wipe.

- Insert needle of syringe with irrigant into injection port.

- Slowly inject irrigant into catheter and bladder.

- Withdraw syringe and remove clamp.

- Allow irrigant to drain into drainage bag.

Δ   Routine Catheter Care

- Equipment

    ◊   Soap and water

    ◊   Wash cloth

    ◊   Gloves

- Procedure

    ◊   Use soap and water at insertion site.

    ◊   Cleanse catheter at least three times/day and after defecation.

    ◊   Monitor patency of the catheter.

        °   The client reports fullness in the bladder area.

        °   Check for kink in tubing.

        °   Check for sediment in tubing.

        °   Check to make sure that the catheter bag/system is above the urethral meatus and not hanging dependent.

Δ   Condom Catheter Application

- Equipment

    ◊   Gloves

    ◊   Condom catheters

    ◊   Elastic tape

    ◊   Leg or Foley bag

- Procedure
  - ◊ Wash hands.
  - ◊ Explain the procedure to the client.
  - ◊ Adjust height of the bed.
  - ◊ Minimally expose the client.
  - ◊ Put on gloves.
  - ◊ Apply skin prep to the skin of the penis.
  - ◊ Hold penis with one hand, and place the condom over the tip allowing 2.5 cm of space between the tip of the penis and the catheter.
  - ◊ Roll down the sides of the condom over the shaft of the penis.
  - ◊ Use elastic tape in a spiral manner to secure if needed.
  - ◊ Attach catheter to leg or Foley bag.
  - ◊ Observe for the presence of urine.
  - ◊ Remove gloves and wash hands.
  - ◊ Lower bed.

Complications and Nursing Implications

Δ **Urinary Tract Infections (UTIs)**

- Factors that increase the risk of UTIs:
  - ◊ Close proximity of urethral meatus in women to their rectal openings
  - ◊ Menopause decreasing estrogen and increasing susceptibility to UTIs
  - ◊ Uncircumcised males
  - ◊ Use of indwelling catheters

- **Nursing implications**
  - ◊ Cleanse female clients from front to back.
  - ◊ Cleanse beneath the foreskin in males.
  - ◊ Provide regular catheter care.

Primary Reference:

Potter, P. A., & Perry, A. G. (2005). *Fundamentals of nursing* (6th ed.). St. Louis, MO: Mosby.

Additional Resources:

NANDA International (2004). *NANDA nursing diagnoses: Definitions and classification 2005-2006*. Philadelphia: NANDA.

Wilkinson, J. M. (2005). *Nursing diagnosis handbook*. Upper Saddle River, NJ: Prentice Hall.

Chapter 79: Urinary Elimination Needs and Specimen Collection

Application Exercises

1. A client with an indwelling catheter reports a need to void. What priority intervention should the nurse perform?

      A. Check to see if the catheter is patent.

      B. Reassure the client that it is not possible for her to void.

      C. Recatheterize the client with a larger-gauge catheter.

      D. Notify the primary care provider.

2. Which of the following interventions is correct when performing a 24-hr urine specimen test?

      A. Ask the client to void and pour the urine into a specimen container.

      B. Ask the client to void first into the toilet and then to stop midstream and finish voiding in the specimen container.

      C. Discard the first voiding.

      D. Keep all voidings for 24 hr in a container at room temperature.

3. Which of the following is the best position for a client to be in to encourage normal elimination?

      A. In left lateral Sims' position

      B. Sitting

      C. Supine

      D. Right side-lying

4. Which of the following interventions is appropriate for the nurse to perform when performing a catheterization on a female client? (Select all that apply.)

      _____ Provide for privacy.

      _____ Darken the room.

      _____ Maintain surgical aseptic technique throughout the procedure.

      _____ Position the client supine with knees bent and apart.

      _____ Ask the client not to talk during the procedure.

Chapter 79: Urinary Elimination Needs and Specimen Collection

Application Exercises Answer Key

1. A client with an indwelling catheter reports a need to void. What priority intervention should the nurse perform?

   A. Check to see if the catheter is patent.

   B. Reassure the client that it is not possible for her to void.

   C. Recatheterize the client with a larger-gauge catheter.

   D. Notify the primary care provider.

   A clogged catheter would cause the bladder to fill and give a sensation to the client of the need to void. Reassuring the client that it is not possible to void is a nontherapeutic response. The patency of the tube would need to be checked before the client's catheter would be replaced. It is not necessary to contact the primary care provider. The nurse can determine if the tube is patent and replace the tube if necessary without a medical order.

2. Which of the following interventions is correct when performing a 24-hr urine specimen test?

   A. Ask the client to void and pour the urine into a specimen container.

   B. Ask the client to void first into the toilet and then to stop midstream and finish voiding in the specimen container.

   C. Discard the first voiding.

   D. Keep all voidings for 24 hr in a container at room temperature.

   The first voiding of the 24-hr urine specimen is discarded, and the time is noted. All voidings are collected after that and kept in a container on ice. If a urinalysis is ordered, ask the client to void and pour the urine into a specimen container. If a culture is ordered, ask the client to void first into the toilet and then to stop midstream and finish voiding in the specimen container. The specimen for a 24-hr collection is stored on ice.

3. Which of the following is the best position for a client to be in to encourage normal elimination?

        A. In left lateral Sims' position

        B. Sitting

        C. Supine

        D. Right side-lying

The most natural and efficient way to void is sitting upright. Left lateral Sims' and right lateral position are not appropriate for being able to collect urine. The supine position makes it difficult to empty the bladder completely.

4. Which of the following interventions is appropriate for the nurse to perform when performing a catheterization on a female client? (Select all that apply.)

        __X__ **Provide for privacy.**

        _____ Darken the room.

        __X__ **Maintain surgical aseptic technique throughout the procedure.**

        __X__ **Position the client supine with knees bent and apart.**

        _____ Ask the client not to talk during the procedure.

It is important to maintain privacy during a catheterization to maintain the dignity of the client. Insertion of a urinary catheter requires surgical aseptic technique, because the catheter is entering a sterile body cavity. Positioning the client supine with knees bent and apart will facilitate insertion of the catheter. It is not necessary to darken the room. Talking will not contaminate the sterile field, so it is not necessary to ask the client not to talk.

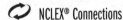

Unit 5

Section:

Supporting Physiologic Needs

Neurosensory Needs

Chapter 80: **Assisting the Client with Sensoriperceptual Alterations**

Contributor: Wendy Buenzli, MN, RN

NCLEX® Connections

Learning Objective: Review and apply knowledge within **"Assisting the Client with Sensoriperceptual Alterations"** in readiness for performance of the following nursing activities as outlined by the NCLEX® test plans:

Δ   Assess/monitor clients for altered sensoriperceptual needs (e.g., hearing impairment, visual impairment).

Δ   Record and report the client's deficits to the primary care provider.

Δ   Plan and/or provide care to assist the client in making accommodations (e.g., hearing aids, dentures, communication devices).

Δ   Identify safety concerns related to the client's sensoriperception alterations.

Δ   Teach/reinforce the proper use of assistive devices to the client.

Δ   Evaluate and document the client's ability to appropriately use assistive devices.

Key Points

Δ   **Sensory perception** is the ability to receive and interpret sensory impressions:

• Consciousness.

• Arousal and awareness.

• Memory.

• Affect.

• Judgment.

• Awareness of reality.

• Language.

Δ   Factors that contribute to loss of vision include presbyopia, cataracts, glaucoma, diabetic retinopathy, macular degeneration, infection, inflammation or injury of the eye, and brain tumor.

Δ   Factors that contribute to conductive hearing loss include obstruction, tympanic membrane perforation, ear infections, and otosclerosis, and to sensorineural hearing loss include exposure to loud noises, ototoxic medications, aging, and acoustic neuroma.

Δ   **Sensory deficit** is a change in perception. Deficits can affect all the senses.

Δ   **Sensory deprivation** is reduced sensory input either from the internal or external environment. Sensory deprivation can be the result of illness, trauma, or isolation.

Δ   **Sensory overload** is excessive and sustained multisensory stimulation.

Key Procedural Factors

Δ   Determine what assistive devices are needed, and plan for their procurement while in the facility/agency and community.

Δ   Assess for communication deficits early on and adjust care accordingly.

Δ   Consult with rehabilitation therapies, as appropriate, for restorative potential.

Δ   Collect equipment necessary to care for assistive devices the client may have (e.g., glasses, hearing aids).

Δ   Do not avoid communicating with a client with sensoriperceptual losses, as these clients tend to withdraw from interactions with others.

NANDA Nursing Diagnoses

Δ   Disturbed sensory perception (Specify auditory, visual, kinesthetic, gustatory, tactile, or olfactory.)

Δ   Disturbed thought processes

Δ   Social isolation

Δ   Risk for injury

Nursing Interventions

Δ   Equipment

- Assistive devices
- Orientation tools (e.g., clocks, calendars)
- Radio, TV, tape/compact disc player
- Large print materials

Δ   Procedures

- Keep the client safe and free from injury.

  ◊   Make sure the call light is readily available.

  ◊   Orient the client to the room.

  ◊   Keep furniture clear from the path to the bathroom.

  ◊   Make IV poles and drainage tubes/bags easy to maneuver.

- Learn the client's preferred alternative method of communication and make accommodations.

- Clients who are hearing impaired:

  ◊   Sit and face the client.

  ◊   Avoid covering mouth while speaking.

  ◊   Have the client use hearing devices.

  ◊   Speak slowly and clearly.

  ◊   Try lowering pitch before increasing volume to be heard.

  ◊   Use brief sentences with simple words.

  ◊   Write things out that are not understood.

  ◊   Minimize background noises.

  ◊   Ask for a sign language interpreter if necessary.

- Clients who are visually impaired:

  ◊   Call the person by name before approaching so as to avoid startling him.

  ◊   Identify yourself.

  ◊   Give specific information about the location of items or areas of the building.

  ◊   Before leaving, inform the client of your departure.

  ◊   Carefully appraise the client's clothing and suggest changes if soiled or torn.

  ◊   Make radio, TV, tape/compact disc player available for the client to use.

  ◊   Describe the arrangement of the food on the tray before departing the room.

- Clients with aphasia:

  ◊   Greet the client and call him by name.

  ◊   Speak clearly and slowly using short sentences.

  ◊   Allow time in between statements to allow the client to understand.

◊ Check for comprehension.

◊ Reinforce verbal with nonverbal communication (e.g., gestures, body language).

◊ Allow plenty of time for the client to respond.

◊ Use methods put in place by speech therapists, such as a picture chart, to improve communication.

◊ Acknowledge any frustration in communicating that the client expresses.

- Disoriented clients

  ◊ Call the client by name and identify yourself.

  ◊ Maintain eye contact at the client's eye level.

  ◊ Use brief, simple sentences.

  ◊ Ask only one question at a time.

  ◊ Allow plenty of time for the client to respond.

  ◊ Give directions one step at a time.

  ◊ Avoid lengthy conversations.

- Encourage the client to verbalize feelings about sensoriperceptual loss.

- Orientate the client to time, person, place, and situation.

  ◊ Keep a clock in the room.

  ◊ Keep a calendar, or write the date where it is visible.

- Provide and/or use assistive devices as needed.

- Provide care the client is not able to do (e.g. reading the menu, opening containers).

- Refer the client to community-based support groups and organizations for additional resources.

Complications and Nursing Implications

Δ Risk for Injury in the Home Environment

- Teach/reinforce with the client ways to reduce hazards at home.

  ◊ Visual – Remove throw rugs to prevent tripping hazards.

  ◊ Auditory – Use flashing lights versus a warning sound from alarms.

  ◊ Olfactory – Make sure smoke detectors and carbon monoxide detectors are functioning to sense odors that are not perceived (e.g., burning food, natural gas).

◊ Gustatory – Read dates on food packing to avoid contaminated or spoiled food that cannot be detected through taste.

◊ Tactile – Protect and inspect body parts that lack sensation (e.g., burns, bed sores, frostbite).

Δ Sensory Deprivation and Overload

• Minimize overall stimuli and provide meaningful stimulation.

◊ Minimize glare.

◊ Provide large print materials or tape/compact disc players for audiobooks.

◊ Amplify phones.

◊ Season foods.

◊ Remove unpleasant odors.

◊ Provide pleasant aromas.

◊ Increase touch with back rubs, holding a hand, range of motion, and caring for a client's hair.

◊ Turn off the TV and minimize the activity surrounding the client's bed when possible.

Primary Reference:

Potter, P. A., & Perry, A. G. (2005). *Fundamentals of nursing* (6th ed.). St. Louis, MO: Mosby.

Additional Resources:

Delaune, S. & Ladner, P. (2006) *Fundamentals of nursing* (3rd ed.). Clifton Park: Thomson Delmar.

NANDA International (2004). *NANDA nursing diagnoses: Definitions and classification 2005-2006*. Philadelphia: NANDA.

Chapter 80: Assisting the Client with Sensoriperceptual Alterations

Application Exercises

1. A nurse is caring for a client with a recent cerebrovascular accident who is exhibiting signs of aphasia. Which of the following interventions will promote communication with this client? . . (Select all that apply.)

   _____ Speak fast and loud.

   _____ Minimize background noise.

   _____ Write things out that are not understood.

   _____ Allow plenty of time for the client to respond.

   _____ Use brief sentences with simple words.

2. A nurse is caring for a client who recently overdosed on amphetamines and is experiencing sensory overload. Which of the following interventions is most important for the nurse to implement?

   A. Immediately complete a thorough assessment.

   B. Put the client in a room with a roommate who is hearing impaired.

   C. Provide a private room and limit stimulation.

   D. Talk loudly to the client and encourage ambulation.

3. A client reports difficulty reading small print and driving, especially at night. She also reports difficulty going up and down steps as they "all seem to blend together." Which of the following nursing diagnoses is a priority?

   A. Sensory-perceptual alteration (auditory) related to social isolation

   B. Risk for injury related to impaired vision

   C. Sensory-perceptual alteration (sensory overload) related to hospitalization

   D. Disturbed thought processes related to hospitalization

4. One form of nonverbal communication that helps to clarify verbal communication to clients is _____.

5. _____ means the client cannot speak or comprehend spoken language.

6. A client experiencing reduced sensory input may experience sensory _____.

Chapter 80: Assisting the Client with Sensoriperceptual Alterations

Application Exercises Answer Key

1. A nurse is caring for a client with a recent cerebrovascular accident who is exhibiting signs of aphasia. Which of the following interventions will promote communication with this client? (Select all that apply.)

   _____ Speak fast and loud.

   __X__ **Minimize background noise.**

   __X__ **Write things out that are not understood.**

   __X__ **Allow plenty of time for the client to respond.**

   __X__ **Use brief sentences with simple words.**

   Writing things out that are not understood, allowing time for the client to respond, and using simple words and brief sentences will promote communication for the client with aphasia. Minimizing background noise will provide a calming environment. The client is not hard of hearing, so speaking loud will not promote communication.

2. A nurse is caring for a client who recently overdosed on amphetamines and is experiencing sensory overload. Which of the following interventions is most important for the nurse to implement?

   A. Immediately complete a thorough assessment.

   B. Put the client in a room with a roommate who is hearing impaired.

   C. Provide a private room and limit stimulation.

   D. Talk loudly to the client and encourage ambulation.

   Minimizing stimuli will assist the client experiencing sensory overload. Immediately completing a thorough assessment will overwhelm the client at this time; therefore, brief assessments done over the course of the shift are preferred. Rooming with a roommate who is hearing impaired and/or talking in a loud voice will increase environmental stimuli.

3. A client reports difficulty reading small print and driving, especially at night. She also reports difficulty going up and down steps as they "all seem to blend together." Which of the following nursing diagnoses is a priority?

    A. Sensory-perceptual alteration (auditory) related to social isolation

    B. Risk for injury related to impaired vision

    C. Sensory-perceptual alteration (sensory overload) related to hospitalization

    D. Disturbed thought processes related to hospitalization

A client with visual deficits is at risk for tripping and falling over unseen obstacles and incurring a serious injury. The client does not report a lack of interactions or sensory overload. The client does not show any signs of confusion.

4. One form of nonverbal communication that helps to clarify verbal communication to clients is _____.

gestures

5. _____ means the client cannot speak or comprehend spoken language.

Aphasia

6. A client experiencing reduced sensory input may experience sensory _____.

deprivation